Veterinary Medical School Admission Requirements

Veterinary Medical School Admission Requirements

2019 EDITION FOR 2020 MATRICULATION

ASSOCIATION OF AMERICAN VETERINARY MEDICAL COLLEGES

PURDUE UNIVERSITY PRESS | WEST LAFAYETTE, INDIANA

COPYRIGHT © 2019 BY THE ASSOCIATION OF AMERICAN VETERINARY MEDICAL COLLEGES.
All rights reserved. Printed in the United States of America.

Compiled by the Association of American Veterinary Medical Colleges;
Tony Wynne, Editor, Director of Admissions and Recruitment Affairs

Paperback ISBN: 978-1-55753-860-4
ePub ISBN: 978-1-61249-574-3
ePDF ISBN: 978-1-61249-575-0
ISSN: 1089-6465

ACCEPTANCE DATE POLICY

In order to grant member schools enough time to complete their admissions processes and to give applicants enough time to consider all offers of admissions, no AAVMC Member Institution will require any applicant to make a decision about admission or financial aid before April 15 of each year. If April 15 falls on a Saturday or a Sunday, the date will be shifted to the following Monday.

To ensure applicants are awareness of this policy, each Member Institution will attach a copy of this policy to all admissions offer letters.

This policy does not apply to:
- Institutions outside the U.S. that do not participate in VMCAS
- Offers of admission for non-VMCAS applicants to institutions outside the U.S.
- Offers of admission for matriculation that is other than August or September

PROCEDURE

The Executive Director will investigate all complaints about alleged violations of this policy and report any findings to the chair of the Admissions and Recruitment Committee.

First Offense: If a Member Institution is found to be in violation of the policy, the Executive Director will send a Warning Letter to the Dean and Admissions Director of the institution and inform the Executive Committee of the Board of Directors.

Second and Subsequent Offenses: If a Member Institution is found to be in violation of this policy after a Warning Letter has been issued, the Executive Director and the chair of the Admissions and Recruitment Committee will report their findings to the Board of Directors and make a recommendation for additional penalties. Penalties may include monetary fines and exclusion from participation in VMCAS for a specified period of time.

Approved by the AAVMC Board of Directors
November 10, 2014

CONTENTS

FOREWORD

Congratulations on your decision to prepare for a career in veterinary medicine. Veterinary medicine is an exciting and rewarding career that provides a diverse array of options for contributing to the health of animals, people, and the planet.

Published annually by the Association of American Veterinary Medical Colleges (AAVMC), this *Veterinary Medical School Admission Requirements (VMSAR)* publication helps prospective students consider an important mix of factors when preparing for a veterinary medical education, including cost, financial aid, special programs, standardized tests, the AAVMC Veterinary Medical College Application Service (VMCAS), and the various colleges' and schools' residency admissions requirements.

> Our profession offers many opportunities beyond the time-honored practice of providing clinical care in general practice.

Where to apply and attend will be one of your initial decisions, and it's an important one, but all of these American Veterinary Medical Association (AVMA)-accredited schools offer great programs. Each one can start you on a rewarding path filled with choices and opportunities. Animal clinical care is an important and popular option in veterinary medicine, but veterinarians also contribute to global health in many other ways, including through careers in public health, research, and specialty practice. You also can prepare yourself for scientific and administrative careers with pharmaceutical, nutrition, and biomedical health corporations, or work in state and federal government. Augmenting your professional degree with advanced graduate work can lead to faculty positions in higher education.

Like other health professions, the pursuit and achievement of a veterinary medical education represents a substantial investment of time, effort, and financial resources. Cost-saving strategies include focusing on in-state veterinary medical schools or states that offer in-state tuition as part of special agreements with neighboring states. Other strategies include focusing on areas of greatest need, such as rural veterinary practice where loan repayment options might be available.

More information can be found on individual college and school websites or on the AAVMC website at www.aavmc.org. Prospective students also can contact the appropriate admissions office at each school or the VMCAS Student and Advisor Hotline, either by e-mail (vmcasinfo@vmcas.org) or by calling VMCAS at (617) 612-2884. The Veterinary Student Engagement System (VSES) is a useful tool as well.

Perhaps no other medical career provides such a broad base of biomedical training and leads to so many different areas of opportunity. The choices can seem overwhelming, but this guide is a great place to start, and step by step, your path will become clear, as it did for me. In my own case, a veterinary medical education led me to service as an officer in the United States Air Force, work in a mixed animal practice, in public health as an official with the U.S. Centers for Disease Control and Prevention, and now, as the chief executive officer of the AAVMC.

All of us at the AAVMC wish you luck and success as you prepare yourself for service in this extraordinary profession.

Dr. Andrew Maccabe
AAVMC Chief Executive Officer

ABOUT THE AAVMC

The Association of American Veterinary Medical Colleges (AAVMC) is a non-profit membership organization working to protect and improve the health and welfare of animals, people, and the environment by advancing academic veterinary medicine. The association was founded in 1966 by the deans of the then-existing eighteen colleges of veterinary medicine in the United States and three in Canada. During the 1970s and 1980s, AAVMC's membership expanded to include departments of veterinary science in colleges of agriculture, and in the 1990s to include divisions or departments of comparative medicine. In 2008, AAVMC began accepting non-accredited colleges and schools of veterinary medicine as affiliate members.

Today, AAVMC provides leadership for an academic veterinary medical community that includes all thirty colleges of veterinary medicine in the United States; nine departments of veterinary science; eight departments of comparative medicine; all five veterinary medical colleges in Canada; thirteen accredited colleges of veterinary medicine in Australia, Grenada, Ireland, Mexico, the Netherlands, New Zealand, St. Kitts, the United Kingdom, and six affiliate members.

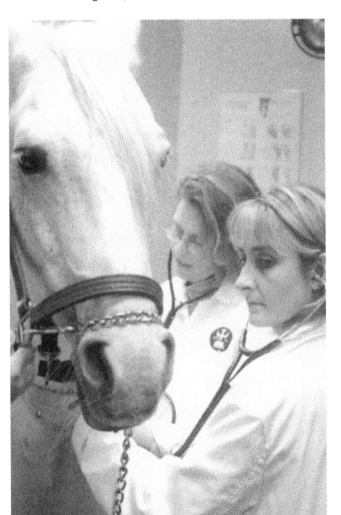

MISSION

AAVMC provides leadership for and promotes excellence in academic veterinary medicine to prepare the veterinary workforce with the scientific knowledge and skills required to meet societal needs through the protection of animal health, the relief of animal suffering, the conservation of animal resources, the promotion of public health, and the advancement of medical knowledge.

AAVMC pursues its mission by providing leadership in:
- Advocating on behalf of academic veterinary medicine;
- Serving as a catalyst and convener on issues of importance to academic veterinary medicine;
- Providing information, knowledge, and solutions to support members' work;
- Facilitating enrollment in veterinary medical schools and colleges; and
- Building global partnerships and coalitions to advance our collective goals.

STRATEGIC GOALS

1. Lead efforts to review, evaluate, and improve veterinary medical education in order to prepare graduates with the competencies needed to address societal needs.
2. Lead efforts to increase the amount of veterinary research conducted and the number of graduates entering research careers.
3. Lead efforts to recruit a student body aligned with the demands for veterinary expertise.
4. Lead efforts to increase the number of racially and/or ethnically underrepresented in veterinary medicine (URVM*) individuals throughout academic veterinary medicine.
5. Lead efforts to develop the next generation of leaders for academic veterinary medicine.
6. Strengthen AAVMC's capacity to better serve its members, partners, and other stakeholders in advancing the AAVMC mission.

*"URVMs are populations of individuals whose advancement in the veterinary medical profession have historically been disproportionately impacted by six specific aspects of diversity (gender, race, ethnicity, and geographic, socio-economic, and educational disadvantage) due to legal, cultural, or social climate impediments." *Definition of Underrepresented in Veterinary Medicine (URVM)*, approved by the AAVMC Board of Directors, July 20, 2008.

Left: A Tufts University Cummings School of Veterinary Medicine student checks out a horse with advice from her professor. Photo courtesy of Andy Cunningham of the Tufts University Cummings School of Veterinary Medicine.

VETERINARY MEDICINE: OPPORTUNITIES AND CHOICES

Veterinarians help animals and people live longer, healthier lives. They serve society through the protection of animal health and welfare, the prevention and relief of animal suffering, the conservation of animal resources, the promotion of public health, and the advancement of medical knowledge. The Doctor of Veterinary Medicine degree can lead to diverse career opportunities and different lifestyles from a solo mixed-animal practice in a rural area to a teaching or research position at an urban university, medical center, or industrial laboratory. The majority of veterinarians in the United States are in private clinical practice, although significant numbers are involved in preventive medicine, regulatory veterinary medicine, military veterinary medicine, laboratory animal medicine, research and development in industry, and teaching and research in a variety of basic science and clinical disciplines.

THE SPECTRUM OF OPPORTUNITIES IN VETERINARY MEDICINE

Veterinarians may choose to become specialists in a clinical area or to work with particular species. The first step on the path toward specialization is usually an internship.

1) FURTHER TRAINING

Internship

Internships are one-year programs in either small- or large-animal medicine and surgery. The most prestigious internship programs are at veterinary medical colleges or at very large private veterinary hospitals with board-certified veterinarians on staff. Since internships are usually at large referral centers, interns are exposed to a larger number of challenging cases than they would be likely to see in a smaller private practice.

Veterinary students in their senior year and veterinary graduates apply for internships through a matching program. Internship applicants and training hospitals rank each other in order of preference, and a computerized system matches each applicant with the highest-ranking teaching hospital that ranked the applicant. Academic performance in the veterinary professional curriculum, as well as recommendations from veterinary school faculty, is considered in the ranking of internship applicants.

Most veterinary interns in the United States receive a nominal salary, and their educational debts, if any, may be postponed in some governmentally subsidized loan programs. Veterinarians can sometimes command a higher starting salary in private practice after completion of an internship. Also, an internship is often the next step, after receiving the veterinary degree, toward residency and board certification.

Residency Training

Residency training is more specialized than an internship. Residency training programs are competitive and most require that the prospective residents complete an internship or equivalent private-practice experience prior to beginning the residency programs. Residency training is available in disciplines as varied as internal medicine, surgery, preventive medicine, behavior, toxicology, dentistry, and pathology.

The programs take two to three years to complete, depending on the nature of the specialty. Successful completion of a residency often is an important step toward attainment of board certification. Some residencies combine research and graduate study, leading to master's or PhD degrees.

Board Certification

Currently, there are twenty-two AVMA-recognized veterinary specialty organizations, comprising forty distinct specialties: anesthesiology, animal behavior, clinical pharmacology, dentistry, dermatology, emergency and critical care, internal medicine, laboratory animal medicine, microbiology, nutrition, ophthalmology, pathology, poultry medicine, private practice, preventive medicine, radiology, surgery, sports medicine and rehabilitation, theriogenology (reproduction), toxicology, and zoological medicine. Veterinarians may become board certified by completing rigorous postgraduate training, education, and examination requirements.

2) PRIVATE AND PUBLIC PRACTICE

The majority of veterinary graduates are engaged in private practice, either as an owner of a solo practice or, more likely, as a partner or associate in a group practice. Increasingly, veterinarians work together as a team, which allows a wider range of services to be provided.

Small-animal veterinarians focus their efforts primarily on dogs and cats but are seeing a growing number of other pets, including other small mammals, birds, reptiles, and fish.

Large-animal veterinarians often place their emphasis on horses, cattle, or pigs, and work both on a farm-call and an in-clinic basis. A mixed-animal veterinarian works with all types of domestic animals.

Public practice provides a variety of opportunities at the international, national, state, county, or city levels. There are exciting career opportunities for veterinarians in food safety, public health, the military, animal disease control, and research. Some veterinarians are employed by zoos and aquariums, wildlife conservation groups, game farms, or fisheries.

3) INDUSTRY

Veterinarians have many opportunities available to them in private industry, particularly in the fields of nutrition and pharmaceuticals. Assisting in the development of new products in the animal industry, conducting research for pharmaceutical companies, diagnosing disease and drug effects as pathologists, or safeguarding the health of laboratory animal colonies are all interesting career possibilities.

4) CONCLUSION

By the very nature of the comparative medical education that veterinarians receive, the many species of animals they care for and work for, and the wide variety of clientele served, the opportunities available to today's veterinarian are abundant.

INFORMATION ABOUT STANDARDIZED TESTS

Most veterinary medical colleges require one or more standardized tests: the Graduate Record Examination (GRE) or the Medical College Admission Test (MCAT). For further information regarding test dates and registration procedures, contact the testing agencies listed below:

GRE Graduate Record Examinations
P.O. Box 6000
Princeton, NJ 08541-6000
(609) 771-7670 (Princeton, NJ)
also: (510) 654-1200 (Oakland, CA)
www.gre.org
Individual school codes: see GRE booklet

MCAT Medical College Admission Test
MCAT Program Office
P.O. Box 4056
Iowa City, IA 52243-4056
(319) 337-1357
www.aamc.org/students/applying/mcat

TOEFL Test of English as a Foreign Language
TOEFL/TSE Services
P.O. Box 6151
Princeton, NJ 08541-6151
(609) 771-7100
www.toefl.org

AAVMC MEMBER INSTITUTIONS AND THE ROLE OF ACCREDITATION

Veterinary Schools join the AAVMC as institutional or affiliate members. A key difference between these two membership categories is whether a college/school of veterinary medicine is accredited by the Council on Education (COE). Only COE-accredited colleges of veterinary medicine may join AAVMC as an institutional (voting) member. Colleges of veterinary medicine that are not COE-accredited may join AAVMC as an affiliate member (non-voting) only. Several of AAVMC's affiliate members (non-COE–accredited institutions) have entered into agreements with AAVMC institutional members for clinical training. It is important for prospective veterinary students to know the different implications of attending and/or graduating from COE-accredited vs. non-COE–accredited colleges of veterinary medicine as it pertains to educational options and eventually seeking and obtaining a license to practice veterinary medicine. AAVMC encourages its affiliate members to become COE-accredited.

ACCREDITATION

The COE accredits DVM or equivalent educational programs. Accreditation through the COE assures that minimum standards in veterinary medical education are met by accredited colleges of veterinary medicine and that students enrolled in these colleges receive an education that will prepare them for entry-level positions in the profession. In the United States, graduation from a COE-accredited college of veterinary medicine is an important prerequisite for application for licensure. Internationally, some veterinary schools have chosen to seek COE accreditation in addition to accreditation by the competent authority in their own regions. COE accreditation of international veterinary schools provides assurance that those programs of education meet the same standards as other similarly accredited schools.

Additionally, COE accreditation assures:

- Prospective students that they will meet a competency threshold for entry into practice, including eligibility for professional credentialing and/or licensure;
- Employers that graduates have achieved specified learning goals and are prepared to begin professional practice;
- Faculty, deans, and administrators that their programs measure satisfactorily against national standards and their own stated missions and goals;

- The public that public health and safety concerns are being addressed; and
- The veterinary profession that the science and art of veterinary medicine are being advanced through contemporary curricula.

*Source: The source for this information and a site recommended for obtaining additional information is as follows: https://www.avma.org /ProfessionalDevelopment/Education/Accreditation /Colleges/Pages/about-accred.aspx

LICENSURE

Licensure in the United States

In the United States, requirements for licensure are set by individual state regulatory boards. The North American Veterinary Licensing Exam (NAVLE) and any additional state exams must be taken by a graduate to become eligible for state licensure. The NAVLE, which is administered by the International Council for Veterinary Assessment (ICVA), fulfills a core requirement for licensure to practice veterinary medicine in all jurisdictions in the United States and Canada. Mexico does not require NAVLE. In addition to the NAVLE, state regulatory boards will have other licensure requirements, which may include state-specific examinations.

To be eligible to take the NAVLE, applicants must have graduated from either a COE-accredited college of veterinary medicine or a non-COE–accredited college (see following details).

Applicants who graduated from a non-COE–accredited college must also have a certification of eligibility, which can come from one of two sources: the Educational Commission for Foreign Veterinary Graduates (ECFVG) Certification Program (www.avma.org /professionaldevelopment/education/foreign/pages /default.aspx) or the Program for the Assessment of Veterinary Education Equivalence (PAVE) (www.aavsb .org/PAVE).

All state regulatory boards accept the ECFVG certification, administered through the American Veterinary Medical Association (AVMA), as meeting in full or in part the educational prerequisite for licensure eligibility. At this time, twenty-eight state regulatory boards also accept PAVE certification, which is administered through the American Association of Veterinary State Boards (AAVSB).

It is important to note that prerequisites for licensure eligibility and requirements for licensure vary amongst state regulatory boards and are subject to periodic modification.

Licensure Outside the United States

Mutual recognition arrangements apply to jurisdictions where there are COE-accredited schools. These specify that graduates of COE-accredited schools in the United States and Canada are permitted to obtain licensure to practice under terms no less favorable than graduates of schools accredited by the competent authority in that jurisdiction.

DECIDING WHERE TO APPLY

There are several factors, as well as the issue of accreditation, that an applicant must consider in identifying school(s) to submit an application for admissions. In addition to licensure issues, there may be economic, educational options, or other differences that students should consider in making decisions on where to apply. This book is intended to provide important information about AAVMC members to assist in informed decision-making for students considering applying to one or more veterinary colleges.

PRE-VETERINARY PROFILE: ME'NISHA JONES

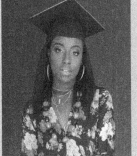

Current School Name
University of Central Florida

What type of veterinary medicine are you interested in pursuing, and why?
As of right now, I want to go into small animal medicine, but I also want to be a well-rounded vet who can help any animal.

What is/was your major during undergraduate school?
Psychology with a pre-veterinary track.

What are your short-term and long-term goals?
My short-term goals are to finish classes and apply to vet school, and my long-term goal is to graduate from vet school.

What are you doing as an applicant/pre-vet to prepare for veterinary school?
I am continuing to take courses that are prerequisites for graduate school, and I am getting jobs in the vet field to keep my dream alive.

What extracurricular activities are you involved in currently?
I was involved in Pre-Vet Society; I was President of First Knights, an organization dedicated to first-generation students; and I was involved SISTUHS Incorporated, dedicated to community service in the community. I was also a brother in the prestigious Alpha Kappa Psi Business Fraternity, and I served as Progressive Black Men's Miss Emerald for the 2016–2017 school year.

How old were you when you first became interested in being a veterinarian?
I was in tenth grade when I watched the sad ASPCA commercial that convinced me to make a difference in the lives of animals and to give them a voice.

Please describe your various experiences in preparation for applying to veterinary school.
I have already accepted my fate that I will be a nontraditional student, which can discourage some students. I have come to terms with the fact that, regardless of how long it takes me to get to vet school, as long as I keep my eye on the prize, nothing will stop me from my ultimate goal.

What characteristics are you looking for in a veterinary school?
II am looking for a challenging, helping vet school that will prepare me for situations that might occur in the real world of practice.

What advice do you have for other pre-veterinary students?
I advise students to never give up. Everyone's journey will not be the same, so don't focus on how everyone else is getting there—focus on what you have to do to get there. With determination and hard work, you can accomplish whatever you put your mind to.

GEOGRAPHICAL LISTING OF AAVMC INSTITUTIONAL (COE ACCREDITED) VETERINARY SCHOOLS AND DIRECTORY OF ADMISSIONS OFFICES

Atlantic Veterinary College at the
  University of Prince Edward Island
  (CANADA)
Registrar's Office
550 University Avenue
Charlottetown PEI C1A 4P3
Canada

Auburn University (USA)
Office for Academic Affairs
College of Veterinary Medicine
217 Goodwin/Overton
Auburn, AL 36849-5536

Colorado State University (USA)
College of Veterinary Medicine and
  Biomedical Sciences
1601 Campus Delivery – Office of
  the Dean
Fort Collins, CO 80523-1601

Cornell University (USA)
Office of Student & Academic Services
College of Veterinary Medicine
S2-009 Schurman Hall
Ithaca, NY 14853-6401

Iowa State University (USA)
Office of Admissions
College of Veterinary Medicine
2270 Veterinary Medicine
P.O. Box 3020
Ames, IA 50010-3020

Kansas State University (USA)
Office of Admissions
College of Veterinary Medicine
101 Trotter Hall
Manhattan, KS 66506-5601

Lincoln Memorial University (USA)
College of Veterinary Medicine
6965 Cumberland Gap Pkwy
Harrogate, TN 37752

Louisiana State University (USA)
Office of Student and Academic Affairs
School of Veterinary Medicine
Skip Bertman Drive
Baton Rouge, LA 70803

Massey University Veterinary School
  (AUSTRALIA)
International Student Affairs
Undergraduate Office
IVABS
Private Bag 11-222
Palmerston North 4442
New Zealand

Michigan State University (USA)
Office of Admissions
College of Veterinary Medicine
784 Wilson Road
F-110 Veterinary Medical Center
East Lansing, MI 48824

Midwestern University (USA)
College of Veterinary Medicine
19555 North 59th Avenue
Glendale, AZ 85308

Mississippi State University (USA)
Office of Student Admissions
College of Veterinary Medicine
P.O. Box 6100
Mississippi State, MS 39762

Murdoch University (AUSTRALIA)
Murdoch International
South Street
Murdoch 6150
Western Australia

North Carolina State University (USA)
Student Services Office
College of Veterinary Medicine
1060 William Moore Drive, Box 8401
Raleigh, NC 27607

The Ohio State University (USA)
Office of Student Affairs
College of Veterinary Medicine
Suite 127 Veterinary Medicine
  Academic Building
1900 Coffey Road
Columbus, OH 43210-1089

Oklahoma State University (USA)
Office of Admissions
112 McElroy Hall
Center for Veterinary Health
  Sciences
College of Veterinary Medicine
Stillwater, OK 74078-2003

Oregon State University (USA)
Office of the Dean
Attention: Admissions
College of Veterinary Medicine
200 Magruder Hall
Corvallis, OR 97331-4801

Purdue University (USA)
Student Services Center
College of Veterinary Medicine
625 Harrison Street
West Lafayette, IN 47907-2026

Ross University School of Veterinary
  Medicine (ST. KITTS)
Office of Admissions
630 US HWY 1
North Brunswick, NJ 08902

Royal Veterinary College
  (UNITED KINGDOM)
Head of Admissions
Royal College Street
London NW1 0TU
United Kingdom

St. George's University (GRENADA)
Office of Admission
c/o The North American Correspondent
University Support Services, LLC
3500 Sunrise Highway
Building 300
Great River, NY 11739

Texas A & M University (USA)
Office of the Dean
College of Veterinary Medicine & Biomedical Sciences
College Station, TX 77843-4461

Tufts University (USA)
Office of Admissions
Cummings School of Veterinary Medicine
200 Westboro Road
North Grafton, MA 01536

Tuskegee University (USA)
Office of Admissions and Recruitment
School of Veterinary Medicine
100 Dr. Frederick Patterson Hall
Tuskegee, AL 36088

Universidad Nacional Autónoma de México (MEXICO)
Office of Undergraduate Studies (Division de Estudios Profesionales)
College of Veterinary Medicine (FMVZ)
Av. Universidad 3000
Circuito Interior
Delegacion Coyoacan
Mexico D.F. 04510

Université de Montréal (CANADA)
Service des Admissions
C.P. 6205
Succursale Centre-Ville
Montréal Québec H3C 3T5 Canada

University of Calgary (CANADA)
Admissions Office
Faculty of Veterinary Medicine
TRW 2D03
3280 Hospital Drive NW
Calgary, AB T2N 4Z6

University of California (USA)
School of Veterinary Medicine
Office of the Dean-Student Programs
One Shields Avenue
Davis, CA 95616

University College Dublin (IRELAND)
Veterinary Medicine Applications
UCD Admissions Office
Tierney Building
Belfield, Dublin 4
Ireland

University of Edinburgh (UNITED KINGDOM)
Admissions Office
Royal (Dick) School of Veterinary Studies
Easter Bush Veterinary Centre
Roslin EH25 9RG
Scotland

University of Florida (USA)
Admissions Office
College of Veterinary Medicine
P.O. Box 100125
Gainesville, FL 32610-0125

The University of Georgia (USA)
Admissions Department
Office for Academic Affairs
College of Veterinary Medicine
Athens, GA 30602-7372

University of Glasgow (UNITED KINGDOM)
Director of Admissions & Student Services Manager
College of Medicine, Veterinary and Life Sciences
School of Veterinary Medicine Undergraduate School
464 Bearsden Road
Glasgow G61 1QH

University of Guelph (CANADA)
Admissions Services
University Centre, Level 3
Guelph Ontario N 1G 2W 1
Canada

University of Illinois (USA)
College of Veterinary Medicine
Office of Academic and Student Affairs
2001 South Lincoln Avenue, Room 2271g
Urbana, IL 61802

University of Melbourne (AUSTRALIA)
Faculty of Veterinary Science
Corner Park Drive and Flemington Road
Parkville
Melbourne 3010
Victoria Australia

University of Minnesota (USA)
Office of Academic and Student Affairs
College of Veterinary Medicine
108 Pomeroy Center
1964 Fitch Ave.
St. Paul, MN 55108

University of Missouri-Columbia (USA)
Office of Academic Affairs
College of Veterinary Medicine
W203 Veterinary Medicine Building
Columbia, MO 65211

University of Pennsylvania (USA)
Admissions Office
School of Veterinary Medicine
3800 Spruce Street
Philadelphia, PA 19104-6044

The University of Queensland–Gatton Campus (AUSTRALIA)
School of Veterinary Science
Gatton, 4343
Queensland, Australia

University of Saskatchewan
   (CANADA)
Admissions Office
Western College of Veterinary
   Medicine
52 Campus Drive
Saskatoon Saskatchewan S7N 5B4
Canada

Sydney School of Veterinary
   Science (AUSTRALIA)
Faculty of Veterinary Science
Sydney, NSW 2006
Australia

University of Tennessee (USA)
Admissions Office
College of Veterinary Medicine
2407 River Drive
Room A-104-C
Knoxville, TN 37996-4550

University of Wisconsin-Madison
   (USA)
Office of Academic Affairs
School of Veterinary Medicine
2015 Linden Drive
Madison, WI 53706-1102

Utrecht University (NETHERLANDS)
Office for International Cooperation
Faculty of Veterinary Medicine
Yalelaan 1
3584 CL Utrecht
The Netherlands

VetAgro Sup (FRANCE)
1, avenue Bourgelat
69280 Marcy l'Etoile
France

Virginia-Maryland College
   of Veterinary Medicine (USA)
Admissions Coordinator
Blacksburg, VA 24061

Washington State University (USA)
Office of Student Services
College of Veterinary Medicine
100 Grimes Way
P.O. Box 647012
Pullman, WA 99164-7012

Western University of Health
   Sciences (USA)
Office of Admissions
College of Veterinary Medicine
309 East 2nd Street
Pomona, CA 91766-1854

GEOGRAPHICAL LISTING OF AAVMC AFFILIATE (NON-COE ACCREDITED) VETERINARY SCHOOLS AND DIRECTORY OF ADMISSIONS OFFICES

University of Adelaide (AUSTRALIA)
The School of Animal and Veterinary Science
Roseworthy Campus
Roseworthy SA 5371
Australia

University of Bristol (ENGLAND)
Beacon House
Queens Road
Bristol, BS8 1QU, UK

Central Luzon State University (PHILIPPINES)
Science City of Munoz
Nueva Ecija 3120
Philippines

City University of Hong Kong (HONG KONG)
5/F, Block 1, To Yuen Building
31 To Yuen Street
City University of Hong Kong
Tat Chee Avenue, Kowloon
Hong Kong

Seoul National University (SOUTH KOREA)
1 Gwanak-ro
Gwanak-gu, Seoul
South Korea

St. Matthew's University (WEST INDIES)
Office of Admissions
12124 High Tech Avenue, Suite 350
Orlando, Fl 32817

United Arab Emirates University (UNITED ARAB EMIRATES) PO Box 15551 Al-Ain, United Arab Emirates

University of Tokyo (JAPAN)
1-1-1, Yayoi, Bunkyo-Ku
Tokyo 113-8657, Japan

University of Veterinary and Animal Sciences - UVAS (PAKISTAN)
Syed Abdul Qadir Jillani (Out Fall) Road, Lahore - Pakistan
UVMP in Košice (Slovak Republic)
Komenského 73
041 81 Košice, Slovak Republic

LISTING OF CONTRACTING STATES AND PROVINCES

Six Canadian provinces and 19 states in the United States have a veterinary school contract with one or more schools to provide access to veterinary medical education for their residents. The state or province, working through the contracting agency, usually agrees to pay a fee to help cover the cost of education for a certain number of places in each entering class. Residents from the contract states then compete with each other for those positions.

Some states contract with more than one school. For example, Arkansas contracts with 5 veterinary schools, and North Dakota contracts with 6 schools. Connecticut, Rhode Island, Vermont, Nebraska, and the District of Columbia presently have no contracts,

so all candidates from these places apply as nonresidents to veterinary schools of their choice.

The educational agreements between contracting agencies and veterinary schools differ. Under some contract arrangements, students pay in-state tuition; in others, they pay nonresident tuition. Some contract states require students to repay all or part of the subsidy that the state provided; others require veterinary graduates to return to practice in the state for a period of time. Applicants should be aware of their obligation to the state before agreeing to participate in a contract program

Following is a list of states and provinces that have educational agreements with schools of veterinary medicine.

UNITED STATES

ARIZONA

Contracts through WICHE* with Colorado State University, Oregon State University, and Washington State University.

ARKANSAS

Contracts through the SREB** with Louisiana State University, University of Missouri, and Oklahoma State University. Contracts not all completed at time of printing; may be some changes.

DELAWARE

Contracts with Oklahoma State University and the University of Georgia.

HAWAII

Contracts through WICHE* with Colorado State University, Oregon State University, and Washington State University.

IDAHO

Contracts with Washington State University.

KENTUCKY

Contracts with Auburn University and Tuskegee University.

MONTANA

Contracts with Washington State University. Contracts through WICHE* with Colorado State University, Oregon State University, and Washington State University.

NEBRASKA

Formal education alliance with Iowa State University allows students admitted into the 2+2 program with the University of Nebraska-Lincoln to pay resident tuition for all 4 years.

NEVADA

Contracts through WICHE* with Colorado State University, Oregon State University, and Washington State University.

NEW MEXICO

Contracts through WICHE* with Colorado State University, Oregon State University, and Washington State University.

NORTH DAKOTA

Contracts with Iowa State University, University of Minnesota, and Kansas State University. Contracts through WICHE* with Colorado State University, Oregon State University, and Washington State University.

SOUTH CAROLINA

Contracts with University of Georgia, Mississippi State University, and Tuskegee University.

SOUTH DAKOTA

Reciprocity with University of Minnesota. Contracts with Iowa State University.

UTAH

Contracts with Washington State University.

* WICHE = Western Interstate Commission for Higher Education (offices in Boulder, Colorado)
**SREB = Southern Regional Educational Board

WEST VIRGINIA

Contracts with Mississippi State University and Virginia-Maryland College of Veterinary Medicine.

WYOMING

Contracts through WICHE* with Colorado State University, Oregon State University, and Washington State University.

CANADA

ALBERTA

Contracts with University of Calgary.

BRITISH COLUMBIA

Contracts with University of Saskatchewan.

MANITOBA

Contracts with University of Saskatchewan.

NEW BRUNSWICK

Contracts with Atlantic Veterinary College at the University of Prince Edward Island and Université de Montréal.

NEWFOUNDLAND

Contracts with Atlantic Veterinary College at the University of Prince Edward Island.

NOVA SCOTIA

Contracts with Atlantic Veterinary College at the University of Prince Edward Island.

* WICHE = Western Interstate Commission for Higher Education (offices in Boulder, Colorado)

PROGRAMS FOR MULTICULTURAL OR DISADVANTAGED STUDENTS

The Association of American Veterinary Medical Colleges affirms the value of diversity within the veterinary medical profession. The membership is committed to incorporating that belief into their actions by advocating for the recruitment and retention of underrepresented persons as students and faculty, and ultimately fostering their success in the profession of veterinary medicine. The Association believes that through these actions, society and the profession will be well served.

Many schools have programs designed to facilitate entry into, and retention by, veterinary programs nationwide. These programs are directed at several levels, from high-school students to the student who has already been accepted by a veterinary college. Most of these programs will accept students from every state, regardless of the school(s) to which an individual might eventually apply or attend.

Following is an alphabetical list of schools by state and a short explanation of their programs:

UNIVERSITY OF CALIFORNIA

Program: Summer Enrichment Program

Description: A 6-week summer program. The purpose of this program is to increase the academic preparedness of disadvantaged students through science-based learning skills development, clinical education, individual advising, and student development.

Eligibility: Educationally and/or economically disadvantaged. Must have completed at least one year of college with a minimum science GPA of 2.8 and demonstrated interest in veterinary medicine.

Program dates: July–August.

Contact: Office of the Dean–Student Programs, School of Veterinary Medicine, University of California, One Shields Avenue, Davis CA 95616; telephone: (530) 752-1383.

Sponsorship: School of Veterinary Medicine, University of California-Davis.

COLORADO STATE UNIVERSITY

Program: Vet Prep

Description: A one-year academic program that serves as a bridge to the Doctor of Veterinary (DVM) program for disadvantaged (cultural, social, economic) applicants who ranked high but were not admitted. Limited to 10 students who upon successful completion are guaranteed admission to the DVM program. Candidates are selected from the current regular admissions applicant pool and do not directly apply to the Vet Prep program.

Eligibility: Disadvantaged students.

Contact: College of Veterinary Medicine and Biomedical Sciences, W102 Anatomy, Colorado State University, Fort Collins CO 80523; telephone: (970) 491-7051; email: DVMAdmissions@colostate.edu.

Sponsorship: College of Veterinary Medicine and Biomedical Sciences, Colorado State University.

CORNELL UNIVERSITY

Program: State University of New York Graduate Underrepresented Minority Fellowships

Description: All matriculating underrepresented minorities are eligible (not restricted by state residency).

Contact: Director of Student Financial Planning, Office of Student & Academic Services, College of Veterinary Medicine, Cornell University, S2-009 Schurman Hall, Ithaca NY 14853-6401; telephone: (607) 253-3766; website: www.vet.cornell.edu/financialaid.

MICHIGAN STATE UNIVERSITY

Program: Enrichment Summer Program (ESP)

Description: The ESP, sponsored by the Michigan State University College of Veterinary Medicine with support of an endowment, provides academic advancement and career knowledge for undergraduate students interested in veterinary medicine. There is no fee to participate in this program.

Eligibility: The program is open to undergraduate students who have selected veterinary medicine as a career choice and plan to apply to a professional program. It focuses on developing well-qualified prospective students from disadvantaged backgrounds. Consideration is given to residents of Michigan who have a cumulative GPA of 3.0 or higher.

Program dates: Early June through late June.

How Do I Apply: The application opens November 1 each year and closes in late January. For more information, visit cvm.msu.edu/esp.

Contact: The Office of Diversity and Inclusion, College of Veterinary Medicine, 784 Wilson Road, F-113 B, Veterinary Medical Center, Michigan State University, East Lansing, MI 48824; telephone: (517) 355-6521; email: cvm.Diversity@cvm.msu.edu.

MISSISSIPPI STATE UNIVERSITY

Program: Board of Trustees of State Institutions of Higher Learning Veterinary Medicine Minority Loan/Scholarship Program

Description: A financial assistance program for Mississippi residents who are underrepresented minorities. The loan to service obligation is one year for each year of scholarship assistance, not to exceed four years.

Contact: Susan Eckels, Program Administrator, Mississippi Institutions of Higher Learning, 3825 Ridgewood Road, Jackson MS 39211-6453; telephone: (800) 327-2980.

Program: Vet Camp

Description: MSU-CVM has been offering Veterinary Camp since 2011. Modeled after the first and second year student experience, our curriculum is heavily hands-on and is taught by our own faculty, with DVM students serving as counselors and leaders. After that first year, the camp grew in the number of students we could serve, the number and types of camps we offered, and the labs and activities we provided. We are proud of the 100% satisfaction rate and willingness to recommend our camp reported by campers, parents, and our own faculty. We love sharing the veterinary profession with young people.

Program: VetAspire

Description: VetAspire is an exciting program designed for students to spend the day at Mississippi State University's College of Veterinary Medicine. Each month, five students will have the opportunity to participate in clinics, lectures, and hands-on activities. The goal of this program is to expose students to the field of veterinary medicine in hopes that they will choose it as a career path. Students will also get to see the real-world impact of math, science, and communications training.

Eligibility: Open to 11th and 12th grade high school students and college freshmen. Must be educationally, economically, and/or socially disadvantaged. All students (11th grade-college senior) will be considered, but priority will be given to students who meet the above criteria.

NORTH CAROLINA STATE UNIVERSITY

Program: UNC Campus Scholarship Program—Graduate Student Component

Description: UNC General Administration funds this program. Eligibility is limited to new or continuing full-time doctoral students who have financial need and who are residents of North Carolina as of the beginning of the award period (as determined under the *Manual to Assist the Public Higher Education Institutions of N.C. in the Matter of Student Resident Classification for Tuition Purposes*). Individuals who have been accepted to a master's degree program in a department offering the doctoral degree and who intend, and will be eligible, to pursue doctoral studies at NC State after completion of the requirements for the master's degree are also eligible. The program provides up to $3,000 annually for North Carolina residents.

Contact: Director of Diversity Affairs, College of Veterinary Medicine, North Carolina State University, 1060 William Moore Drive, Box 8401, Raleigh, NC 27607; telephone: (919) 513-6262; website: www.cvm.ncsu.edu.

Program: Diversity Graduate Assistant Grant

Description: Funded by the North Carolina State University Graduate School, recipients must be full-time, new or continuing students pursuing master's and doctoral degrees at North Carolina State University. The program provides up to $3,000 annually. Both resident and nonresident students are eligible to apply.

Contact: Director of Diversity Affairs, College of Veterinary Medicine, North Carolina State University, 1060 William Moore Drive, Box 8401, Raleigh, NC 27607; telephone: (919) 513-6262; website: www.cvm.ncsu.edu.

Note: North Carolina residents are encouraged to apply for both programs. However, the annual maximum award for these grant programs is a combined $3,000 (with an option of $500 in additional support for study in the summer). The grant is awarded on an annual basis. Awardees must reapply each year.

THE OHIO STATE UNIVERSITY

Program: Buckeye Veterinary Camp

Description: In this summer residential camp, high school students will learn more about veterinary school and the profession.

Eligibility: Scholarships are available for those who qualify.

Program dates: Application typically opens in September-January. Dates of the camp are at the end of June.

Sponsorship: the State of Ohio and The Ohio State University.

Program: Summer Research Opportunities Program (SROP)

Description: The Summer Research Opportunities Program (SROP) at Ohio State is designed to help historically underrepresented students explore opportunities for graduate study and academic careers. Over the course of eight weeks during the summer, Ohio State SROP participants will conduct research with a faculty mentor on a topic of mutual interest, and participate in activities crucial to preparation for graduate school, including workshops on research skills, seminars on topics related to graduate education, and professional development events. At the end of the summer program, participants present their research at a campus summary conference and a regional conference.

Eligibility: All historically underrepresented undergraduates who are U.S. citizens and who meet the criteria listed in the qualifications section below are eligible to participate in the program. The selection process targets groups underrepresented in graduate education. Priority is given to those students who have not participated in SROP previously.

Contact: Graduate Student Recruitment, 614-247-6377, gradrecruit@osu.edu. Website: https://gradsch.osu.edu /research/summer-research-opportunities-program. SROP is overseen by the Big Ten Academic Alliance.

PURDUE UNIVERSITY

Program: Vet Up!™ National HCOP Academy for Veterinary Medicine

Description: Vet Up!™! provides opportunities and support for equity-minded individuals from disadvantaged backgrounds to enter the veterinary profession and serve society by advancing public health, ensuring food safety, or serving rural areas. Vet Up!™ consists of three programs with a competitive selection process for admissions: Vet Up! Champions; Vet Up! College; and Vet Up! DVM Scholars. Vet Up! Champions integrates face-to-face and interactive online learning to provide a 12-month structured curriculum to a cohort of 26 students each year comprised of rising high-school juniors/seniors, adult/nontraditional learners including veterans, and first or second year undergraduate students. Champions will prepare for entry into veterinary college by receiving mentorship, financial and cultural competence training, and gaining exposure to veterinary careers. The Vet Up! College program is a six-week-long residential summer program at the Purdue University College of Veterinary Medicine for 26 educationally or economically disadvantaged undergraduate students each year that will prepare students to be competitive in the DVM applicant pool. Vet Up! College is geared towards rising college juniors and seniors. Vet Up! College replaces Purdue Veterinary Medicine's Access to Animal-Related Careers (A2RC) 2-week-long summer program which has been discontinued. The Vet Up! DVM Scholars program provides academic, social, and financial support post-matriculation to five educationally or economically disadvantaged Purdue University College of Veterinary Medicine D.V.M. degree students per year, to support them from matriculation to a timely graduation from their veterinary medical degree program and employment in a veterinary shortage area.

Eligibility: Vet Up! is open to individuals who are: U.S. citizens, Non-citizen nationals, and Foreign nationals who possess a visa permitting permanent residence in the United States. Participants must also establish an educationally or economically disadvantaged background by meeting two or more of the following criteria:

- The individual is an underrepresented minority with respect to race or ethnicity.
- The individual is from a rural background.
- The individual is the first-generation in their family to attend college (neither parent nor legal guardian completed a Bachelor's degree or higher).
- The individual graduated from (or last attended) a high school that, based on the most recent annual data available, had:
- Less than 60% of seniors receiving a high school diploma; or
- Less than 60% of graduates going to college the first year after graduation; or
- Over half of the enrolled students eligible for free or reduced-price lunches.
- Low family annual income based the 2018 Poverty Guidelines and validated by federal income tax return.

Program dates: Dates vary by program.

Contact: Website: www.PurdueVetUp.org; Email: vetup@purdue.edu; Purdue Veterinary Medicine Office for Diversity and Inclusion, (765) 496-1908;

Sponsorship: This program is supported by the Health Resources and Services Administration (HRSA) of the U.S. Department of Health and Human Services (HHS) as part of an award totaling $3.18 million.

UNIVERSITY OF TENNESSEE

Program: Veterinary Summer Experience for Tennessee High School Students

Description: The College of Veterinary Medicine offers an eight-week program that provides high school students an opportunity to gain experience working with veterinarians at a veterinary practice in their home towns for seven weeks during the summer. During the eighth week of this summer experience, students will be guests of the College of Veterinary Medicine on the campus of The University of Tennessee in Knoxville. Students will attend clinical rotations in the Equine, Farm Animal, Small Animal, and Avian and Exotic Animal (including zoo medicine) Hospitals in the Veterinary Medical Center. Students will also attend special educational functions related to veterinary medicine.

Eligibility: To qualify for this summer program, a student must be a Tennessee resident and be at least 16 years of age by June 1, be enrolled as a senior or junior in a Tennessee high school, and have earned a minimum 3.0 high school GPA. Applicants must also have an interest in veterinary medicine as a potential career. Preference will be given to applicants who will contribute greatly to the diversity of the summer program and, potentially, to the veterinary profession. Students receive a financial stipend for satisfactory performance in the eight-week program.

Program dates: Summer.

Contact: Dr. William Hill, The University of Tennessee, College of Veterinary Medicine, 2431 Joe Johnson Drive, 339 Ellington Plant Science, Knoxville TN 37996, telephone: (865) 974-5770. E-mail: wahill@utk.edu.

UNIVERSITY OF MINNESOTA

Program: Veterinary Leadership in Early Admissions for Diversity (VetLEAD)

Description: VetLEAD creates a pathway into the DVM program for high-ability students at underrepresented serving partner schools, including Florida Agricultural and Mechanical University (FAMU).

Eligibility: Any high-achieving student enrolled in the Animal Science program at FAMU may apply for an early admissions decision at the end of their sophomore year of undergraduate studies. Eligible students have past experience working or volunteering in a veterinary related setting, a FAMU cumulative GPA of 3.4 with coursework consistent with required prerequisite courses, and strong letters of references.

Contact: Karen Nelson, Director of Admissions, dvminfo@umn.edu

TUSKEGEE UNIVERSITY

Program: Tuskegee University Summer Enrichment and Reinforcement Program (SERP)

Description: This is an exclusive program available only to accepted first year students. The SERP five-week program is a great introduction to the highly anticipated veterinary curriculum. It is an opportunity to strengthen the student's performance, surrounded by others who share their passion for animals, health, and science. The program focuses on the following key areas: critical thinking, analysis and application of clinical information, and learning strategies.

Eligibility: Participation is restricted to first year students accepted to the Tuskegee University College of Veterinary Medicine.

Program dates: May 30 - June 28, 2019

Contact: Kheri Spence, Assistant Director for Student Success/Counselor, College of Veterinary Medicine, Patterson Hall, 1200 W. Old Montgomery Road, Tuskegee Institute, Al 36088, telephone (334) 724-4247, email: kspence@tuskegee.edu.

Program: Veterinary Science Training, Education and Preparation Institute (Vet STEP)

Description: A residential program designed to introduce underrepresented minority high school students to exciting careers in veterinary medicine. Students spend a week on the campus of Tuskegee University learning about what it takes to be a veterinarian while attending stimulating academic classes. The all inclusive tuition for Vet STEP is $500.00.

Eligibility: Participation in Vet STEP I is restricted to high school students in 9th and 10th grade. Participation in Vet STEP II is restricted to high school students in 11th and 12th grade.

Contact: LaTia McCurdy, Coordinator of Veterinary Recruitment, Tuskegee University College of Veterinary Medicine, Patterson Hall, 1200 W. Montgomery Road, Tuskegee Institute, Al 36088. Telephone: (334) 727-8309, email: lmccurdy@tuskegee.edu.

VIRGINIA-MARYLAND COLLEGE
OF VETERINARY MEDICINE

Program: VetTRAC Summer Program

Description: A weeklong program, VetTRAC aims to teach, inspire, mentor, engage, excite, and enlighten students from underrepresented populations with respect to the field of veterinary medicine to promote diversity and inclusion within the VA-MD College of Veterinary Medicine and the veterinary profession. Only undergraduate students are accepted.

Contact: DVM Admissions Office at Blacksburg campus.

UNIVERSITY OF WISCONSIN

Program: Pre-College Enrollment Opportunity Program for Learning Excellence (PEOPLE)

Description: This program began in the summer of 1999 as a partnership between the Milwaukee Public Schools and the UW-Madison with a group of students who had just completed the ninth grade. Partner schools now also include Madison high schools as well as a number of Northern Wisconsin high schools. The program is designed with a precollege track and a bridge program to undergraduate work and continues through a student's undergraduate career at University of Wisconsin-Madison. The main purposes are to promote academic preparation, increase enrollment in postsecondary institutions, and improve retention and graduation rates of minority and disadvantaged students.

Eligibility: PEOPLE is designed for students with strong academic potential who are U.S. citizens or permanent residents who are also African American, American Indian, Asian American (with an emphasis on Southeast Asian American), Chicano/a, Puerto Rican, Latino/a, or low-income students. Priority for admission will be given to students eligible for the free and reduced hot lunch program.

Program dates: June–July summer residential programs and year-round nonresidential programs.

Contact: PEOPLE Program, 1305 Linden Drive, University of Wisconsin-Madison, Madison, WI 53706.

FINANCIAL AID INFORMATION

Financing your veterinary medical education requires careful planning, good money management skills, and a willingness to make short-term sacrifices to achieve long-range goals.

Many of you will apply for and receive some type of financial assistance during your undergraduate education. This will help you become somewhat familiar with the process, and to know that the rules and regulations governing programs can and do change periodically.

> Don't live the lifestyle of a DVM until you have completed your education. Get in the habit of being thrifty.

As a professional student, you will be entering a partnership with the financial aid office, which will require you to complete the appropriate financial aid forms accurately, meet required deadlines, and submit any additional information that may be requested. In return, the financial aid office will determine your aid eligibility and make awards based on the available programs. Your financial aid eligibility takes into account the cost of your education minus any other available resources. Amounts of assistance and the school policies for awarding assistance vary from one veterinary medical school to another and from year to year.

Any questions or concerns that you may have about this topic need to be directed to each of the appropriate financial aid offices to ensure that you receive accurate information and guidance.

FINANCING YOUR VETERINARY MEDICAL EDUCATION

Your education is one of the biggest investments you will make in your lifetime, and one of your most important goals should be to maximize the return on all of your investments. To reach this goal, you must take an active role in managing your financial resources. You need to understand and implement good financial practices. To get you started, here are some good financial habits you should adopt:

- Do not use credit cards to extend your lifestyle. Deciding not to use credit cards except in emergencies is one of the most important decisions you can make, and one that will reduce your stress while you are pursuing your education.
- Budget your money just as carefully as you budget your time. Contact a financial aid administrator to help you set up a budget that will be easy to follow.
- Distinguish between wants and needs. Before you make any purchase, you should ask yourself, "Do I need this, or do I want it?"
- Be a well-informed borrower. If you have not previously taken an active role in understanding the differences between various student loan programs, now is the time to do it. You need to know these differences in order to avoid high-interest loans and to borrow wisely.
- Borrow the minimum amount necessary in order to maximize the return on your educational investment.
- Be thrifty. Live as cheaply as you can. Remember, you are a student. You'll enjoy a more comfortable lifestyle once you are a DVM.
- Pay any interest that accrues on student loans if you can afford to do so, rather than let the interest accrue and capitalize. Any amount you pay while you're a student will save you money once you enter repayment.

What is the most important piece of advice for making the most of your educational investment? Don't live the lifestyle of a DVM until you have completed your education. Get in the habit of being thrifty. If you live like a DVM while you are in school, you may have to live like a student when you are a DVM.

FEDERAL LOAN PROGRAMS

Please note that subsidized loans are not available beginning fall 2012.

	William D. Ford Unsubsidized Stafford Loan	Perkins Loan	Health Professions Student Loan	Loan for Disadvantaged Students	Grad Plus Loans for Graduate/ Professional Students
Lender	Federal Loan Program	Federal Loan Program	Federal Loan Program	Federal Loan Program	Federal Loan Program
Financial Need	No	Yes	Yes	Yes	No
Citizenship Requirement	U.S. Citizen, U.S. National, or U.S. Permanent Resident	U.S. Citizen, U.S. National, or U.S. Permanent Resident	U.S. Citizen, U.S. National, or U.S. Permanent Resident	U.S. Citizen, U.S. National, or U.S. Permanent Resident	U.S. Citizen, U.S. National, or U.S. Permanent Resident
Borrowing Limits	Cost of attendance minus other aid; $189,125 aggregate undergraduate and graduate	$6,000/year; $40,000 aggregate undergraduate and graduate	Cost of attendance at participating school	Federal Loan Programs	Cost of attendance minus other aid
Interest Rate	Fixed; capped at 6.8%	5%	5%	5%	7%
Interest Accrues While Enrolled in School	Yes	No	No	No	Yes
Deferments	Yes	Yes	Yes	Yes	Yes
Grace Period	Yes	Yes	Yes	Yes	No

A GUIDE TO PREPARING FOR VETERINARY SCHOOL

Maybe you already know that you have a strong interest in veterinary medicine, but you don't know where to start. It's never too early to begin preparing. Below are a few guidelines to help you plan your coursework and get in touch with mentors and other professionals who can help you along the way.

HIGH SCHOOL STUDENTS

- Take science and math classes, including chemistry, biology, and algebra. If available, take Advanced Placement (AP) coursework. Note, AP courses may not always satisfy vet college prerequisite coursework, but they will give you the highest level of preparation. Consult with the vet colleges to understand if AP credit in high school will satisfy a prerequisite course requirement.
- Talk to people in the field. Call local veterinarians or contact a veterinary society in your city or town to find people who can help answer your questions.
- Gain animal experiences. These will give you a good understanding of working with animals and excellent references when you seek a volunteer experience or internship with a veterinarian. Examples include volunteering at a humane society, cleaning stables and grooming horses, doing an internship at a zoo, volunteering at a nature or wildlife center, or getting involved with 4-H, just to name a few.
- Visit veterinary college websites and perhaps make a visit during one of their admissions presentations or during an open house. The more you know early on, the better prepared you will be.
- Get on the veterinary college's mailing lists for admissions updates and invitations to programs.

COLLEGE YEAR 1

Fall semester

- Obtain a copy of the *AAVMC Veterinary Medical School Admission Requirements* (*VMSAR*) to review the veterinary schools' requirements with your advisor.
- Meet with an advisor and plan coursework. Take the list of prerequisite courses on the AAVMC website or in *VMSAR* for planning purposes. Not all vet colleges require the exact same courses, but most will want courses in the areas of biology, chemistry, and physics. That's a good place to start until you narrow down your list of vet colleges to apply to.
- Start working on the prerequisite coursework. Most vet colleges require quite a few biology and chemistry courses. Starting out right away in these introductory courses will allow you to move forward quickly.

Spring semester

- Think about summer volunteer or employment opportunities in veterinary medicine, such as shadowing a veterinarian or volunteering in an animal shelter.
- Continue working on the introductory courses and register for the fall semester.
- Research preveterinary enrichment programs at ExploreHealthCareers.org. Preveterinary enrichment programs can help you decide if a career in veterinary medicine is a good fit and help prepare you for the application process.

Summer

- Complete an internship or volunteer program.
- Attend summer school, if necessary. Note, many vet colleges prefer the prerequisite coursework be taken in a full-time load during the academic year. If possible, take general education or major courses during the summer.

COLLEGE YEAR 2

Fall semester

- Meet with your advisor to discuss your progress.
- Attend preveterinary activities.
- Join your school's preveterinary society, if one is available.
- Continue working on prerequisite coursework.
- Explore community service opportunities through your school (they don't necessarily need to be animal-related). If possible, continue activities throughout undergraduate career.

Spring semester

- Look into paid or volunteer veterinary-related research opportunities.
- Complete second semester coursework and register for the fall.

Summer

- Complete a summer research or volunteer veterinary-related program.
- Attend summer school, if necessary.
- Prepare for the Graduate Record Examination (GRE).

- Visit veterinary colleges. Meet with someone from the admissions office or attend an admissions presentation and take a tour.

COLLEGE YEAR 3

Fall semester

- Meet with your preveterinary advisor.
- Discuss veterinary schools.
- Register for spring semester.
- Visit the AAVMC's website (www.aavmc.org) to learn about applying to veterinary schools.
- Place your order for the *AAVMC Veterinary Medical School Admission Requirements*.
- Research schools.

Spring semester

- Identify individuals (veterinarian, faculty member or advisor, supervisor of animal experiences, research faculty) to write letters of recommendation.
- Take the GRE during late spring or early summer.
- Prepare to submit your vet school applications.
- Register for the fall semester.
- Schedule a volunteer or paid veterinary medicine-related activity.

Summer

- Take the GRE if you have not done so already.
- Budget time and finances appropriately to attend interviews.
- Participate in a volunteer or paid opportunity.
- Attend summer school, if necessary.
- Work on and submit your applications. Most vet colleges have a supplemental application, so be very careful to meet **all deadlines** for the VMCAS application, supplemental application, and getting in supporting documentation and letters.

COLLEGE YEAR 4

Fall semester

- Meet with your advisor.
- Attend interviews with schools.
- Notification of acceptances begins December 1.

Spring semester

- Apply for federal financial aid.
- April 15 deadline to let the vet colleges where you have been admitted know your decision.

Summer

- Attend school's orientation.
- Prepare to relocate, if necessary.

VETERINARY MEDICAL COLLEGE APPLICATION SERVICE (VMCAS)

The Veterinary Medical College Application Service is a centralized application service sponsored by the Association of American Veterinary Medical Colleges. Applicants use VMCAS to apply to most of the AVMA-accredited colleges in the United States and abroad.

VMCAS collects, processes, and ships application materials to veterinary colleges designated by the applicant, and responds to applicant inquiries about the application process. This service is the data collection, processing, and distribution component of the admission process for colleges participating in VMCAS. VMCAS, however, does not take part in the admissions selection process.

Twenty-nine (29) of the thirty (30) U.S. veterinary institutions participate in VMCAS, along with two (2) Canadian, two (2) Scottish, one (1) English, one (1) Irish, two (2) Australian, and one (1) New Zealand veterinary institutions. Application material deadlines, prerequisite courses, and other aspects of the admissions process differ from school to school. Applicants are responsible for being informed of all instructions provided by VMCAS and the associated member colleges. Questions about using VMCAS should be directed to the VMCAS Student and Advisor Hotline.

APPLICATION CYCLE TIMELINE

VMCAS launch: May 9, 2019
VMCAS Application Deadline: September 17, 2019, 11:59 PM Eastern Time
AAVMC Acceptance Deadline: April 16, 2020
Please be sure to verify individual school deadlines

KEY ONLINE RESOURCES

General Information Chart

A one-stop comparison of school info such as location, tuition, seat availability, etc.
http://aavmc.org/data/files/vmcas/geninfochart.pdf

Prerequisite Comparison Chart

A course requirement comparison chart of all AAVMC member schools.
http://aavmc.org/data/files/vmcas/prereqchart.pdf

Fee Structure

VMCAS fees broken down by number of designations.
http://aavmc.org/Applicant-Responsibilities/Fees.aspx

Evaluation Requirements

Individual recommendation requirements by school.
www.aavmc.org/Applicant-Responsibilities/Evaluations.aspx

VMCAS

655 K Street, NW Suite 725
Washington, DC 20001
Telephone: (617) 612-2884
Fax: (617) 612-2051
vmcasinfo@vmcas.org
www.aavmc.org

VETERINARY MEDICAL SCHOOLS IN THE **UNITED STATES**

COE Accredited

AUBURN UNIVERSITY

Email: admissions@vetmed.auburn.edu
Website: www.vetmed.auburn.edu

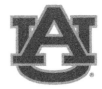

AUBURN UNIVERSITY
COLLEGE OF VETERINARY MEDICINE

SCHOOL DESCRIPTION

The College of Veterinary Medicine at Auburn University is located in south central Alabama off Interstate 85 between Montgomery and Atlanta. The college is known for its friendly small-campus atmosphere.

Veterinary medicine began as a department at Auburn in 1892 and became a college in 1907. Today it is situated on 330 acres one mile from the main Auburn campus that serves more than 28,000 students. In addition, the college has a 700-acre research farm five miles from its campus. The college is fully accredited by the American Veterinary Medical Association.

PROGRAM DESCRIPTION

Health & Wellness:

Auburn University's Health Promotion and Wellness Services strives to support student learning and academic success through evidence-based and theory-driven health promotion and prevention services. Health Promotion and Wellness Services serve as health and wellness advocates for the Auburn Family and strive to foster a campus atmosphere that helps cultivate and support healthy lifestyle choices. Health Promotion and Wellness Services work in collaboration with our diverse campus population to create positive transformational health opportunities.

Diversity & Disadvantaged / Accommodations:

Auburn University recognizes and values the considerable educational benefits emanating from diversity as we prepare our students for life and leadership in a multicultural world. Students who interact with and learn about people from a variety of backgrounds are more apt to understand, appreciate, and excel in the community they inhabit. In this context, diversity is aligned with Auburn University's land-grant mission

of providing its students with a superior education in service to the needs of Alabama, the nation, and the world.

Students who require accommodations must schedule a meeting with a representative of Auburn University's Office of Accessibility.

- Class Size
  - Resident #: 41 Alabama residents
  - Non-Resident #: 51
  - Contract # and where: 38 Kentucky
  - International Seats # 0
- Applicant Pool (prior year)
  - Resident #: 110
  - Non-Resident #: 867
  - Contract #: 117 from Kentucky
- International School: No
- Accepts International Applicants: No
- VMCAS Participant: Yes

ENTRANCE REQUIREMENTS
- Pre-Requisite Chart Update
  - Date pre-reqs must be completed: June 15 prior to matriculation
  - Pre-requisite required grade: C- or better
- VMCAS application: Yes
- Supplemental application: No
- Transcript Requirements
  - AP Policy: must appear on official college transcripts and be equivalent to the appropriate college-level coursework.
  - WES Report Required: Yes
- Test Requirements
  - GRE Test Deadline: September 1 of application year
- Experiences

- o Requirements statement
  - A minimum 500 hours of veterinary experiences are required at the time of application submission in addition to having experience working with large & small animals
- Letters of Recommendation (eLOR)
  - o Letters Guidance Statement
    - Minimum number required: 3
    - Veterinarian Required: Yes
- Bachelor's degree required: No
- Academic Statement
  - o Required minimum cumulative GPA: 2.5 for Alabama and Kentucky residents, 3.0 for non-residents.
  - o Required Grades: C- or better for any required course.
  - o Preferred GRE score: 300 or higher
- Interview Required: Yes

ADMISSIONS PROCESS & DEADLINES
- Admissions Process Statement
  - o Applications undergo review after the VMCAS application deadline. Applications not verified by VMCAS are not typically reviewed. Invitations to interview are sent 4-6 weeks prior to interview dates.
  - o Deadlines:
    - Application Open Date: May 9, 2019
    - Application Deadline Date: September 17, 2019
    - Transcripts Received Date: September 17, 2019
    - eLOR Received Date: September 16, 2019
    - GRE Scores Received Date: September 16, 2019
  - o Interviews held:
    - Non-resident invitations sent: mid-December
      Interviews: February
    - Alabama/Kentucky invitations sent: late-January
      Interviews: March
  - o Interview format statement: Qualified applicants will be invited to an on-site 30-minute interview with multiple members of the Admissions Committee. The purpose of this interview is to optimize the committee's understanding of the applicant's communication skills, depth and breadth of experience working with veterinarians, and professional potential.
  - o Offers released: Within 12 days following interviews

- o Orientation held: Week prior to the start of classes
- o Deposit required: No
- o Defers granted: No
- o Transfers accepted: No

EVALUATION CRITERIA
*If applicable, please enter percentage weighted
- Academic History
- Science GPA
- Organic Chemistry/Physics/Biochemistry GPA
- Cumulative GPA
- Last 60 hours GPA (trend GPA)
- GRE Scores
- eLORS
- Experiences
- Personal Essays
- Communication Skills
- Professional Potential
- Readiness to Matriculate
- Employment History
- Interview

ACCEPTANCE DATA (PRIOR YEAR)
- GRE Average: 306 (combined verbal and quantitative)
- GPA Average: 3.67
- Number of applications: 1094
- Number interviewed: Approximately 500
- Number matriculated: 120

TUITION / COST OF ATTENDANCE
*For current year (2018 matriculation)
- Resident (Alabama/Kentucky)
  - o $20,588 - tuition
  - o Fees – tuition amount reflects tuition and fees
  - o $43,421 – cost of attendance (includes tuition, fees, and estimated expenses)
  *First-year students are required to purchase a laptop computer through the College of Veterinary Medicine's tablet computer program.
- Non-Resident (out-of-state)
  - o $48,244 – tuition
  - o Fees – tuition amount reflects tuition and fees
  - o $71,077 – cost of attendance (includes tuition, fees, and estimated expenses)
  * First-year students are required to purchase a laptop computer through the College of Veterinary Medicine's tablet computer program.

EDUCATION / RESEARCH

- Special programs statement:
  Through the Office of Research and Graduate Studies, the Auburn University College of Veterinary Medicine offers students enrolled in the DVM program the opportunity to complete Master of Public Health (MPH), Master of Science (MS), or Doctor of Philosophy (PhD) programs while continuing their veterinary education.

  Applicants wanting to learn more about dual degree options should visit https://www.vetmed.auburn.edu/education/dual-degree-programs/

- Curriculum Statement:
  The Doctor of Veterinary Medicine (DVM) curriculum is a rigorous four-year program which provides a broad-based education to all students. This prepares them to enter a variety of career opportunities within veterinary medicine. Students take 20 to 24 credit hours per term. This course load requires an average of 36 hours per week in the classroom or laboratory for students seeking to become a doctor of veterinary medicine.

  The curriculum is designed as a modified "systems approach." The first year deals primarily with structure and function of the normal animal. This year includes gross and microscopic anatomy, imaging, physiology, and other related courses. During the first semester of the second year, several principles courses are taught, such as immunology, infectious diseases, and pathology. Students then begin courses based on a body system (for example, gastrointestinal or cardiovascular systems). Each system includes appropriate pathology, diagnostic techniques, and therapeutic measures for both large and small animal diseases. Each semester also includes a case-based course related to topics currently being taught.

  All students are required to take at least four hours of electives. Most take one elective course per semester beginning with the second semester. The clinical year begins March of students' third year in the program.

Q&A

- Top 10 FAQs

Q: Do you accept transfers to your program?
A: Curricula between programs rarely align in a way that proves to be beneficial to students. As a result, the program currently does not accept transfer students.

Q: Do you accept international students to the DVM program at Auburn?
A: Auburn University College of Veterinary Medicine currently does not accept international students to the program. U.S. citizens and permanent residents may be accepted to the program.

Q: My school does not offer "cellular biology", may I use my microbiology/genetics/or other science course to fulfill this requirement?
A: Applicants may not use other science courses to fulfill the cellular biology requirement. You may submit a detailed course syllabus to the College for review if you believe a course that you have taken or are considering taking fulfills the cell biology requirement. Only after reviewing the course syllabus can a decision about that course be made.

Q: My school does not offer animal nutrition. May I take this course online?
A: You may take animal nutrition online or as a correspondence course.

Q: Do you accept online courses?
A: Applicants who complete prerequisite courses through online mediums are eligible for admission. However, we strongly encourage applicants to complete science-specific prerequisite courses through traditional, in-person classwork.

Q: May I be considered an in-state resident for tuition purposes after living in the State of Alabama for one year?
A: No, there is not a process by which a student may change their residency once admitted. All questions concerning matters of residency should be directed to Auburn University's Office of the Registrar by sending an email to residency@auburn.edu.

Q: If I am offered a seat in the class, am I required to secure my seat with a deposit?
A: No. No deposit is required to secure a seat in the class. However, students entering the class are required to purchase their tablet computer through our tablet computer program by May 31.

Q: Other schools show that my GRE scores have been received. How do I know if Auburn University has received my GRE scores?
A: Since GRE scores are sent directly to Auburn University (using school code 1005), VMCAS does not reflect receipt of your GRE scores. Be sure to keep a copy of your GRE score request receipt. The admissions coordinator will contact you *if* your scores have not been received.

Q: Is there any benefit to submitting my VMCAS application early?

A: Applicants are encouraged to begin working on their applications as soon as the application becomes available. Applicants are also encouraged to take their time, submitting their applications only after they have carefully reviewed it. VMCAS encourages applicants to submit applications by August 15 to ensure they undergo verification in a timely manner. There is no preference to applicants who submit their applications early in the application cycle.

Q: Who should I contact if I have questions about specific courses/requirements that may not be outlined on the website or VMSAR?

A: You should contact the coordinator of admissions if you have specific questions about courses and/or requirements. The coordinator of admissions can be reached by sending an email to admissions@vetmed.auburn.edu.

PREREQUISITES FOR ADMISSION

Course Requirements	Number of Semester Hours
Written composition#	6
* Literature#	3
Fine Arts#	3
Humanities/fine arts elective#	6
* History#	3
Social/behavioral science electives#	9
Mathematics—precalculus with trigonometry#	3
Biology I with lab	4
Biology II with lab	4
***Cellular Biology	3
Fundamentals of chemistry with lab	8
Organic chemistry 1 with lab; Organic chemistry 2	6
Physics I	4
Biochemistry	3
Science electives**	6
Animal Nutrition##	3

* Students must complete a 6-semester-hour sequence either in literature or in history.
** Science electives must be two of the following: genetics, microbiology, physics II, comparative anatomy, histology, reproductive physiology, mammalian or animal physiology, parasitology, embryology, or immunology.
*** The cellular biology course, beyond an introductory biology course, should focus on the molecular biology of cells, membranes, cytoplasm, and organelles as well as energy, transport, motility, cell division, signaling, transcription, and translation. Microbiology, genetics, physiology, or other courses may not be used to fulfill the cell biology requirement.
# These requirements will be waived if the student has a bachelor's degree.
Will accept web based or correspondence course. Animal nutrition must focus on large animal, small animal, monogastric, and ruminant species.

UNIVERSITY OF CALIFORNIA

Email: admissions@vetmed.ucdavis.edu
Website: www.vetmed.ucdavis.edu

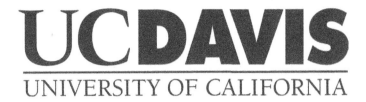

SCHOOL DESCRIPTION

The University of California, Davis (UC Davis) campus is one of 10 campuses of the University of California system. It is the largest campus, with 5,300 acres. The Davis campus is located in Yolo County in the Central Valley of Northern California. Davis is situated 11 miles west of Sacramento, 385 miles north of Los Angeles, and 72 miles northeast of San Francisco. Davis is surrounded by open space, including some of the most productive agricultural land in the state. The terrain is flat and the City of Davis is a friendly college town that cares about sustainability and welcoming newcomers. Ranked as one of the best towns to live in in the nation, Davis is also considered the most bike-friendly city in the nation. The Central Valley climate can be described as Mediterranean. The mild temperate climate means enjoyment of outdoors all year long. During the hot, dry, sunny summers, temperatures on some days can exceed 100 degrees F; however, more often summer temperatures are in the low 90s. Spring and fall has some of the most pleasant weather in the state. Winters in Davis are usually mild. UC Davis is an outstanding research and training institution with over 35,000 undergraduate, graduate and professional students. The Davis campus has four undergraduate colleges, graduate studies in all schools and colleges, and six professional programs carried out in the schools of Education, Law, Management, Medicine, Nursing, and Veterinary Medicine.

Since 1948 the School of Veterinary Medicine serves the people of California by providing educational, research, clinical service, and public service programs of the highest quality to advance the health and care of animals, the public, and the environment. School of Veterinary Medicine faculty members have earned a reputation for their broad expertise and shared commitment to solving some of society's most persistent health problems. The school's impact is

evident in the accomplishments of clinicians who have developed novel treatments and basic scientists who continue to make major discoveries in animal, human and environmental health. We address the health of all animals, including livestock, poultry, companion animals, captive and free-ranging wildlife, exotic animals, birds, aquatic mammals and fish, and animals used in biological and medical research. Our expertise also encompasses related human health concerns.

To carry out this mission, we focus on students in our professional Doctor of Veterinary Medicine program, Master of Preventive Veterinary Medicine program, graduate clinical residency program and graduate academic MS and PhD programs. The school is fully committed to recruiting students with diverse backgrounds.

The School of Veterinary Medicine is home of the William R. Pritchard Veterinary Medical Teaching Hospital, Veterinary Medicine Teaching and Research Center, California Animal Health and Food Safety Laboratory, UC Veterinary Medical Center-San Diego and Centers of Excellence-fostering research, teaching and service focused on species interests and multidisciplinary themes. There are many other centers and innovative programs at UC Davis. Our statewide mission includes 28 research and clinical programs including continuing education; extension; and community outreach.

PROGRAM DESCRIPTION

The professional curriculum at UC Davis is a four-year program of academic study and clinical skills training leading to the Doctor of Veterinary Medicine degree. Each student is provided with a broad foundation of knowledge and skills in comparative veterinary medicine, before choosing a species-specific stream in small or large animal. Following this, the flexible design allows students to focus on careers in small animal, large animal, equine, livestock, zoologic or mixed animal practices as well as poultry, laboratory animal, aquatic medicine, pathology, public health or research.

PROGRAM DESCRIPTION
- Health & Wellness: https://www.vetmed. ucdavis.edu/student-life/career-leadership-wellness/wellness-counseling-services
- Diversity & Disadvantaged / Accommodations: https://www.vetmed.ucdavis.edu/student-life/diversity/diversity-initiatives
- Class Size: 150 available
  - Resident #: varied
  - Non-Resident #: varied
  - Contract #: 0
  - International Seats #: considered non-resident
- Applicant Pool (prior year) 2017-18?
  - Resident #: 493
  - Non-Resident #: 553
- International School: No
- Accepts International Applicants: Yes
- VMCAS Participant: Yes

ENTRANCE REQUIREMENTS
- Pre-Requisite Chart Update
  - Date pre-reqs must be completed: June 30, 2020
  - Minimum grade of C in all pre-requisite courses.
- VMCAS application: Yes
- Supplemental application: Yes
  - Through VMCAS: No
  - External: Yes
- Transcript Requirements
  - AP Policy: Credit must appear on official college transcript with course name and units awarded and must be equivalent to the prerequisite course being satisfied.
  - International Transcripts Required unless attached to WES report
  - WES Report Required: Yes
- Test Requirements
  - GRE Test Deadline: August 31
  - TOEFL Test Deadline: August 31
  - OTHER Test Deadlines: N/A
- Experiences
  - Requirements statement
  - A minimum of 180 hours of *veterinary experience* are required by the application deadline (September 17 of current application year) to have your application considered for admission. https://www.vetmed.ucdavis.edu/admissions/criteria-admission
    - Minimum hours requirements 180
- Letters of Recommendation (eLOR)
  - Letters Guidance Statement: https://www.vetmed.ucdavis.edu/admissions/criteria-admission
    - Minimum number required: 3
    - Veterinarian Required: Yes
- Bachelor's degree required: Yes
- Academic Statement
  - Required minimum cumulative GPA: 2.5
  - Required minimum science GPA: 2.50
- Interview Required: Yes
  - Type of interview MMI

ADMISSIONS PROCESS & DEADLINES
- Admissions Process Statement: https://www.vetmed.ucdavis.edu/admissions/application-process-timeline
  - Deadlines:
    - Application Open Date: May 9, 2019
    - Application Deadline Date: September 17
    - Supplemental Open Date: After the VMCAS application has been Verified, applicants will have access to the supplemental application
    - Supplemental Deadline Date: Mid-October
    - Transcripts Received Date: September 17
    - eLOR Received Date: September 17
    - GRE Scores Received Date: September 17
  - Interviews held: December
    - https://www.vetmed.ucdavis.edu/admissions/criteria-admission
    - Interviews are conducted using the Multiple Mini Interview (MMI) technique. The MMI is a series of short, structured interviews used to assess personal traits/qualities. Each mini interview provides a candidate with a few minutes to read a question/scenario and mentally prepare before entering the interview room. Upon entering, the candidate has several minutes of dialogue with one interviewer/assessor/rater

(or, in some cases, a third party as the interviewer/assessor observes). At the conclusion of the interview, the interviewer/assessor has a few minutes to evaluate while the candidate moves to the next scenario. This pattern is repeated through a circuit of 10 stations.

- Offers released: Mid-January
- Orientation held: Mid-August
- Classes being: Mid-August
- Deposit required: No
- Defers granted: Reviewed on a case-by-case basis for unexpected medical reasons or extenuating circumstances beyond the control of the student
- Transfers accepted: Yes

EVALUATION CRITERIA

https://www.vetmed.ucdavis.edu/admissions/application-process-timeline

*If applicable, please enter percentage weighted

- Science GPA
- Academic History Science GPA
- Last 45 GPA semester/68 quarter units
- GRE Quantitative Scores
- eLOR Composite score of three eLORs
- Veterinary Experience
- Leadership Skills
- Personal Essays
- Contribution to diversity
- Non-cognitive skills
- Readiness to matriculate
- Employment history
- Interview
- Letters of Recommendation

ACCEPTANCE DATA (PRIOR YEAR) 2017-18

https://www.vetmed.ucdavis.edu/admissions/application-statistics-class-2022

- GRE Average and Range Quantitative: 73%
- GPA Average and Range: Mean Cumulative: 3.7
- Number of applications: 1046
- Number interviewed (or N/A): 239
- Number selected: 184
- Number accepted into class: 150
- Number matriculated: 150

TUITION / COST OF ATTENDANCE

https://financialaid.ucdavis.edu/graduate/vet/cost
*For current year (2020 matriculation) unknown. 2019 matriculation approx.:

- Resident (in-State)
  - $ 36,452 includes mandatory health insurance unless waived
- Non-Resident (out-of-state)
  - $ 48,697 includes mandatory health insurance unless waived

EDUCATION / RESEARCH

- Special programs / entrance pathways statement
- Combined Programs statement
  - Veterinary Scientist Training Program (VSTP) Combined DVM/PhD graduate degree program. https://www2.vetmed.ucdavis.edu/vstp/index.cfm
- Curriculum Statement
  - https://www.vetmed.ucdavis.edu/dvm/dvm-curriculum The curriculum utilizes block scheduling which provides all students with a comparative approach integrating normal and abnormal anatomy and physiology centered on body systems rather than disciplines. Recognizing that students learn in different ways, it utilizes a variety of methodologies such as problems, cases, lectures, small groups discussions and laboratories. It is learner-centered allowing students to take ownership of their education and designed such that students are allotted time to work in small groups researching information and solving problems.
  - Clinicals begin: 4th-year clinics are 58 weeks and begin in late April through the following May.
  - https://www.vetmed.ucdavis.edu/admissions/research-opportunities

Q&A

- Top 10 FAQs: https://www.vetmed.ucdavis.edu/admissions/frequently-asked-questions

PREREQUISITES FOR ADMISSION

Course Description	Number of Hours/Credits	Necessity
General chemistry (with laboratory)	Two semesters (3 quarters) w/lab	Required
Organic chemistry (with laboratory)	Two semesters (2-3 quarters) w/lab	Required
Physics	Two semesters (2-3 quarters)	Required
General biology (with laboratory)	Two semesters (3 quarters) w/lab	Required
*Systemic physiology	One semester/quarter	Required
*Biochemistry (bioenergetics and metabolism)	One semester/quarter	Required
*Genetics (genes and gene expression)	One semester/quarter	Required
Statistics	One semester/quarter	Required

*courses must be taken at the upper division level at a four-year university.

COLORADO STATE UNIVERSITY

Email Address: dvmadmissions@colostate.edu
Website: csu-cvmbs.colostate.edu/dvm-program
/Pages/DVM-Program-Entrance-Requirements.aspx

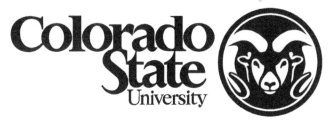

Colorado State University

DOCTOR OF VETERINARY MEDICINE PROGRAM

SCHOOL DESCRIPTION

Colorado State University (CSU) is located in Fort Collins, a city of about 165,000 in the eastern foothills of the Rocky Mountains approximately 65 miles north of Denver. Fort Collins has a pleasant, seasonal climate and offers many cultural and recreational activities. Many world-class ski areas lie within a short driving distance. The nearby river canyons and mountain parks are scenic attractions and provide opportunities for hiking, fishing, photography, camping, and biking. The College of Veterinary Medicine and Biomedical Sciences (CVMBS) is made up of four academic departments: Biomedical Sciences, Clinical Sciences, Environmental and Radiological Health Sciences, and Microbiology, Immunology, and Pathology. Clinical specialists, research scientists, and graduate educators from all four departments provide instruction and mentorship to DVM students. The college is renowned for programs in infectious disease, oncology, equine surgery and reproduction, and professional communication, among others. Prospective students may choose to apply to combined programs, including the MPH-DVM, MBA-DVM, MS Toxicology-DVM, MS Animal Sciences-DVM, and PhD-DVM. The CSU Veterinary Medical Center houses 28 clinical specialties; every year, 42,000 patients are served by over 350 veterinary caregivers. The Clinical Sciences department boasts a variety of clinical and research units, including the internationally acclaimed Robert H. and Mary G. Flint Animal Cancer Center, Integrated Livestock Management Program, Gail Holmes Equine Orthopaedic Research Center, and C. Wayne McIlwraith Translational Medicine Institute. The uniquely designed Diagnostic Medicine Center houses the CVMBS Veterinary Diagnostic Laboratory (VDL), the University's Extension Veterinarian, the Clinical Pathology Laboratory, and the Animal Population Health Institute.

PROGRAM DESCRIPTION

Health & Wellbeing

We provide mentorship, education and individual counseling in the areas of mental health and wellbeing. One-on-one confidential counseling, small group workshops, and large group educational sessions are offered at no cost throughout the semester. Seeking help is not a sign of weakness or vulnerability, it is, in fact, a sign of strength and maturity. Having a robust system of supportive individuals, tools, and healthy practices can be vital to staying on track and balancing the demands of a rigorous professional program. Wellbeing is more than freedom from illness, it is a conscious, self-directed and evolving process of achieving one's full potential.

Diversity & Disadvantaged / Accommodations

Diversity: The CSU College of Veterinary Medicine and Biomedical Sciences (CVMBS) fosters a college climate that welcomes diverse populations of students, faculty, and staff. The CSU CVMBS Veterinary Admissions Committee strives to admit a class of veterinary students who will successfully complete the program and actively contribute to the diverse and dynamic needs of the veterinary profession.

Disadvantaged: Vet Prep is a one-year program that serves as a bridge to the Doctor of Veterinary Medicine (DVM) program for disadvantaged (cultural, social, economic) applicants who ranked high but were not admitted. This program is limited to 10 candidates who upon successful completion are guaranteed admission to the DVM program. Candidates are selected from the regular admissions applicant pool and do not directly apply to the Vet Prep program.
http://csu-cvmbs.colostate.edu/dvm-program/Pages/DVM-Special-Programs.aspx

Accommodations: Our Student Disability Center (SDC) encourages students, family members, and faculty to engage in learning more about the resources and accommodations offered. The SDC will work with students who have chronic physical/mental illnesses or conditions that impact their ability to be an optimally successful student. Their goal is to provide accommodations and support that will contribute to student learning and success within the educational program and beyond. https://disabilitycenter.colostate.edu

- Class Size
  - Resident #: 70
  - Non-Resident #: 40-50
  - Contract # and where: 20-30 WICHE: AZ, HI, MT, ND, NM, NV, WY
  - UAF/CSU: 10
- Applicant Pool (prior year)
  - Resident #: 200
  - Non-Resident #: 1900
  - Contract # and where: 140 WICHE: AZ, HI, MT, ND, NM, NV, WY
- International School: No
- Accepts International Applicants: Yes
- VMCAS Participant: Yes

ENTRANCE REQUIREMENTS
- Pre-Requisite Chart Update
  - Date pre-reqs must be completed: July 15 of the year you would matriculate
  - Pre-requisite required grade: C- or better and must be taken for credit
- VMCAS application: Yes
- Supplemental application: Yes
  - Through VMCAS: No
  - External: Yes, https://dvmadmissions.colostate.edu/apply/
- Transcript Requirements
  - AP Policy: must appear on official transcript
  - International Transcripts: a WES Report is required (course-by-course evaluation)
  - WES Report Required: Yes
- Test Requirements
  - GRE Test Deadline: Tuesday, September 17, 2019 @ 11:59 pm EDT
  - TOEFL Test Deadline: September 17, 2019
- Experiences
  - Requirements statement
    - We do not have a required minimum number of hours for veterinary experience. We look for quality of experience rather than the number of hours. A suggested target is 300-500 hours of veterinary experience.
- Letters of Recommendation (eLOR)
  - We suggest having the following as references: one from a veterinarian, one from an academic source, one from an employment/personal source – but ultimately selecting recommenders with whom you are most comfortable – with at least one being from a veterinarian. Recommendations that can speak to academic and non-academic experiences will provide valuable insights. These can be from faculty, advisers, supervisors as some examples.
    - Minimum number required: 3
    - Veterinarian Required: Yes
- Bachelor's degree required: No
- Academic Statement:
  - The admissions committee strives to admit candidates who will successfully complete the program and actively contribute to the current and future needs of the veterinary profession. The admissions committee a holistic approach to evaluate each and every applicant's file in it's entirety, including the candidate's academic history, veterinary experiences, life experiences, and their potential as a successful veterinarian. Unique attributes that may positively impact future professional success are considered on an individual basis. Our holistic evaluation does not use calculated gpa's; required minimums/threshholds for any category.
- Interview Required: Yes
  - Type of interview: Multiple Mini Interview (MMI)

ADMISSIONS PROCESS & DEADLINES
- Admissions Process Statement
  - CSU requires the VMCAS Application; the Colorado Supplemental Application; GRE scores; three LORs. Note: International transcripts must be evaluated by WES (the course-by-course evaluation).
  - Deadlines:
    - VMCAS application Open Date: May 2019
    - VMCAS application Deadline Date: September 17, 2019
    - Supplemental Open Date: July 2019

- Supplemental Deadline Date: September 17, 2019
- Transcripts Received Date: at VMCAS by September 17, 2019
- eLOR Received Date: at VM-CAS by September 17, 2019
- GRE Scores Received Date: September 16, 2019
  - Interviews held: January 2020
    - The MMI interview format consists of six timed scenarios; is about one hour in length; each scenario is eight minutes in length.
  - Offers released: late January-February 2020
  - Orientation held: late August
  - Deposit required: None required
  - Defers granted: Case by case basis
  - Transfers accepted: Yes

EVALUATION CRITERIA
CSU does not assign points to any category. Admissions decisions are based on a combined rank of the application rank and the interview rank (50/50).
- Academic History
- Science GPA
- Science pre-requisite GPA
- Cumulative GPA
- Last 45 GPA
- GRE Scores
- eLORS
- Experiences
- Leadership Skills
- Personal Essays
- Contribution to diversity
- Non-cognitive skills
- Readiness to matriculate
- Employment history
- Interview 50%
- Other (please list) Application Folder 50%

ACCEPTANCE DATA (PRIOR YEAR)
- GRE Average and Range:
  - Verbal and Quantitative Average: mid-150's
  - Verbal and Quantitative Range: 140-170
  - Analytical Average: 4.25
  - Analytical Range: 2.5-6.0
- GPA Average and Range:
  - GPA Average: 3.60
  - GPA Range: 2.8-4.0
- Number of applications: 2284
- Number interviewed: 400-450
- Number selected: 148
- Number accepted into class: 148
- Number matriculated: 148

TUITION / COST OF ATTENDANCE
*For current year (2018 matriculation)
- Resident (in-State)
  - Establishing domicile (residency) https://financialaid.colostate.edu/in-state-tuition-requirements
  - $33,000 Tuition
  - $3,000 Fees
  - $20,000 COA
- Non-Resident (out-of-state)
  - $57,000 Tuition
  - $3,000 Fees
  - $20,000 COA

EDUCATION / RESEARCH
- Special programs / entrance pathways – see Combined Programs
  - Combined Programs: CSU offers the following combined/special programs, *please see individual webpages for **program-specific** requirements.*
  - FAVCIP (for CSU undergrads): http://csu-cvmbs.colostate.edu/dvm/Pages/DVM-Special-Programs.aspx
  - MBA/DVM: http://csu-cvmbs.colostate.edu/dvm-program/Pages/DVM-MBA.aspx
  - MPH/DVM: http://csu-cvmbs.colostate.edu/dvm-program/Pages/DVM-MPH.aspx
  - MSA/DVM (Animal Science): http://csu-cvmbs.colostate.edu/dvm-program/Pages/dvm-msansci.aspx
  - MST/DVM (Toxicology): http://csu-cvmbs.colostate.edu/dvm-program/Pages/DVM-MST.aspx
  - PhD/DVM: http://csu-cvmbs.colostate.edu/dvm-program/Pages/DVM-PhD.aspx
  - UAF (Alaska)/CSU: http://csu-cvmbs.colostate.edu/dvm-program/Pages/uaf-csu-collaborative-veterinary-program.aspx
- Other Academic Programs statement
  - Vet Prep is a one-year academic program that serves as a bridge to the DVM program for disadvantaged (cultural, social, economic) applicants who ranked high but were not admitted. This program is limited to ten candidates who upon successful completion are guaranteed admission to the DVM program. Candidates are selected from the regular admissions applicant pool and do not directly apply to the Vet Prep program. http://csu-cvmbs.colostate.edu/dvm-program/Pages/DVM-Special-Programs.aspx

- CSU participates in the Veterinary Scholars Summer Program. http://csu-cvmbs.colostate.edu/dvm-program/Pages/Veterinary-Scholars-Program.aspx
- CSU supports additional Young Investigator Grant Programs for research projects. http://csu-cvmbs.colostate.edu/vth/veterinarians/research/companion-animals/Pages/student-projects.aspx
- Curriculum Statement
  - The curriculum allows flexibility for each individual to pursue elective courses and clinical experiences consistent with one's professional aims. Additionally, each student chooses a track (i.e. small animal, large animal, general) in the spring of the third year. There is ample flexibility in the fourth year to emphasize training in a clinical specialty in-house or to participate in experiences outside of CSU.
  - Fourth year practicums are determined by track per above, with five core rotations common to all students.
  - Educational delivery is primarily by didactic lectures, laboratories, problem-based learning, case based learning, and clinical rotations within our Veterinary Teaching Hospital (VTH).
  - Students in years one and two include comprehensive biomedical veterinary sciences education, case-based learning, and hands-on laboratory experiences on the main CSU campus.
  - Students in years three and four work side-by-side with exceptional clinicians at the CSU VTH through a series of specialty rotations. Students are team members, not bystanders. Development of communication and interpersonal skills are emphasized.
- Clinicals begin
  - Students in the third year spend mornings in laboratories and clinics, and afternoons in the classroom, with spring coursework determined by student-selected track (i.e. small animal, large animal, general). Fourth year students are in clinics full time,

with rotations also determined by chosen track. During their time at the VTH, students rotate through a series of specialty and primary care rotations, serving as important team members in meeting with clients, evaluating patients, and developing diagnostic and treatment plans under the supervision of faculty clinicians. Throughout the program, course and clinical electives allow students to tailor their education to align with professional aims.

- Highlights
  - A Financial Education Specialist providing financial education and individual advisement, free of charge, to DVM students
  - Nationally renowned for programs in oncology; equine surgery, sports medicine, and reproduction; infectious disease; and communication.
  - Ample research opportunities in laboratories lead the nation in veterinary research funding
  - Combined programs that allow students to obtain your DVM in tandem with another advanced degree
  - Clinical faculty board-certified in 28 specialties to include Zoo Medicine, Theriogenology, Surgery, Radiology, Pathology, Ophthalmology, Internal Medicine, Emergency and Critical Care, Dermatology, and Dentistry among others
  - More than 35 active student veterinary clubs
  - Unique international and off-site learning opportunities

Q&A
- How does the admissions committee review applications?
  - The admissions committee uses a holistic approach in the review of every application. Each component helps build the full 360 degree picture of who you are and your story. Each piece, GPA, GRE, quality/hours of experience, classes, personal statement, and letters of recommendation are all looked at individually and as a whole when reviewing an applicant to help them select a candidate who will not only be able to handle the academic rigor of a veterinary program but also will contribute to the veterinary profession.

- What is CSU's DVM program best known for?
  - Nationally renowned for programs in oncology; equine surgery, sports medicine and reproduction; infectious disease; and communication
  - Ample research opportunities and leads the nation in veterinary research funding
  - Combined programs that allow you to obtain your DVM in tandem with another advanced degree
  - Unique international and off-site learning opportunities
  - Clinical faculty are board-certified in 28 specialties to include Zoo Medicine, Theriogenology, Surgery, Radiology, Pathology, Ophthalmology, Internal Medicine, Emergency and Critical Care, Dermatology, and Dentistry among others.
  - More than 35 active student veterinary clubs
- Is there a minimum GPA to apply to the program? No
  - We have admitted students in the past with an average GPA of less than 3.0. While the average GPA of previously accepted students is 3.6, please know this represents a range of average GPA's. The admissions committee will look closely at courses taken and grades received as they are looking for upward academic trends and evidence the applicant can handle a rigorous upper division biomedical science curriculum.
  - We have an early academic review of applications with a cumulative gpa of 3.2 or lower. While some applications may be early denied, others are returned to the pool and move forward to the DVM review. Some of these applicants have received offers in the past.
- How many hours of veterinary experience are required?
  - We do not have a required minimum number of hours for veterinary experience. We look for quality of experience rather than the number of hours. A suggested target is 300-500 hours of veterinary experience.
- Do all prerequisite courses have to be completed at the time of application? Does my course meet your requirement?
  - You can apply to our DVM program and be admitted under provisional admission before completing all required prerequisite courses. Please keep in mind the admissions committee will only be able to evaluate completed courses at the time of application.
  - If you are not sure your course content will meet our requirement, please submit a course substitution request. This request should be submitted by SEP 1. http://csu-cvmbs .colostate.edu/Documents/dvm -course-substitution-request-form.pdf
- Do prerequisites become out-dated?
  - We highly recommend that your courses be completed within the past 10 years. (However, biochemistry and genetics are two classes that we suggest be more recently completed.) You can have classes that are older than ten years and they can be used to fulfill our prerequisites. However, the challenge with classes completed many years ago is that the admissions committee doesn't have recent evidence of your ability to handle a rigorous biomedical science curriculum.
- How does the admissions committee view retaking a course?
  - If you retake a course, both the original grade and the new grade will be considered, so they will essentially average out. We suggest only retaking prerequisite courses where you have not received a "C" or higher. Taking additional upper level science classes will raise your GPA more and will better show the admissions committee your ability to handle multiple higher division science classes rather than retaking prerequisite courses.
- How is course load viewed?
  - Credit load, grades, and work/volunteer hours are considered on a per semester basis. Stronger loads are greatly valued. Work/volunteer hours are closely looked at and are also strongly valued when done in tandem with higher credit loads/grades.
- Is there a preferred major?
  - While there are no preferred nor recommended majors for someone who wants to go to veterinary school, many majors offer excellent preparation for veterinary school and eventual work as a doctor of veterinary medicine. It is recommended to select

a major because you are interested in the course of study and because it can provide a good alternate plan for a career in case they change their mind about veterinary medicine. We do not require a specific degree for admission, simply completion of our prerequisite courses.

- What is tracking/when do you start?
  - Our students select a specialty track (small animal/large animal/general) during third year. All tracks provide core experiences required for all students while allowing room to tailor their education to their area of interest.

PREREQUISITES FOR ADMISSION

Course Description	Number of Semester Credits	Necessity
Biochemistry (that requires Org Chem)	3	Required
Genetics (that requires biology)	3	Required
Physics (with a laboratory)	4	Required
Statistics	3	Required
Lab associated with a biology course	1	Required
Lab associated with a chemistry course	1	Required
English Composition (or completion of four-year degree)	3	Required
Social sciences and humanities	12	Required
Electives	30	Required
Upper level biomedical sciences		Recommended

VETERINARIAN PROFILE: JAMES GAFFNEY

YEAR OF GRADUATION
2016

PLACE OF EMPLOYMENT
Veterinary Corps, United States Army
(Public Health Activity - Italy)

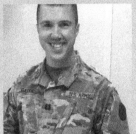

What is your favorite aspect of being a veterinarian?
I enjoy the ability to work on a variety of species across multiple disciplines while being in the same profession -- each day in the clinic is different which prevents things from getting stagnant. As an Army veterinarian, I also get to manage my own clinic and the staff/soldiers that are in it which allows me to develop as a leader in the profession.

What type of veterinary medicine do you practice?
Army veterinarians support the warfighter in a number of ways. We provide care to Military Working Dogs as well as pets owned by service members and retirees. In addition, we conduct audits of commercial food establishments and inspect military facilities where food is stored and/or prepared to ensure that food is safe to eat. We also serve as subject matter experts of zoonotic diseases and the Human Animal Bond. Although the Veterinary Corps is small in size across the Active and Reserve Components, we provide diverse support to all branches of the Military.

Where did you attend veterinary school?
Cornell University College of Veterinary Medicine (CUCVM)

How long have you been practicing as a veterinarian?
1.5 years

What advice do you have for those considering a career in veterinary medicine?
Being able to 'flex-ecute' is important -- you will encounter cases where you may not have all of the tests or medications you'd like and the patient may not present with a 'classic' case of a disease. Being able to creatively manage the case despite the limitations is important. That aside, don't be afraid to ask for help as two (or more) minds are always better than one! Many cases can be managed by an involved general practitioner that knows their limitations.

What challenges have you faced while practicing veterinary medicine?
The human element is the least predictable part of our profession at times. People will question your medical judgement, the cost of your services, and the need for treatment -- it can be enough to drive you crazy! Nonetheless, it is important to be an empathic listener and maintain your professionalism. Surprisingly enough, some of my 'toughest' clients have been the ones to write nice comment cards after the appointment.

CORNELL UNIVERSITY

Email Address: vet_admissions@cornell.edu
Website: www.vet.cornell.edu

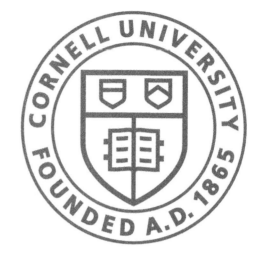

SCHOOL DESCRIPTION

Cornell is located in Ithaca, a college town of about 30,000 in the Finger Lakes region of upstate New York, a beautiful area of rolling hills, deep valleys, scenic gorges, and clear lakes. Established in 1894 with over 5,000 graduates our Veterinary College has 7 teaching hospitals, 5 academic departments, 4 research centers and 43 clinical specialties. Our students pass rate for the NAVLE (licensing exam) was 100% last year.

Through evidence-based, learner-centered education, we prepare our students in all facets of veterinary medicine. Our innovative veterinary curriculum includes small and large group learning, lectures, discussion and laboratories building on a strong foundation of biomedical and clinical knowledge. Students work with live animals the first week of classes, fostering sound clinical and medical decision-making skills along with critical thinking through problem solving. Our internationally renowned faculty, state of the art technology, and extensive educational facilities provide students with an unparalleled educational experience and preparation for a most rewarding career in veterinary medicine. Opportunities and access to research allows our students to be on the forefront of discovery and enhances their educational experience.

PROGRAM DESCRIPTION

Health & Wellness: CVM Wellbeing Program Mission: "Through proactive programming, education, and evidence-based initiatives the Wellbeing Program supports and develops the individual and community wellbeing of faculty, staff, and students at the College of Veterinary Medicine."

- Diversity- Cornell is committed to fostering a welcoming climate that provides rich opportunities for learning and engagement.

- Accommodations- Cornell provides reasonable accommodations for students with qualifying disabilities that apply to the classroom, examination situations, and activities based in the Hospital for Animals.
- Class Size
  - Resident #: 66
  - Non-Resident #: 54
  - Contract # and where: 0
- International School: No
- Accepts International Applicants: Yes
- VMCAS Participant: Yes

ENTRANCE REQUIREMENTS

- Prerequisite Chart Update
  - Date prereqs must be completed: Can apply with up to 12 semester credits (18 quarter credits) of prerequisite course work in progress; all prerequisite course work must be completed by the end of the Spring Term prior to enrolling.
  - Prerequisite required grade: C- or better
- VMCAS application: Yes
- Supplemental application: Yes (embedded in VMCAS)
  - Through VMCAS: Yes
  - External: No
- Transcript Requirements
  - AP Policy: Accepted for physics and general or inorganic chemistry with a score of 4 or higher.
  - International Transcripts
  - WES Report Required: Yes

- Test Requirements
  - GRE Test Deadline: September 17
  - TOEFL Test Deadline: September 17
  - OTHER Test Deadlines: September 17 (MCAT)
- Experiences
  - Requirements statement
    - Minimum hours requirements (recommended 400 hours in veterinary medicine and some breadth of experience)
- Letters of Recommendation (eLOR)
  - Guidelines for Evaluators
    - Minimum number required: 3
    - Veterinarian Required: Yes
- Bachelor's degree required: No (minimum of 60 semester credits and all prerequisite courses completed)
- Academic Statement
  - Required minimum cumulative GPA: None
  - Required Grades- C- for prerequisite courses
  - Required minimum of last 45
  - Required minimum science GPA
  - Required minimum GRE score
  - Other GPA requirements
- Interview Required: No

ADMISSIONS PROCESS & DEADLINES
- Admissions Process Statement
  - Deadlines:
    - Application Open Date: May 9, 2019
    - Application Deadline Date: September 17
    - Supplemental Open Date May 9, 2019
    - Supplemental Deadline Date (embedded in VMCAS with September 17 deadline)
    - Transcripts Received Date: VMCAS deadline of September 17
    - eLOR Received Date: VMCAS deadline of September 17 GRE Scores Received Date: VMCAS deadline of September 17
  - Interviews held: Dates
    - Interview format statement
  - Offers released: January
  - Orientation held: Dates
  - Deposit required: Yes
    - If YES, amount: $500
  - Defers granted: Yes
  - Transfers accepted: Yes

EVALUATION CRITERIA
*If applicable, please enter percentage weighted
- Academic History included in 5% quality of academic program
- Science GPA included in 5% quality of academic program
- Science prerequisite GPA included in 5% quality of academic program
- Cumulative GPA 25%
- Last 45 GPA
- GRE Scores 25%
- eLORS included in several parts of the application review
- Experiences 20%
- Leadership Skills included in 10% all other experiences
- Personal Essays 5%
- Contribution to diversity
- Non-cognitive skills 10%
- Readiness to matriculate
- Employment history
- Interview
- Other (please list) 10% other achievements

ACCEPTANCE DATA (PRIOR YEAR)
- GRE Average and Range 317
- GPA Average and Range: 3.67; Range 3.16-4.0
- Number matriculated: 120

TUITION / COST OF ATTENDANCE
*For current year (2020 matriculation)
- Resident (in-State)
  - $37,136
- Non-Resident (out-of-state)
  - $54,744

EDUCATION / RESEARCH
- Special programs / entrance pathways statement: Cornell BS/DVM Accelerated Program; Early Acceptance Program for Sophomores
- Combined Programs statement: Combined DVM/PhD
  - Combined DVM/PhD- The Combined DVM/PhD Degree Program seeks to integrate the most rigorous basic scientific and clinical training so that our graduates will be at the forefront of biomedical science and the veterinary profession in academic research, medicine and teaching; government service and public health; or the bio-technology/pharmaceutical industry.
- Curriculum Statement
- Our innovative veterinary curriculum includes small and large group learning, lectures, discussion and laboratories. Students work with live animals the first week of classes, pursue

interests, and tailor their learning to meet their interests. Goals include Critical thinking through problem solving; Sound clinical judgment and medical decision-making skills; an understanding of the interactions among animals, people, and the environment; and unparalleled professionalism.

- Clinicals begin: Clinical Rotations and Pathways begin Spring term of the Junior Year (after the March White Coat Ceremony). Students have access to baby rotations earlier in the program.

  - o Other educational and research opportunities include Expanding Horizons; Veterinary Investigators Program; Leadership Program; Aquavet;
  - o Summer Dairy
- Highlights
  - o Business and Entrepreneur Program-Cornell Center for Veterinary Entrepreneurship and Innovation

PREREQUISITES FOR ADMISSION

Course Description	Number of Semester Credits	Necessity
English composition/writing-intensive courses (full year)	6	Required
Biology or zoology, full year with laboratory	6	Required
Physics, full year with laboratory	6	Required
Inorganic (or general) chemistry, full year with laboratory	6	Required
Organic chemistry, one semester	3	Required
Biochemistry, half year required; full year preferred	4	Required
Advanced Life Science course	3	Required
Non-prerequisite elective credits needed	26	Required

UNIVERSITY OF FLORIDA

Email Address: studentservices@vetmed.ufl.edu
Website: www.vetmed.ufl.edu

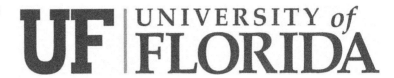

SCHOOL DESCRIPTION
The University of Florida is located in Gainesville, a college town of approximately 132,000 in north central Florida. Winter is mild and summer permits year-round participation in outdoor activities. The College of Veterinary Medicine is part of the Institute of Food and Agricultural Sciences and is a member of the Health Science Center that encompasses five other colleges (Dentistry, Public Health and Health Professions, Medicine, Nursing, and Pharmacy). Our students spend the first two years learning physical examinations and diagnosis, radiology, and basic skills in the Clinical Skills Laboratory. During the last two years of their DVM education, students actively participate in clinical rotations, externship opportunities and specialized electives.

PROGRAM DESCRIPTION
- o Four Professional Certificate Programs (Aquatics, Food Animal, Shelter and Veterinary Business)
- o Combined DVM/MPH Degree
- o Clinical Skills Laboratory
- Health & Wellness
  - o Yoga Classes
  - o Monthly educational and developmental events
  - o On-site Licensed Psychologist
  - o Health initiatives integrated in our curriculum
- Diversity & Disadvantaged / Accommodations
  - o Diversity & Inclusion Committee
  - o Disability Resource Center
- Class Size
  - o Resident: 94
  - o Non-Resident: 26
  - o International Seats: N/A
- Applicant Pool (prior year)
  - o Resident: 390
  - o Non-Resident: 884

- International School: No
- Accepts International Applicants: Yes
- VMCAS Participant: Yes

ENTRANCE REQUIREMENTS
- Pre-Requisite Chart Update
  - o All prerequisite courses must be completed by the end of Spring term prior to the start of veterinary school. We strongly recommend 80% of Science and Math pre-requisites completed by VMCAS application deadline.
  - o Pre-requisite required grade: C or higher (C- must be repeated)
- VMCAS application: Yes
- Supplemental application: Yes
  - o Through VMCAS: No
  - o External: Yes
- Transcript Requirements
  - o AP Policy: Must be listed in official college/university transcript with course and credit equivalency
  - o International Transcripts: Yes
  - o WES Report Required: Yes
- Test Requirements
- Experiences
  - o Requirements statement: Significant hours of veterinary experience under the supervision of a licensed veterinarian, legitimate animal experience and strong letters of recommendation. Documented research is a valuable form of experience.
- Letters of Recommendation (eLOR)
  - o Requirement of three strong letters of recommendation with at least one from a veterinarian. Letters of recommendation from family members are not accepted.

- Minimum number required: 3
- Veterinarian Required: Yes
- Bachelor's degree required: No
- Academic Statement
  - Recommended cumulative GPA: 3.0
  - Required Grades: N/A
  - Recommended last 45: 3.0
  - Recommended science GPA: 3.0
  - Required minimum GRE score: N/A
  - Other GPA requirements: N/A
- Interview Required: Yes
  - Type of interview: Behavioral/Situational Judgement Interview

ADMISSIONS PROCESS & DEADLINES
- Admissions Process Statement
  - Deadlines:
    - Application Open Date: May 9, 2019
    - Application Deadline Date: September 17, 2019
    - Supplemental Open Date: Same as VMCAS
    - Supplemental Deadline Date: Same as VMCAS
    - Transcripts Received Date: Same as VMCAS
    - eLOR Received Date: N/A
    - GRE Scores Received Date: Same as VMCAS
  - Interviews held: January-February
    - Interview format statement: 45-minute behavioral interview
  - Offers released: Early March
  - Orientation held: August
  - Deposit required: No
  - Defers granted: Requires admissions approval
  - Transfers accepted: Yes

EVALUATION CRITERIA
*If applicable, please enter percentage weighted
- Academic History
- Science GPA
- Cumulative GPA
- Last 45 GPA
- GRE Scores
- eLORS
- Experiences
- Leadership Skills
- Short Essays
- Contribution to diversity
- Non-cognitive skills
- Self and Social Awareness
- Readiness to matriculate
- Employment history

- Knowledge of issues affecting the veterinary profession
- Interview

ACCEPTANCE DATA (PRIOR YEAR)
- GRE Average: 64.5%
- GPA Average: 3.69
- Number of applications: 1274
- Number interviewed: 289
- Number selected: 182
- Number accepted into class: 116
- Number matriculated: 116

TUITION / COST OF ATTENDANCE
*For current year (2018-2019 academic year)
- Resident (in-State)
  - Tuition and fees: $28,790
  - COA: $25,060
- Non-Resident (out-of-state)
  - Tuition and fees: $45,500
  - COA: $25,060

EDUCATION / RESEARCH
- Special programs / entrance pathways statement: N/A
- Combined Programs statement
  - DVM/MPH Degree
- Other Academic Programs statement
  - Opportunities to engage in research through:
    - Florida Veterinary Scholars Program
    - Phi Zeta Research
- Curriculum Statement
  - 9-semesters of combined didactic and practical clinical core and elective experiences
- Clinicals begin
  - End of the second year DVM program
- Highlights
  - Professional Certificate Programs
  - Multiple Student Club Opportunities
  - Clinical Skills Laboratory
  - State-of-the-art Small and Large hospitals on campus
  - One Health collaboration with five other affiliated health science colleges
  - Renowned faculty and research
  - Diversity and Inclusion Initiatives
  - Holistic Admissions Process

Q&A
- Top 10 FAQs

Do you require a bachelor's degree?
No we do not require a bachelor's degree.

Is there a preference or recommended major?
No preference is given to any major. We recommend a major that you enjoy as this will result in your best academic performance.

If I retake a class, will it replace the first class taken or do you count both grades?
No, it will not replace the first class grade. Both grades will be counted in our GPA calculations.

What are your minimum hours of veterinary experience?
There is not a minimum requirement hours. A successful applicant would have gained significant veterinary/clinical experience for a consistent period of 10 months or longer at one designated location. Employed experiences are desirable but shadow and volunteer hours are acceptable. Documented research is a valuable form of experience.

How many letters of reference you require?
We require a minimum of three letters of reference. We suggest a fourth reference to ensure the required three references are received by VMCAS.

Can I use veterinarians from the same clinic as references?
Our admissions committee prefers references from different clinics.

Do you accept AP credits?
We accept AP credits. They must be listed in official college/university transcript with course and credit equivalence.

My major does not require microbiology and Biochemistry. What should I take to satisfy these pre-requisites?
These two courses are usually offered as electives for Biology/Science majors and most students are able to take them as electives. These courses are not typically offered at community colleges. A nursing microbiology will not satisfy our microbiology pre-requisite.

Do you require a deposit?
No, we do not require a deposit.

Do you offer in state tuition for out-of-state students during the second year of studies?
No, we do not offer in state tuition for out-of-state students during the second year of studies. Out-of-state students are charged a fixed rate that remains the same for the four years of education.

PREREQUISITES FOR ADMISSION

Course Description	Number of Hours/Credits	Necessity
Biology (general, genetics, microbiology)	15	Required
Chemistry (inorganic, organic, biochemistry)	19	Required
Physics	8	Required
Mathematics (statistics)	3	Required
Humanities	9	Required
Social sciences	6	Required
English (composition, writing or literature)	6	Required
Recommended Electives	9	Required

UNIVERSITY OF GEORGIA

Email: dvmadmit@uga.edu
Website: www.vet.uga.edu/admissions

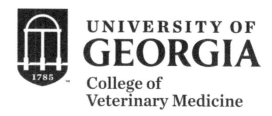

UNIVERSITY OF
GEORGIA
College of
Veterinary Medicine

SCHOOL DESCRIPTION

The University of Georgia is located in Athens-Clarke County, with a population of over 100,000. Georgia's Classic City is a prospering community that reflects the charm of the Old South while growing in culture and industry (www. visitathensga.com). Athens is just over an hour away from the north Georgia mountains and the metropolitan area of Atlanta, and just over 5 hours away from the Atlantic coast.

In 1785, Georgia became the first state to grant a charter for a state-supported university. In 1801 the first students came to the newly formed frontier town of Athens. The University of Georgia has grown into an institution with 16 schools and colleges and more than 3,045 faculty members and 37,606 students.

The University of Georgia College of Veterinary Medicine, founded in 1946, is dedicated to training future veterinarians, providing services to animal owners and veterinarians, and conducting investigations to improve the health of animals as well as people. The college benefits pets and their owners, food-producing animals, and wildlife by offering the highest quality hospital and diagnostic laboratory services. Equipped with the most technologically advanced facilities located on a university campus, the college is dedicated to safeguarding public health by studying emerging infectious diseases that affect both animal and human health.

PROGRAM DESCRIPTION

- Class Size
  - Resident #: 80
  - Non-Resident #: 15
  - Contract # and where: 19, Delaware and South Carolina
- International School: No
- Accepts International Applicants: Yes
- VMCAS Participant: Yes

ENTRANCE REQUIREMENTS

- Pre-Requisite Chart Update
  - Date pre-reqs must be completed: The end of the Spring semester prior to Fall matriculation
  - Pre-requisite required grade: C or better
- VMCAS application: Yes
- Supplemental application: Yes
  - Through VMCAS: No
  - External: Yes
- Transcript Requirements
  - AP Policy: AP credits must appear on official college transcripts and be equivalent to the appropriate college-level coursework.
  - International Transcripts
  - WES Report Required: Yes
- Test Requirements
  - GRE Test Deadline: must be completed within the 5 years immediately preceding the deadline for receipt
  - TOEFL Test Deadline: Application Deadline
- Experiences
  - Requirements statement
    - A minimum of 250 veterinary experience hours is required for all applicants. The 250 hours must be completed at the time the VMCAS application is submitted. To count toward veterinary experience, you must be under the direct supervision of a veterinarian. If you are not under the supervision of a veterinarian, the experience is considered animal experience.

- Letters of Recommendation (eLOR)
  - Letters Guidance Statement: Letters of Recommendation should be completed by references who are familiar with you on a personal level. Letters should include, but are not limited to, information pertaining to your abilities, character, communication skills, intellectual curiosity, decision making, interpersonal relations, leadership, and professional demeanor.
    - Minimum number required: 3
    - Veterinarian Required: Yes
- Bachelor's degree required: No
- Academic Statement
  - Required minimum cumulative GPA: 3.0 or a combined score on the verbal and quantitative portions of the GRE of 308 or greater
- Interview Required: No

ADMISSIONS PROCESS & DEADLINES
- Admissions Process Statement
  - Deadlines:
    - Application Open Date: May 9
    - Application Deadline Date: September 17
    - Supplemental Open Date September 17
    - Supplemental Deadline Date: September 17
    - Updated Fall Transcripts Received Date: February 3
    - eLOR Received Date September 17
    - GRE Scores Received Date September 17
  - Offers released: early–middle February
  - Orientation held: Early-August
  - Deposit required: Yes
    - If YES, amount: $500; $750 for non-resident, non-contract students.
  - Defers granted: Yes, on a case by case basis
  - Transfers accepted: Yes, based on seats becoming available

ACCEPTANCE DATA (PRIOR YEAR)
- GRE Average 310 (V&Q); 4.0 (AW)
- GPA Average 3.65
- Number of applications 1136
- Number accepted into class 114
- Number matriculated 114

TUITION / COST OF ATTENDANCE
Cost of tuition and fees for the 2018-19 academic year
- Resident (in-State)
  - Tuition and fees: $19,448
- Non-Resident (out-of-state)
  - Tuition and fees: $48,528
For more information pertaining to tuition/fees and cost of attendance, please visit: vet.uga.edu/academic-affairs/financing

EDUCATION / RESEARCH
- Special programs / entrance pathways statement
- Combined Programs statement
  - DVM/PhD
  - DVM/MPH
For more information pertaining to combined programs, please visit: vet.uga.edu/graduate/vmstp
- Other Academic Programs statement
  - FAVIP: The "Food Animal Veterinary Incentive Program" was created to recruit and train future food animal veterinarians for under-served communities, central to the future of safe and successful food animal production. This program is offered to incoming freshman attending undergrad at the University of Georgia College of Agricultural and Environmental Sciences. For further information on this program, please visit: http://www.caes.uga.edu/students/undergraduate-programs/preprofessional-studies/pre-vet/favip.html
- Curriculum Statement
  - For information pertaining to curriculum overview please visit: vet.uga.edu/academic-affairs/program-overview
- Clinicals begin
  - The fourth year program allows veterinary students some flexibility to concentrate their interests in specific areas. The program begins immediately following the conclusion of Year 3 (approximately early March) and continues for 14 months.
  - Each course in the fourth year is taught as a 2 or 3 week block. Students take each course as a separate block. Students select clinical rotations with guidance from faculty advisors. A student may concentrate their attentions toward small or large animal rotations, or they may pursue a general, mixed-animal course of study.

- Highlights
  - Health & Wellness: The Academic Affairs Wellness Program is committed to creating a healthy DVM community through the development of wellness initiatives, education, counseling, and curriculum. Please visit vet.uga.edu/academic-affairs/health-and-wellness for more information.
  - Council for Inclusion, Diversity and Awareness (CIDA): The Council for Inclusion, Diversity and Awareness is a college-wide committee of faculty, staff, and students committed to fostering a diverse and inclusive environment for everyone in the College of Veterinary Medicine. Please visit vet.uga.edu/academic-affairs/diversity for more information.
  - International Certificate: The mission of the UGA College of Veterinary Medicine International Certificate is to help students, faculty and administrators of the College make meaningful contributions to the understanding of international veterinary medicine and the inter-relatedness of animal health globally. Please visit vet.uga.edu/academic-affairs/international-program for more information.

Q&A

- Top 10 FAQs

Is there a minimum GPA or GRE requirement?
In order to be considered for admission, you must have a cumulative grade point average of 3.0 or greater or a combined score on the verbal and quantitative portions of the GRE of 308 or greater. Applicants must meet one or the other of these two criteria to be considered, it is not required to meet both. Overall GPA is calculated using ALL courses taken at the undergraduate level (this includes all repeated courses).

If I retake a class, how is GPA calculated?
We consider three different GPAs in our review process. Retaken courses are factored in the following way:
Overall GPA: All courses (even those repeated) are considered in the Overall GPA calculation.
Science GPA: We consider all science prerequisite courses in the Science GPA. If a student repeats any prerequisite, the higher grade for this course is considered.
Last 45hours GPA: Starting with the most recently completed coursework (including graduate level) counting backwards to the nearest semester.

What undergraduate major should I pursue?
An applicant can study any major as long as the prerequisite requirements for our program are met. Typically accepted students major in the life sciences including Biology, Biological Sciences, Animal Science, etc. as these majors can better prepare students for the veterinary science coursework in our program.

Where should I go for my undergraduate degree?
You can attend any accredited institution including 4 year universities and community colleges. However, the admissions committee does take into consideration the rigor of an institution and chosen program of study. If an applicant takes prerequisite coursework at multiple institutions, they must send all transcripts to VMCAS to be included on their application.

Do you have to complete all prerequisites before you can apply?
No. Prerequisite coursework may be in progress at the time of application, but courses must be completed by the end of spring term with a grade of C (2.00) or better prior to fall matriculation.

Are applicants allowed to take some prerequisites at a community college or technical college?
Yes, as long as the community college or technical college is accredited. Please understand that many community college and technical programs do not offer the rigor expected for our upper level prerequisites. We recommend that students taking courses communicate with our office to confirm that we will accept coursework from these institutions.

Do you accept Veterinary Technical Courses?
No. We do not accept veterinary technician courses to fulfill prerequisite requirements.

Will UGA CVM accept GRE scores that were sent to the undergraduate or graduate program at UGA?
No. We require all applicants to send their GRE directly to the College of Veterinary Medicine code 5752.

When should I take the GRE?
Generally speaking, the GRE should be taken during the Fall, Spring, or Summer before the anticipated application cycle. Scores must be received by the application deadline.

Are there scholarships available at the UGA CVM?
The College of Veterinary Medicine at the University of Georgia provides many opportunities for students to receive scholarships throughout

their four years of veterinary medical education. Each academic year, enrolled DVM students will be strongly encouraged to complete the CVM scholarship application, which will allow them to be considered for the bulk of the scholarship money available. Students MUST complete this form to qualify for all of our CVM internal scholarships. Current students will receive information on how to apply via email. The College has a Scholarships and Awards Committee that determines the recipients of our various scholarships based on the criteria set forth by the scholarship donor. Most of our internal UGA-CVM scholarships are awarded in April at our annual Honors and Awards Banquet. This gives students a chance to meet the donors who make these scholarships possible and thank them for their support.

ADDITIONAL INFORMATION

Combined DVM-graduate degree programs are available:

DVM-MPH Veterinarians in Public Health

DVM/PhD Veterinary Medical Scientist Training Program

Online Courses:
As of April 4, 2016 we will accept Biochemistry and Advanced Biology courses from an online program that is regionally accredited. We do, however, still highly recommend that you complete these courses in the traditional lecture style, if possible. We will not accept online courses for any of our other science prerequisites (General Biology, General Chemistry, Organic Chemistry, or Physics).

PREREQUISITES FOR ADMISSION

Course Description	Number of Hours/Credits	Necessity
General Biology with lab	8	Required
General Chemistry with Lab	8	Required
Advanced Biology courses (300/3000 or higher)	8	Required
Organic Chemistry with lab	8	Required
Biochemistry (lecture hours only)	3	Required
Physics with lab	8	Required
English	6	Required
Humanities or Social studies	14	Required

UNIVERSITY OF ILLINOIS

Email: admissions@vetmed.illinois.edu
Website: vetmed.illinois.edu

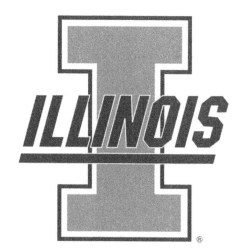

SCHOOL DESCRIPTION

The University of Illinois is in Urbana-Champaign, a community of 100,000 people located 140 miles south of Chicago. It is served by airports in Champaign, Chicago, Indianapolis, and St. Louis, 3 interstate highways, bus, and rail. The twin cities and university make a pleasant community with easy access to all areas and facilities. The university has 45,000 students and more than 11,000 faculty and staff members. It is known for its high-quality academic programs and its exceptional resources and facilities. It is the first university to have established a division of student disability resources. The university library has the largest collection of any public university and ranks third among all U.S. academic libraries. The university also has outstanding cultural and sports facilities and activities.

The College of Veterinary Medicine is located at the south edge of the campus. In addition to over 500 veterinary students, the college has about 100 graduate students plus a full complement of residents and interns. There are more than 100 full-time faculty with research interests in a variety of biomedical sciences and clinical areas. This research activity offers a broad variety of experiences for students. The college also offers students a dynamic, integrated core-elective curriculum to prepare for careers in almost any area of the profession.

PROGRAM DESCRIPTION

- Class Size
  - Resident #: 70
  - Non-Resident #: 60
  - Contract # and where: 0
  - International Seats #: None reserved
- International School: No
- Accepts International Applicants: Yes
- VMCAS Participant: Yes

ENTRANCE REQUIREMENTS

- Pre-Requisite Chart Update
  - Date pre-reqs must be completed: No more than 2 pending in spring
  - Pre-requisite required grade: C- or better done in summer
- VMCAS application: Yes
- Supplemental application: Yes
  - Through VMCAS: Yes
  - External: Yes
- Transcript Requirements
  - AP Policy: AP credit is allowed to meet the 8 s.h. physics prerequisite requirement if a student is awarded the full 8 s.h. AP credit is allowed for biology and chemistry if it is followed up by more advanced college-level courses in those science areas.
  - International Transcripts
  - WES Report Required: Yes, must be WES verified
- Test Requirements
  - GRE Test Deadline: Before September 1. Test dates must be between August 1, 2017 and September 1, 2019.
  - TOEFL Test Deadline: Before matriculation
  - OTHER Test Deadlines: None
- Experiences
  - Requirements statement
    - Minimum hours requirements: 60 s.h.
- Letters of Recommendation (eLOR)
  - Letters Guidance Statement
    - Minimum number required: #3
    - Veterinarian Required: Yes
- Bachelor's degree required: No

- Academic Statement
    - Required minimum cumulative GPA: 2.75
    - Required Grades: C- or better
    - Required minimum Illinois science GPA 2.75
    - Required minimum GRE score not specified
    - Other GPA requirements: None
- Interview Required: Yes
    - Type of interview: Behavioral

ADMISSIONS PROCESS & DEADLINES
- Admissions Process Statement
    - Deadlines:
        - Application Open Date: May 9, 2019 VMCAS
        - Application Deadline Date: September 17 VMCAS
        - Supplemental Open Date: VMCAS
        - Supplemental Deadline Date: VMCAS
        - Transcripts Received Date: VMCAS
        - eLOR Received Date: VMCAS
        - GRE Scores Received Date: VMCAS
    - Interviews held: Mid-February
        - Interview format: Behavioral
    - Offers released: Late February
    - Orientation held: August
    - Deposit required: Yes
        - If YES, amount: $500
    - Defers granted: Yes
    - Transfers accepted: Yes, only into 2nd year

EVALUATION CRITERIA
*If applicable, please enter percentage weighted We do not specify any of this in VMSAR
- Academic History
- Illinois Science GPA
- Science pre-requisite GPA NO
- Cumulative GPA
- Last 45 GPA NO
- GRE Scores
- eLORS
- Experiences

- Leadership Skills
- Personal Essays
- Contribution to diversity NO
- Non-cognitive skills NO
- Readiness to matriculate NO
- Employment history
- Interview
- Other (please list) NO

ACCEPTANCE DATA (PRIOR YEAR)
- GRE Average: 63%
- GPA Average: 3.59
- Number of applications: 1,163 verified
- Number interviewed (or N/A): 338
- Number accepted into class: 130
- Number matriculated: 130

TUITION / COST OF ATTENDANCE
*For current year (2020 matriculation)
- Resident (in-State)
    - Tuition: $27,578
    - Fees: $3,000
- Non-Resident (out-of-state)
    - Tuition: $49,402
    - Fees: $3,000

EDUCATION / RESEARCH
- Special programs / entrance pathways statement
    - 3 and 4 joint degree program with Augustana College and Elmhurst College
- Combined Programs statement
    - Combined DVM/PhD programs may be available.
    - DVM/MPH with concurrent enrollment at University of Illinois at Chicago School of Public Health are available.
- Other Academic Programs statement
    - 3 and 4 joint degree program with Augustana College and Elmhurst College
- Curriculum Statement
    - With 8 weeks of clinics in years 1, 2, and 3
- Clinicals begin 9th week of class for first year students
- Highlights
    - See website

PREREQUISITES FOR ADMISSION

Course Description*	Number of Hours/Credits	Necessity
Biological Science (with laboratories)	8	Required
Chemical Sciences (with laboratories)	16	Required
Physics (with laboratories)	8	Required

With a bachelor's degree completed before matriculation in veterinary school. Without a bachelor's degree, all above must be taken; additional prerequisites are required in English Composition (3 hrs), Speech/Communication (3 hrs), Humanities/Social Science (12 hrs); 12 hrs of junior/senior/graduate level science courses.

PRE-VETERINARY PROFILE: ANA CALOMINO

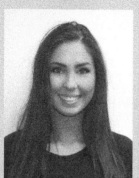

Current School Name
Kansas State University

What type of veterinary medicine are you interested in pursuing, and why?
I am very interested in pursuing small animals. I have worked with large, small, equine, and exotics and although I love all I feel companions are the best fit for me. I love working with owners that feel as though their pet is part of the family allowing me to help not only the animal but the family as well.

What is/was your major during undergraduate school?
Animal Science Pre-vet

What are your short-term and long-term goals?
Some of my short term goals as a sophomore standing now are; work underneath a large animal vet in Sweden this summer, obtain a position on the pre-vet club board, and successfully apply and make it into vet school this upcoming summer. Some of my long term goals would be; graduate at the top of my class from vet school, open my own practice, and make all the clients that I tend to understand how passionate I really am about my field and the animals I am caring for.

What are you doing as an applicant/pre-vet to prepare for veterinary school?
For the past 9 months I am working as a veterinarian technician in a clinic in Kansas City working with small and exotic animals as well as working underneath a large animal vet once a week. Last summer I flew to Cambodia to work in an elephant rehabilitation program. I hold a board position as head of adoptions at a humane society, and foster animals from there as well. I have volunteered at multiple shelters since I was young and still currently do. This upcoming semester I will be a Teaching Assistant for the anatomy and physiology course in the animal science program.

What extracurricular activities are you involved in currently?
I am a part of my Universities pre vet and wildlife club. I am also a part of the Greek system as a chi Omega.

How old were you when you first became interested in being a veterinarian?
I have always wanted to become a veterinarian for as long as I can remember. I believe I was born to do it and my career path has not been altered the 19 years I have been on this earth. My mom told me once that I refused to play with dolls as a little girl, instead, I would only play with stuffed animals pretending to nurse them back to life.

Please describe your various experiences in preparation for applying to veterinary school.
This summer will be my first year applying to vet school. I have began studying for the GRE and plan to take my first trial within a week or so. I am working one on one with my counselor to make sure I have put myself in the best possible position I can be in prior to the application process.

What characteristics are you looking for in a veterinary school?
I want a school that will challenge me, push me outside my comfort zone, and support me along the way. I want classes that will force me to understand and comprehend the material versus memorizing for a test. I want to be given the opportunity for hands on outside experience to help me grow and learn as a student.

What advice do you have for other pre-veterinary students?
If you love something don't ever let anyone else tell you you can't do it. People are always going to want to see you fail, I have already had many personal experiences of this, but never loose site of your goal and your dream. Write down your goals next to your bed. Every night before you go to bed or when you wake up read them and remind yourself why you started.

IOWA STATE UNIVERSITY

Email Address: cvmadmissions@iastate.edu
Website: www.vetmed.iastate.edu

IOWA STATE UNIVERSITY
College of Veterinary Medicine

SCHOOL DESCRIPTION

Iowa State University is located in Ames which has a population of 66,000, and is approximately 30 miles north of Des Moines. The College of Veterinary Medicine is located southeast of main campus. The veterinary medicine campus houses the state's only fully accredited Veterinary Diagnostic Laboratory, the Lloyd Veterinary Medical Center with its state-of-the-art Small and Large Animal Hospitals, Wildlife Care Clinic, the nation's only dedicated Swine Medicine Education Center, Center for Food Security and Public Health, Iowa Center for Neurotoxicity, and the Institute for International Cooperation in Animal Biologics. Central to our mission is the hands-on education and training provided to our students, from day one of the professional program. Iowa State's veterinary program is designed with your career at the center, providing students with the flexibility to add experiences throughout the four years.

PROGRAM DESCRIPTION

Health & Wellness - The CVM is dedicated to a community that supports health and wellness. The College has two-half time clinical therapists on site that are available to students for individual and group counseling and educational seminars for faculty and staff. The CVM has a 24/7 on site fitness room containing free weights, treadmills and other fitness equipment. The College houses Biofeedback equipment and a relaxation room. Recreational Stress Relief and Revolution Wellness, groups under the SAVMA umbrella, provide opportunities for students, faculty and staff to participate in activities ranging from hockey games to Zumba, Yoga, and offers in conjunction with the clinical therapist, educational opportunities addressing healthy lifestyles.

Diversity & Disadvantaged / Accommodations - The CVM is committed to enhancing diversity in the veterinary profession. There is a full time admissions recruiter on staff who does outreach and recruitment at venues with large populations of underrepresented groups. Because the Admissions Committee recogniz-es that a community is only as strong as the richness that accompanies diversity, it strives to admit qualified applicants who will bring that strength through their varied backgrounds, ethnicities and experiences.

Accommodations for DVM students is coordinated through a partnership with Iowa State University Student Accessibility Services and the CVM liaison to that office. The CVM liaison is an advocate who assists students with navigating the process of meeting with faculty regarding their accommodations, to provide education/assistance to faculty and to reserve testing rooms.

- Class Size
  - Resident #: 60
  - Non-Resident #: 60
  - Contract #: 36, North Dakota, South Dakota, and Nebraska
  - International Seats: Included in non-resident group
- Applicant Pool (prior year)
  - Resident #: 138
  - Non-Resident #: 1,355
  - Contract #: 93, North Dakota – 16, South Dakota – 20, Nebraska – 57
- International School: No
- Accepts International Applicants: Yes
- VMCAS Participant: Yes

ENTRANCE REQUIREMENTS
- Pre-Requisite Chart Update
  - Date pre-reqs must be completed, all but 2 required sciences completed in the fall semester of date of application.
  - Pre-requisite required grade, C (2.0) or better
- VMCAS application: Yes
- Supplemental application: Yes
  - Through VMCAS: Yes (partial)
  - External: Yes (partial)
- Transcript Requirements
  - AP Policy: must be documented by original scores submitted to the

university, and must meet the university's minimum requirement in the appropriate subject area. CLEP (College-Level Examination Program) credits accepted only for the arts, humanities, and social sciences.

- International Transcripts: Accepted
- WES Report Required: Yes

- Test Requirements
  - No GRE required
  - TOEFL Test Deadline: September 17
- Experiences
  - Requirements statement
    - Minimum hours requirements – 200 hours animal, veterinary and/or research
- Letters of Recommendation (eLOR)
  - Letters Guidance Statement
    - Minimum number required: 3
    - Veterinarian Required: No
- Bachelor's degree required: No
- Academic Statement
  - Required minimum cumulative GPA: 2.5 (cumulative undergraduate GPA)
  - Required Grades, C (2.0) or better
  - Required minimum of last 45: N/A
  - Required minimum science GPA: Determined yearly
  - Required minimum GRE score: N/A
  - Other GPA requirements
- Interview Required: No
  - Type of interview

ADMISSIONS PROCESS & DEADLINES

- Admissions Process Statement
  - Deadlines:
    - Application Open Date: May 9, 2019
    - Application Deadline Date: Monday, September 17, 2019 at 12 Midnight Eastern Time
    - Supplemental Open Date: May 9, 2019
    - Supplemental Deadline Date: September 17, 2019 at 12 Midnight Eastern Time (11:00 pm Central Time)
    - Transcripts Received Date: Due on VMCAS published date
    - eLOR Received Date: September 17, 2019
  - Interviews held: N/A
  - Interview format statement
    Offers released: approximately February 15
  - Orientation held: late August
  - Deposit required: Yes
    - If YES, amount: $500

- Defers granted: Yes
- Transfers accepted: Yes

EVALUATION CRITERIA
Iowa State University College of Veterinary Medicine
- 2.5-Minimum undergraduate cumulative GPA required to apply
- Academic Review-50%
  - Required science courses GPA
  - Last 45 credits GPA
- Committee Review-50%
  - eLORS
  - Veterinary/Animal/Research Experience
  - Personal Essays
  - Employment history
  - Personal Development
  - Extracurricular and leadership activities

University of Nebraska Lincoln Professional Program in Veterinary Medicine
- 2.5-Minimum undergraduate cumulative GPA required to apply
- Academic Review-50%
  - Required science courses GPA
  - Last 45 credits GPA
- Committee Review-25%
  - eLORS
  - Veterinary/Animal/Research Experience
  - Personal Essays
  - Employment history
  - Personal Development
  - Extracurricular and leadership activities
- Interview-25%

ACCEPTANCE DATA (PRIOR YEAR)
- Required science GPA: Mean 3.48
- Last 45 credit GPA: 3.67
- Number of applications: 1248
- Number selected: 262
- Number accepted into class: 157
- Number matriculated: 157

TUITION / COST OF ATTENDANCE
*For current year (2020 matriculation – not yet determined – These amounts are for 2018-19)
- Resident (in-State)
  - $23,288
  - $1,249
  - $37,872
- Non-Resident (out-of-state)
  - $51,254
  - $1,249
  - $65,838

EDUCATION / RESEARCH
- Special programs / entrance pathways statement: N/A

- Combined Programs statement
  - The College of Veterinary Medicine offers DVM/MPH, DVM/MBA programs as well as DVM/MS and DVM/PhD combined programs.
- Other Academic Programs statement
  - The College of Veterinary Medicine offers a number of educational and internship opportunities for veterinary students including **SMARI (Swine Medicine Applied Research Internship), DVIP (Dairy Veterinary Internship Program), SVIP (Swine Veterinary Internship Program)** and the **Summer Scholar Research Program.**

- Curriculum Statement
  3 year discipline based pre-clinical curriculum employing a mixture of didactic and interactive lectures, in-class discussion (including team based learning and other flipped modalities), laboratories, and case based learning.
- Clinicals begin
  Clinical rotations begin in May of the fourth year.

HIGHLIGHTS
- The **Swine Medicine Education Center** is dedicated to providing veterinary students and practicing veterinarians from across the United States and around the world with extensive hands-on experiences and education in swine health and production.
- The **Great Plains Veterinary Educational Center** (GPVEC) provides education to veterinary students and practitioners through a cooperative agreement between Iowa State University College of Veterinary Medicine, the University of Nebraska and the U.S. Meat Animal Research Center. The teaching program is primarily in food animal health and production management of beef cattle.
- Iowa State University's College of Veterinary Medicine has a cooperative program with the **Blank Park Zoo** in Des Moines, which provides educational experiences for veterinary students, enabling them to work with all types of exotic animals. Students can take four-week elective rotations where they work with exotic animal and wildlife medicine. The College of Veterinary Medicine and the Blank Park Zoo share a veterinarian position, who oversees the clinical rotation at the zoo.
- The **Center for Food Security and Public Health (CFSPH)** was established with funding from the Centers for Disease Control and Prevention (CDC) in 2002 at the Iowa State University College of Veterinary Medicine. The CFSPH was designated as a World Organization for Animal Health (OIE) Collaborating Centre for Day-One Veterinary Competencies and Continuing Education in 2016.
- **The One Health program** embraces translational medicine in research, outreach, and learning. The College of Veterinary Medicine has been **significantly engaged in the university-wide research effort** including ISU's High Impact Hire Initiatives, which hired new college faculty researching infectious diseases; developing more animal models for human diseases; and using Big Data analysis. These areas support the future focus of the University healthy lives research theme that seeks to position ISU as one of the best universities in the world that provides transformative science-based solutions to pursuing a healthy lifestyle by recognizing the interdependencies of human, animal, and plant health.

Q&A

Q: How do I know veterinary medicine is the right career for me?
A: In addition to a sincere concern for animals, an aptitude for science, and good people skills, applicants must have a realistic understanding of the veterinary profession. It is expected that the applicant will have exposure to the profession through experiences with practicing veterinarians and/or veterinary researchers. Exploring the profession through these experiences is the best way to learn and understand what is involved in the veterinary profession and whether veterinary medicine is the right career for you.

Q: What should I major in as an undergraduate?
A: There is no preference for any particular major. We encourage applicants to major in an area of their choice so they have a Plan B if they are not admitted to veterinary school.

Q: Do I have a better chance of admission if I attend Iowa State University for my undergraduate education?
A: Undergraduate coursework, including the required pre-veterinary courses, may be taken at any accredited institution. Preference is not given to applicants who have attended Iowa State University.

Q: How may I obtain Iowa residency?
A: The College of Veterinary Medicine does not determine residency. Residency is determined by the Iowa State University Registrar's Office. For further information, please visit the residency webpage at http://www.registrar.iastate.edu/forms/residency

Q: How are repeated courses used in calculating the GPAs?
A: The most recent grade for a repeated course is used in calculating the GPA. The previous grade is no longer used.

Q: Will pursuing a graduate degree improve my GPA?
A: Didactic graduate coursework may be used in calculating the last 45 credit GPA. Seminar, internships, thesis, and research is not used.

Q: May I take required courses Pass/Fail?
A: All required courses must be taken for a grade. Any required course taken as Pass/Fail or similar systems will not fulfill the requirement.

Q: Can required courses be waived?
A: No pre-veterinary requirements will be waived. A course taken for a grade or AP credit is required. The exceptions to this are the English composition and oral communication requirements. If you will have a bachelor's degree by the end of the Spring term prior to matriculation and have met your primary institution's general education requirements for English composition and oral communication, 3 credits of the English composition and the oral communication requirement will be met. The primary institution must state that these competencies are goals of their general education curriculum.

Q: May I apply before I have completed all the required pre-veterinary coursework?
A: You may apply while still completing pre-veterinary coursework during the Fall and Spring terms prior to matriculation. You may take no more than two Iowa State College of Veterinary Medicine required science courses during the Spring term prior to matriculation. All other required coursework must be completed by the end of the Spring term prior to matriculation. You may not take any required coursework the Summer term prior to matriculation.

Q: Will it be helpful to my application if I send more than three confidential letters of recommendation?
A: Up to six letters of recommendation will be accepted through VMCAS. Applicants are encouraged to ask for more than the three required letters of recommendation in case an evaluator is not able to provide the evaluation by the deadline.

PREREQUISITES FOR ADMISSION

Course Description	Semester Hours/Credits	Necessity
General chemistry (1 year series w/lab)	7	Required
Organic chemistry	4	Required
(Organic Chem I & lab – first semester of a 2 semester series)		
Biochemistry	3	Required
Biology (1 year series w/labs)	8	Required
Genetics or Animal Breeding (Upper level)	3	Required
Mammalian anatomy and/or physiology	3	Required
Oral communication	3	Required
(interpersonal, group or public speaking)		
English composition	6	Required
Social Science/Humanities	6	Required
Physics	4	Required
(Physics 1 & lab - first semester of a 2 semester series with mechanics)		
Electives	8	Required

KANSAS STATE UNIVERSITY

Email: admit@vet.k-state.edu

Website: www.vet.k-state.edu

KANSAS STATE
U N I V E R S I T Y

SCHOOL DESCRIPTION

The Kansas State University College of Veterinary Medicine, located in Manhattan, KS is dedicated to scholarship through innovation and excellence in teaching, research, and service to promote animal and human health for the public good. We are committed to creating an environment that is fulfilling and rewarding, being recognized for professional communication, productive collaboration, mutual respect, diversity, integrity, honesty, and inclusivity. Established in 1905, K-State has one of the first veterinary medicine programs in the United States, and proudly claims over 7,000 Doctor of Veterinary Medicine graduates. We pride ourselves in a rich history of tradition, innovation, and a focus on the future.

Manhattan, KS is located in the center of Kansas, within the Animal Health Corridor. The region boasts 56% of the total worldwide animal health, diagnostics and pet food sales. The Corridor is home to more than 300 animal health companies, representing the largest concentration in the world. Students at Kansas State University College of Veterinary Medicine attend a veterinary program anchored in this region allowing a vast variety of unique experiences and opportunities.

PROGRAM DESCRIPTION

- Health/wellness and diversity
  - Two full time Marriage and Family Therapists available to all students, faculty, staff and clientele. Unlimited visits and free of charge.
  - Yoga offered twice a week, 24/7 access to in-house gym.
  - Vet Med ROCKS (Recruitment and Outreach Club of Kansas State) offers both merit-based and need-based scholarships to campers attending summer camp and participate in veterinary labs and hands-on activities.

This club also participates in outreach activities as they occur or are created.
  - This is How We "Role" program is provided to K-4 students through the Boys and Girls Club of Manhattan.
- Class Size
  - Resident #: 50
  - Non-Resident #: 62
  - Contract 5 with North Dakota
  - Contract International Seats #: 1
- Applicant Pool (prior year)
  - Resident #: 111
  - Non-Resident #: 969
  - Contract #: 6 ND
- International School: No
- Accepts International Applicants: Yes
- VMCAS Participant: Yes

ENTRANCE REQUIREMENTS

- Pre-Requisites remain the same
  - Date pre-reqs: Prerequisite courses must be completed by the end of the spring term of the year in which admission is sought.
  - Prerequisite Science courses must be completed within 6 years of application.
  - Pre-requisite required grade: KSU CVM accepts a C- or better on all prerequisite courses.
- VMCAS application: Yes
- Supplemental application: Yes
  - Through VMCAS: No
  - External: Yes
- Transcript Requirements
  - AP Policy: AP credits must appear on official college transcripts and be equivalent to the appropriate college-level coursework.

- o International Transcript
- o WES Report Required: Yes
- Test Requirements
  - o GRE Test Deadline: VMCAS deadline
  - o TOEFL Test Deadline: VMCAS deadline
- Experiences
  - o Requirements statement
    - ▪ KSU CVM does not have a minimum requirement for veterinary hours. Veterinary hours should be time spent working alongside a veterinarian and provide the applicant insight into the everyday life of veterinary practice and a broad knowledge of opportunities in veterinary medicine.
- Letters of Recommendation (eLOR)
  - o Minimum number required: 3
  - o Veterinarian Required: Yes
  - o Veterinarian, academic or pre-professional advisor, professor or other professional; non-family member.
- Bachelor's degree required: No
- Academic Statement
  - o Required minimum cumulative GPA: 2.8
  - o Required Grades: C-or higher on all prerequisite courses on a transcript at the time of application.
  - o Required minimum of last 45: 2.8
  - o Required minimum science GPA: 2.9
- Interview Required: Yes
  - o Traditional, personal and behavioral interview by a team of faculty and KVMA members.

ADMISSIONS PROCESS & DEADLINES
- Admissions Process Statement
  - o Deadlines:
    - ▪ Application Open Date: May 9, 2019
    - ▪ Application Deadline Date: September 17, 2019
    - ▪ Supplemental Open Date: Adhere to VMCAS dates Supplemental Deadline Date : Adhere to VMCAS dates
    - ▪ Transcripts Received Date: September 17, 2019
    - ▪ eLOR Received Date: September 17, 2019
    - ▪ GRE Scores Received Date: September 17, 2019
  - o Interviews held: Mid December-February
    - ▪ Applicants invited for interviews will meet a team of faculty and KVMA members

for a personal and behavioral interview. The interview team will have reviewed each application.
- o Offers released: Within 6 weeks after interview.
- o Orientation held: One week prior to the beginning of classes in August.
- o Deposit required: Yes
  - ▪ If YES, amount: $500
- o Defers granted: Yes, under extraordinary circumstances
- o Transfers accepted: Yes

EVALUATION CRITERIA
*If applicable, please enter percentage weighted:
Academics
Academics include Prerequisite Science GPA, Last 45 semester credit hour GPA and GRE scores.
Non-Academic and Interview
Non-academic includes veterinary experience, animal experience; extracurricular and leadership activity; employment, research, industrial and biomedical experience; references; personal statement/essay question; and overall application impression.
Top applicants ranked on the above criteria will be invited to participate in personal and behavioral interviews on campus. A combination of the Academic, non-academic and interview scores will determine offers.
- Academic History
- Science GPA
- Science pre-requisite GPA
- Cumulative GPA
- Last 45 GPA
- GRE Scores
- eLORS
- Veterinary Experiences
- Leadership Skills
- Personal Essays
- Contribution to diversity
- Non-cognitive skills
- Readiness to matriculate
- Employment history
- Interview
- Other (please list)

ACCEPTANCE DATA (PRIOR YEAR)
- GRE Average and Range: V: 69%, Q: 56%, AW: 70%
- GPA Average and Range:
  - o Avg. Science GPA: 3.64
  - o Avg. Overall GPA: 3.64
  - o Avg. Last 45 hr GPA: 3.69
- Number of applications: 1,086
- Number interviewed: 468
- Number selected: 112
- Number accepted into class: 112
- Number matriculated: 112

TUITION / COST OF ATTENDANCE
*For current year (2020 matriculation)
- Resident (in-State)
  - Tuition: $24,974
  - Books and supplies: $1,027
  - Total cost of attendance: $43,464
- Non-Resident (out-of-state)
  - Tuition: $54,366
  - Books and supplies: $1,027
  - Total cost of attendance: $72,856

EDUCATION / RESEARCH
- Combined Programs statement
  - DVM/MPH
  - DVM/MS
  - DVM/PhD
- Early Admissions Program for Pre-Veterinary Scholars recruits exceptional candidates for admission to the CVM. Focused mentoring allows for career focus, experiences, clinical and research training to produce the future leaders in veterinary medicine. High school seniors scoring a 29 or higher on the ACT are considered for this program. Evaluation of qualified applicants will include unweighted high school GPA, extracurricular activities, veterinary experiences, and letters of reference. Students will be selected for interviews based on these criteria. Interviews occur on the KSU CVM campus. Students accepted into the program must maintain a 3.3 Science GPA and complete all other activities required by KSU CVM Early Admission Pre-Veterinary Scholars Program.
- Curriculum Statement
  - The Doctor of Veterinary Medicine program at the Kansas State College of Veterinary Medicine is a four-year program with three years of pre-clinical classroom instruction followed by one year of clinical training in the Veterinary Health Center. Students have many opportunities to hone their veterinary skills through mentorships, internships and externships. Graduates of the doctoral program in Veterinary Medicine will: demonstrate competency in knowledge, skill, values, attitudes, aptitude and behaviors in the practice of medicine and surgery applicable to a broad range of species in the context of ever-changing societal expectations and life-long learning.
- Clinicals begin
  - Clinical skills training begins the first semester and is a required course each semester until students enter clinical rotations.
  - Anesthesia and Surgery courses and labs of small and large animals occur during the 3rd year.
  - KSU CVM provides a broad classroom and clinical education for students. Clinical rotations during the 4th year include Ophthalmology, Small Animal Medicine and Surgery, Equine Medicine and Surgery, Small Animal Emergency, Food Animal Local Practice, Food Animal Medicine and Surgery, Diagnostic Imaging, Clinical Anesthesiology, Diagnostic Medicine and Dentistry. Elective rotations in 4th year allow students specialization. Students graduate with the excellent skills and broad knowledge to facilitate practice on a wide variety of patients and in multiple areas of interest.
- Highlights
  - An excellent elective course offered to 4th year students is the Shelter Medicine Mobile Surgery Unit 2 week rotation. Students travel to area Animal Shelters and Humane Societies to spay and neuter dogs and cats and address medical issues at the facilities. Each student on the rotation will average 50 surgical procedures.
  - The National Bio and Agro-defense Facility: A $6.1 million grant from the US Department of Agriculture's Animal and Plant Health Inspection Service is funding five graduate students from the KSU College of Veterinary Medicine through the NBAF Scientist Training Program Fellowship. Students receive tuition, stipends and funds for supplies and travel.
  - Multiple construction projects have been completed and are being planned to enhance educational experiences and student life. Recently completed projects include a new $5.1 million anatomy lab and Student Success Center for 1st year students, a spacious Student Success Center for 2nd and 3rd year students, a state-of-the-art Clinical Skills Lab, a 24/7 access in-house gym, and a beautiful Equine Performance Testing Center. Future projects include an expanded Pet Health Center in the Veterinary Health Center, a modernized Large Animal Receiving, and a spacious lecture hall.

- Beef Cattle Institute: The purpose of the Beef Cattle Institute is to create a collaborative environment at KSU to tackle today and tomorrow's issues facing the beef cattle industry through education, research and outreach. Biosecurity Research Institute is the home of comprehensive infectious disease research to address threats to plant, animal and human health, including food-borne pathogens.
- KSU College of Veterinary Medicine boasts an Exotic and Zoo Animal Service that provides excellent, professional care of exotic pets and zoo animals. Dr. James Carpenter, named one of the 15 Most Influential Veterinarians in 2016 by veterinarianedu. org, leads this extraordinary service.
- The Kansas State Veterinary Diagnostic Laboratory is dedicated to serving clients in a variety of ways including, but not limited to, disease diagnosis, field investigation, expert consultation, health surveillance, and regulatory testing. We possess testing capabilities in the areas of pathology, microbiology, clinical pathology, virology, molecular diagnostics and many more. Our rabies laboratory is the largest in the nation providing both animal and human testing services. Our mission also includes training veterinary students and residents pursuing board certification in multiple disciplines. The Center of Excellence for Emerging and Zoonotic Animal Diseases develops innovative countermeasures against high-priority foreign, emerging and zoonotic diseases that threaten human and animal health.
- The Veterinary Health Center at Kansas State University is a full service veterinary hospital providing routine, specialty and emergency care. Our mission is to provide superior veterinary medical education, quality patient care and exceptional customer service in a caring environment.
- Students attending KSU CVM enjoy the hospitality of Manhattan, KS with national rankings by Princeton Review including No. 3 for Town-Gown relations, No. 4 for best quality of life and one of the top 10 college towns in the nation. In 2018, The KSU College of Veterinary Medicine was ranked No. 4 by College Magazine.

Q&A

Q: Do you offer tracking at Kansas State University?
A: Kansas State University College of Veterinary Medicine does not offer tracking. All students receive education on all major species. All students also practice on all major species. KSU CVM believes this system produces well educated, well rounded students. Students choose electives each semester in their areas of interest. Students also select three elective clinical rotations during the 4th clinical year. The elective courses and rotations allow students to specialize in their areas of interest while receiving a broad core education. The Class of 2018 had a NAVLE pass rate of 99%! KSU CVM historically had a pass rate 4 points higher than the national average likely due to the outstanding faculty and broad education they receive during the DVM program.

Q: Can I establish residency after beginning the DVM program at Kansas State University?
A: Students accepted into the program will sign a 4 year contract stating they are responsible for non-resident tuition through the course of the program.

PREREQUISITES FOR ADMISSION

Course Description	Number of Hours/Credits	Necessity
Expository Writing I and II	6	Required
Public Speaking	2	Required
Chemistry I and II	8	Required
General Organic Chemistry w/lab	5	Required
General Biochemistry	3	Required
Physics I and II	8	Required
Principles of Biology or General Zoology	4	Required
Microbiology w/lab	4	Required
Genetics	3	Required
Social Sciences and/or Humanities	12	Required
Electives	9	Required

LINCOLN MEMORIAL UNIVERSITY

Email: veterinaryadmissions@LMUnet.edu
Website: vetmed.lmunet.edu

LMU
Lincoln Memorial University

SCHOOL DESCRIPTION

Lincoln Memorial University (LMU) is an accredited, nonprofit university founded in 1897 through Abraham Lincoln's desire to provide an outstanding university for the people of Appalachia. The LMU main campus is located in Harrogate, Tennessee, beautifully situated at the foot of the historic Cumberland Gap and occupies more than 1,000 wooded acres with modern educational facilities that include classrooms and laboratories equipped with smart technology. Preclinical courses are taught at both the main Harrogate campus and at the DeBusk Veterinary Teaching Center (DVTC), utilizing state-of-the-art technology and clinical facilities about 15 minutes away from main campus in Ewing, Virginia.

The goal of our innovative curriculum is to produce confident, competent, practice-ready veterinarians by emphasizing clinical and professional skills. All students receive a well-rounded education in small animal medicine, bovine and equine medicine as well as exposure to avian and exotic animal medicine.

Features of the LMU-CVM program:
- Hands-on animal and clinical or professional skills-based experiences start in the first semester and continuing throughout the entire curriculum.
- The large animal component of the DVTC provides a working farm environment with a large cattle and horse herd.
- Clinical Year Hybrid Distributive Education program prepares students by providing experience working in both primary care and specialty private practice environments. Students have flexibility through clinical electives to focus on the facets of veterinary medicine that interest them the most such as small animal, equine, or exotics.

- Veterinary research opportunities offer students valuable experience in this important facet of the profession. A diverse range of opportunities are available at LMU-CVM and with our partnership with the University of Kentucky.
- Case simulation labs teach professional and communication skills in an exam room environment with standardized patients in case scenarios.
- Students, staff, and faculty serve the health and wellness needs of people, animals, and the environment in Appalachia and beyond with an emphasis on the One Health approach.
- Our Shelter Outreach to the Appalachian Region (SOAR) program provides small animal spays and neuters for the Appalachian region while providing valuable learning expertise for veterinary students.

Outside of classes, LMU-CVM students have the opportunity to participate in student clubs and activities. LMU is centrally located between Knoxville, TN, and Lexington, KY, two major cities that offer many cultural and recreational opportunities. The Cumberland Gap National Park is a favorite location for students to hike, run, bicycle, and relax between classes.

PROGRAM DESCRIPTION
- Class Size: 115
- International School: Yes
- Accepts International Applicants: Yes
- VMCAS Participant: Yes

ENTRANCE REQUIREMENTS
- Pre-Requisite Chart Update
  - Date pre-reqs must be completed: By the end of the spring 2020 semester
  - Pre-requisite required grade: C-

61

- VMCAS application: Yes
- Supplemental application: Yes
  - Through VMCAS: No
  - External: Yes
- Transcript Requirements
  - AP Policy: AP courses are accepted if they are specifically listed on an official college transcript and are equivalent to the appropriate college-level coursework.
  - International Transcripts
  - WES Report Required: Yes
- Test Requirements
  - GRE Test Deadline: September 17, 2019
- Experiences
  - Requirements statement
- Letters of Recommendation (eLOR)
  - Minimum number required: 3
  - Veterinarian Required: Yes
- Bachelor's degree required: No
- Academic Statement
  - Required minimum cumulative GPA: 2.8
  - Required Grades, C- or higher
- Interview Required: Yes
  - Type of interview: Multi-mini format

ADMISSIONS PROCESS & DEADLINES
- Admissions Process Statement
  - Deadlines:
    - Application Open Date: May 9, 2019
    - Application Deadline Date: September 17, 2019
    - Supplemental Open Date: May 9, 2019
    - Supplemental Deadline Date: September 17, 2019
    - Transcripts Received Date
    - eLOR Received Date
    - GRE Scores Received Date: September 17, 2019
  - Interviews held: September through February
  - Offers released: March
  - Deposit required: Yes
    - If YES, amount: $1,250
  - Transfers accepted: Yes

EVALUATION CRITERIA
Each completed application will receive a holistic review based on both academic and non-academic factors. Considerations include but are not limited to the following:
- Overall GPA, Science GPA, GPA in last two years of study, Graduate GPA
- GRE Scores
- Leadership Skills
- Well-rounded life experience that demonstrates a judicious balance of academic achievement, community service and personal interests
- Experience in and knowledge of the veterinary profession
- Written communication skills as seen in essay responses
- Letters of recommended provided via VMCAS

TUITION / COST OF ATTENDANCE
*For current year (2022 matriculation)
- $47,638
- $212

Requirements	Semester Hours	Quarter hours
General Biology with lab	8	12
Genetics[1]	3	4
Biochemistry	3	4
Upper Division Science Electives (300 level or higher)[2]	8	12
Organic Chemistry with lab	6	9
General Chemistry with lab	6	12
Physics	3	4
English	3	4
Social and Behavioral Sciences	3	4

[1] Animal breeding/reproduction courses must be approved by LMU-CVM
[2] Upper Division coursework (300 level or higher) including Anatomy, Cell Biology, Immunology, Microbiology, Molecular Biology, Physiology, Virology

FIRST-YEAR PROFILE: VICTORIA ROBERTSON

Current School Name
Cornell University College of Veterinary Medicine

Why do you want to be a veterinarian?
As a veterinarian, I will have the opportunity to touch people's lives by helping their animals.

What are your short-term and long-term goals?
My short-term goals are completing vet school with the long-term goal of opening and owning my own private practice.

What did you do as an applicant to prepare for applying to veterinary school?
I began preparing for veterinary school as a freshman. This allowed me to complete the required classes and determine which schools matched most with my learning style before the application cycle.

What advice would you give to applicants or those considering applying to veterinary school?
I highly suggest that applicants truly determine that veterinary medicine is their passion. It is a difficult field for students who do not have the grit to continue and part of that determination comes from a passion for veterinary medicine.

What helped make the transition to veterinary school easier for you?
It was helpful for me to continue staying involved in clubs and sports. It is easy to get bogged down in trying to learn everything possible when in reality your brain needs time to process the information. Activities outside of studying can really help make studying more effective.

What is your advice on student debt?
Work when you have time to work, try to pay interest as you go (I pay my loan interest every semester to keep it from capitalizing), and apply for external scholarships during breaks.

What are you most excited about learning in veterinary school?
I want to learn how to put my veterinary knowledge into action and act quickly in emergency situations.

LOUISIANA STATE UNIVERSITY

Email: svmadmissions@lsu.edu
Website: www.lsu.edu/vetmed

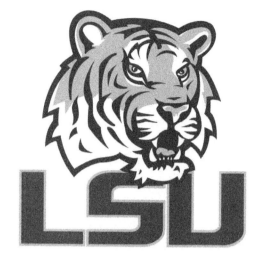

SCHOOL DESCRIPTION

The Louisiana State University campus is located in Baton Rouge, which has a population of more than 500,000 and is a major industrial city, a thriving port, and the state's capital. Since it is located on the Mississippi River, Baton Rouge was a target for domination by Spanish, French, and English settlers. The city bears the influence of all three cultures and offers a range of choices in everything from food to architectural design. Geographically, Baton Rouge is the center of south Louisiana's main cultural and recreational attractions. Equally distant from New Orleans and the fabled Cajun bayou country, there is an abundance of cultural and outdoor recreational activities. The LSU campus encompasses more than 2,000 acres in the southern part of Baton Rouge and is bordered on the west by the Mississippi River. The Veterinary Medicine Building, occupied in 1978, houses the academic departments, the veterinary library, the Louisiana Animal Disease Diagnostic Laboratory, the Wildlife Hospital of Louisiana, and the Veterinary Teaching Hospital. The school is fully accredited by the American Veterinary Medical Association. The curriculum is four years in length and includes a lock-step phase 1 lecture and laboratory portion that is 5 semesters in length and covers all species. The clinical phase 2 portion of the curriculum is a year and a half and allows the students to choose a concentration that focuses on the area of veterinary medicine they plan to go into. The school focuses on wellness with a state of the art recreation center and onsite counseling and values diversity as exemplified by having an Associate Dean of diversity, an active VOICE and Broad Spectrum chapter, and an engaged diversity committee.

PROGRAM DESCRIPTION
- Class Size
  - Resident #: 60-65
  - Non-Resident #: 30-40
  - Contract # and where: 9 (Arkansas)
  - International Seats #: included in non-resident
- Applicant Pool (prior year)
  - Resident #: 145
  - Non-Resident #: 589
  - Contract # and where: 40 (Arkansas)
- International School: No
- Accepts International Applicants: Yes
- VMCAS Participant: Yes

ENTRANCE REQUIREMENTS
- Pre-Requisite Chart Update
  - Date pre-reqs must be completed Must be completed by June 1 prior to matriculation
  - Pre-requisite required grade C or above
- VMCAS application: Yes
- Supplemental application: Yes
  - Through VMCAS: Yes
  - External: No
- Transcript Requirements
  - AP Policy Credit earned through advanced standing is acceptable, although it is not used in the computation of the grade point average. Official credit earned from the AP exam must be reflected on your undergraduate transcripts.
  - International Transcripts: Yes with WES evaluation
  - WES Report Required: Yes
- Test Requirements
  - GRE Test Deadline: August 15
  - TOEFL Test Deadline: N/A
  - OTHER Test Deadlines: N/A

- Experiences
  - Requirements statement
    - Minimum hours requirements: The minimum requirement of 66 semester hours, including 20 hours of elective courses, may be completed in a minimum of two years.
- Letters of Recommendation (eLOR)
  - Letters Guidance Statement
    - Minimum number required: 3
    - Veterinarian Required: Yes
- Bachelor's degree required: No
- Academic Statement
  - Required minimum cumulative GPA: 3.0
  - Required Grades: 3.0 - Required courses GPA: In addition to the specific prerequisite courses, any other Animal Science, Physical Science or Biological Science courses that are taken and in which an "A" grade is earned are factored into the GPA.
  - Required minimum of last 45: 3.0
- Interview Required: Yes (for Louisiana and Arkansas residents)
  - Type of interview: Blinded interview

ADMISSIONS PROCESS & DEADLINES
- Admissions Process Statement
  - Deadlines:
    - Application Open Date: May 9, 2019
    - Application Deadline Date: September 17
    - Supplemental Open Date Part of Webadmit
    - Supplemental Deadline Date Part of Webadmit
    - Transcripts Received Date October 1
    - eLOR Received Date October 1
    - GRE Scores Received Date: October 1
  - Interviews held: February
    - Interview format statement: When conducted, interviews feature a three-member panel consisting of a member of the Admissions Committee, an LSU SVM faculty member, and an outside professional practitioner.
  - Offers released: December for out of state applicants; late February/Early March for Louisiana and Arkansas applicants

- Orientation held: Early to mid-August
- Deposit required: Yes
  - If YES, amount: $500
- Defers granted: Case by case
- Transfers accepted: Yes

EVALUATION CRITERIA
*If applicable, please enter percentage weighted
- Academic History part of Folder Review (15%)
- Science GPA
- Science pre-requisite GPA 29%
- Cumulative GPA
- Last 45 GPA 18%
- GRE Scores 18%
- eLORS part of Folder Review (15%)
- Experiences part of Folder Review (15%)
- Leadership Skills part of Folder Review (15%)
- Personal Essays part of Folder Review (15%)
- Contribution to diversity part of Folder Review (15%)
- Non-cognitive skills part of Folder Review (15%)
- Readiness to matriculate part of Folder Review (15%)
- Employment history part of Folder Review (15%)
- Interview 10%
- Other (please list) 10% (Committee Holistic Evaluation)

ACCEPTANCE DATA (PRIOR YEAR)
- GRE Average and Range: 304 (Average), 283–324 (Range)
- GPA Average and Range: 3.75 (Average), 3.36–4.00 (Range)
- Number of applications 774
- Number interviewed (or N/A) NA
- Number selected NA
- Number accepted into class 174
- Number matriculated 97

TUITION / COST OF ATTENDANCE
*For current year (2020 matriculation)
- Resident (in-State)
  - $27,400
  - Fees NA
  - COA $53,000
- Non-Resident (out-of-state)
  - $56,500
  - Fees NA
  - COA $82,000

EDUCATION / RESEARCH
- Special programs / entrance pathways statement NA
- Combined Programs statement Concurrent DVM/PhD and DVM/MPH are available

- Curriculum Statement
  - Traditional lock-step curriculum with electives that utilizes lecture/lab, clinical skills, and PBL. Clinical phase of the curriculum is a 1.5 years and is a core/elective curriculum that allows the students to choose one of six concentrations (Small Animal; Mixed Animal; Equine; Food Animal; Exotics, Zoo Animal, and Wildlife; and Public Practice)
- Clinicals begin: The clinical phase of the curriculum begins in spring semester of year 3 and is year round from that point.
  - A summer research experience is available to students between their first and second or second and third years.
- Highlights
  - (Anything you would like to highlight about your DVM program) The DVM program provides a well-rounded exposure to all domestic species. Signature programs include Equine Health Studies, Exotic and Wildlife Medicine, Shelter Medicine, Integrative Medicine, and Comparative Biomedical Research

Q&A

- Top 10 FAQs

1. What does the Admission Committee use as criteria to select applicants admitted to the DVM program? Academic and non-academic qualifications are considered in the selection process. Selection for admission is based on the sum of two scores: an objective score which comprises approximately 65 percent of the final calculation and a holistic score which comprises the remaining 35 percent.

2. Are my chances of being admitted to the LSU School of Veterinary Medicine better if I attend LSU as an undergraduate and/ or take the required science courses there? No. The pre-veterinary requirements may be completed at LSU or at any other accredited college or university offering courses of the quality and content of those prescribed in the LSU General Catalog. No preference is given to one school over another; however the caliber of the school(s) attended may be looked at during the folder reviews.

3. What should I choose as an undergraduate major? We do not give preference to one area of study over another; however we strongly encourage all applicants to pursue a degree path in the event an applicant is not accepted after numerous application attempts. The majority of our applicants pursue studies in the sciences. However, an applicant may study or possess a degree in any major provided the prerequisite courses are taken. Students who take the majority of their course work in the sciences, may be better prepared for the veterinary curriculum.

4. Is a bachelor's degree required to be admitted to veterinary school? No. While approximately 75% of students have a bachelor's degree, an applicant must only have completed 66 semester hours at an accredited college prior to entering the DVM program (requirements are listed on the school web site under "Course Prerequisites"), but does not need to earn a degree in order to apply.

5. Do all of the requirements need to be complete before I submit an application? No. However, we prefer that applicants have most of the required course work completed at the time of application. Required course work in the process of completion at the time of application must be complete by the end of the spring semester prior to matriculation. (e.g., If you apply for matriculation into the fall '20 semester, all prerequisites must be completed by the end of the spring '20 semester.)

6. Is it advantageous to take extra science courses in addition to the required course work? Additional coursework is beneficial in preparation for the professional DVM program; courses such as Animal Science, Biological Science, Physical Science, and/or Business courses.

7. How are the Required Course GPA and Last 45 Credit Hour GPA calculated? Grades earned after the VMCAS deadline will not count towards the Required Course GPA and Last 45 Credit Hour GPA for any applicants. In fact, no grades not verified by VMCAS will count towards the Required Course GPA and Last 45 Credit Hour GPA.

The LSU SVM does not use an overall cumulative GPA when computing an overall score. The Required Course GPA is computed by using all of the specific 46 required prerequisite courses (or equivalents). In addition to the specific prerequisite courses, also factored into the Required Course GPA are any other Animal Science, Physical Science or Biological

Science courses that are taken and in which an "A" grade is earned. Social science, humanities, business, kinesiology, and any general education courses are not calculated into the Required Course GPA; however these courses (with the exception of kinesiology courses) will still be used for the Last 45 Credit Hour as seen below.

The Last 45 Credit Hour GPA is computed by using the most recent 45-60 semester hours of course work, with the exception of kinesiology courses. The entire last semester is included when calculating the Last 45 Credit Hour GPA. (If only 3 more credit hours is needed from one semester during which 18 credit hours were taken, all 18 credit hours would be factored into the Last 45 Credit Hour GPA.)

Applicants may choose to re-take a course to better master the subject at any point or to try to improve upon their Required Courses GPA or Last 45 Credit Hour GPA. If a course that is more than six years old is retaken, the most recent grade will be used in calculating the Required Course GPA, otherwise the two grades will be averaged together when computing grade point averages. (If a course is taken more than twice within the past six years, all grades/credit hours will be used.) If a course substitution is approved by the Admissions Office, the course being used as the prerequisite will be calculated into the Required Course GPA. (Note: Course Substitutions are on a case-by-case basis and are not guaranteed.)

8. How much veterinary experience is required? Hands on veterinary or animal handling experience is not required but is strongly recommended. We are looking for the vision that an applicant has of how they see themselves fitting into the profession. Generally, the more experiences an applicant has and the more varied those experiences are (small animal, large animal, exotic, etc.) the better the vision of the applicant will be.

9. How many letters of evaluation do I need? A minimum of three letters of evaluation are required. One or two of the evaluations should be from veterinarians with whom you have worked and who can evaluate your potential as a veterinarian. Letters of evaluation MUST be submitted via the VMCAS application. Please carefully follow the application instructions for more details.

10. Am I required to have health insurance to be in the DVM program? Yes. All students in veterinary medicine are required to have sickness and accident insurance protection either through enrollment in the Student Accident & Sickness Insurance Plan or through proof of participation in any other equal or better program. Additionally, all students need to be vaccinated for Rabies.

PREREQUISITES FOR ADMISSION

Course Description	Number of Hours/Credits	Necessity
General Biology (w/lab)	8	Required
Microbiology (w/lab)	4	Required
Physics	6	Required
General Chemistry (w/lab)	8	Required
Organic chemistry	3	Required
Biochemistry	3	Required
English Composition	6	Required
Mathematics	5	Required
Electives	17	Required

MICHIGAN STATE UNIVERSITY

Email: admiss@cvm.msu.edu
Website: http://www.cvm.msu.edu

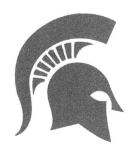

MICHIGAN STATE
U N I V E R S I T Y

SCHOOL DESCRIPTION

Michigan State University's campus is bordered by the city of East Lansing, which offers sidewalk cafes, restaurants, shops, and convenient mass transit. The campus is traversed by the Red Cedar River and has many miles of bike paths and walkways. This park-like setting provides an ideal venue in which MSU's 49,00 students may enjoy outdoor concerts and plays, canoeing, and cross-country skiing. The campus is located in East Lansing, three miles east of Michigan's capitol in Lansing. It sits on a 5,200-acre campus with 2,100 acres in existing or planned development. There are 532 buildings which include 103 academic buildings.

PROGRAM DESCRIPTION

- College Mission: Learn. Discover. Heal. Protect.
- College Vision: The MSU College of Veterinary Medicine is the trusted leader in animal health, delivering unparalleled solutions to serve an ever-evolving world.
- College Values: Accountability, Compassion, Diversity, Excellence, Innovation, Integrity and Teamwork
- Class Size
  - Resident #: 78
  - Non-Resident #: 37
  - International Seats #: Included in 37 non-resident seats
- Applicant Pool (prior year)
  - Resident #: 324
  - Non-Resident #: 875
  - Contract # and where
- International School: No
- Accepts International Applicants: Yes
- VMCAS Participant: Yes

ENTRANCE REQUIREMENTS

- Pre-Requisite Chart Update
  - Date pre-reqs must be completed – July 1, 2020
  - Pre-requisite required grade – 2.0
- VMCAS application: Yes
- Supplemental application: No
- Transcript Requirements
  - AP Policy: AP credit(s) must appear on an official transcript and be equivalent to appropriate college-level coursework.
  - International Transcripts: International transcripts must be evaluated by World Education Services (WES) and submitted to VMCAS. It is recommended that transcript(s) be submitted to the translation service at least one month prior to the deadline of Monday, September 16, 2019.
  - WES Report Required: Yes
- Test Requirements
  - TOEFL Test Deadline: September 16, 2019
- Experiences
  - Requirements statement
    - Minimum hours requirements: 150 Veterinary hours recommended, though not required.
- Letters of Recommendation (eLOR)
  - Letters Guidance Statement
    - Minimum number required: 3
    - Veterinarian Required: Yes – 1 must be from a veterinarian
- Bachelor's degree required: No
  Academic Statement
  - Required Grades – Pre-requisites – 2.0

- o Required minimum of last 45: 3.0
- o Required minimum science GPA: 3.0
- o Other GPA requirements
- Interview Required: Yes
  - o Type of interview: MMI

ADMISSIONS PROCESS & DEADLINES
- Admissions Process Statement
  - o Deadlines:
    - ▪ Application Open Date: May 15
    - ▪ Application Deadline Date: September 17
    - ▪ Transcripts Received Date: September 17
    - ▪ eLOR Received Date: September 17
  - o Interviews held: November through February
    - ▪ Multi-mini Interview
  - o Offers released: December through February
  - o Orientation held: Dates – August 14, 2019 – August 16, 2019
  - o Deposit required: Yes
    - ▪ If YES, amount: $500.00 for residents; $1,000.00 for non-residents
  - o Defers granted: Yes, rare.
  - o Transfers accepted: No

EVALUATION CRITERIA
*If applicable, please enter percentage weighted
- Science pre-requisite GPA
- Last 45 GPA
- eLORS
- Experiences
- Leadership Skills
- Personal Essays
- Contribution to diversity
- Non-cognitive skills
- Readiness to matriculate
- Employment history
- Interview
- Other (please list)

ACCEPTANCE DATA (PRIOR YEAR)
- GPA Average : 3.60 Last 3 semesters, 3.43 Science Pre-reqs
- Number of applications: 1,199
- Number interviewed: 348
- Number selected: 187
- Number accepted into class: 115
- Number matriculated: 115

TUITION / COST OF ATTENDANCE
*For current year (2020 matriculation)
- Resident (in-State)
  - o Tuition: $31,008
  - o Fees: Included in tuition
  - o COA: $21,000 estimated annual living expenses
- Non-Resident (out-of-state)
  - o Tuition: $56470
  - o Fees: Included in tuition
  - o COA: $21,000 estimated annual living expenses

EDUCATION / RESEARCH
- Special programs / entrance pathways statement
- Combined Programs statement
  - o Combined DVM-MPH degree program possible
  - o Combined online DVM/MS in Food Safety possible
- Other Academic Programs statement
- Curriculum Statement
  - o Flipped classroom
- Clinicals begin: Spring semester of the 3rd year
- Highlights
  - o 1.5 years clinical experience
  - o New curriculum focused on active learning
  - o Veterinary Diagnostic Laboratory
  - o Veterinary Technology Program on site

Q&A
- Top FAQs
  - o Do you require the GRE? No
  - o Do you have a supplemental application? No
  - o Do you have a supplemental Fee? No
  - o Do you have interviews? Yes, multi-mini interviews
  - o Are interviews in person? Yes
  - o Do you have a dual degree program? It is possible to do a dual degree
  - o What is your requirement for Veterinary hours? No requirement but we recommend 150 hours

TOP DISTINCTIONS
The College of Veterinary Medicine is fortunate to have an outstanding faculty, all of whom hold the doctor of veterinary medicine degree and/or the doctor of philosophy degree. Nearly all of the specialty boards recognized by the American Veterinary Medical Association are represented on the faculty. Many of these faculty members are leaders in their fields, both nationally and internationally.

Today, the College includes four biomedical science departments—microbiology and molecular genetics, pathobiology and diagnostic investigation, pharmacology and toxicology, and physiology; two clinical departments—large-animal clinical sciences and small animal clinical sciences; two service units—the Veterinary Diagnostic Laboratory and Veterinary Medical Center.

MSU has a long-standing commitment to equal opportunity, affirmative action, and multiculturalism. The College has attained national recognition for its leadership in programs for the encouragement of underrepresented groups at the preprofessional, professional, and advanced studies levels, as well as for increased diversity in its faculty.

DUAL DEGREE PROGRAMS

PREREQUISITES FOR ADMISSION

Course Description	Number of Hours/Credits	Necessity
English Composition	3	Required
Social and Behavioral Sciences	6	Required
Humanities	6	Required
General Inorganic Chemistry (with Laboratory)	3	Required
Organic Chemistry (with laboratory)	6	Required
Biochemistry (upper division)	3	Required
General Biology (with laboratory)	6	Required
College Algebra and Trigonometry	3	Required
College Physics (with laboratory)	8	Required
Upper Level Biology Elective Course	3	Required

For the most accurate information about the prerequisites, please contact the Office of Admissions at admiss@cvm.msu.edu

MIDWESTERN UNIVERSITY

Email Address: admissaz@midwestern.edu
Website: www.midwestern.edu

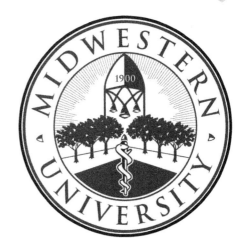

SCHOOL DESCRIPTION

The Midwestern University College of Veterinary Medicine (MWU-CVM) presents to its students a four-year program leading to the Doctor of Veterinary Medicine (DVM) degree. The first 8 quarters are a mix of classroom lectures, laboratories, simulation lab exercises with virtual clients and patients, and small group, student-centered learning experiences. Hands-on live animal contact begins in the first quarter and continues throughout the program. Quarters 9-13 involve diverse clinical training, both on campus (about 85%) and at external sites (about 15%). Three new buildings, including a 111,000 square foot small animal Veterinary Teaching Hospital and a roughly 36,000 square foot large animal/pathology facility, insure our students will begin their careers in state-of-the-art surroundings.

Midwestern University CVM is fully accredited through the American Veterinary Medical Association's Council on Education (AVMA – COE).

PROGRAM DESCRIPTION

- Class Size #: 120
  - Resident #: 15
  - Non-Resident #: 105
  - International Seats #: 0
- Applicant Pool (prior year)
  - Resident #: 75
  - Non-Resident #: 911
- International School: No
- Accepts International Applicants: Yes
- VMCAS Participant: Yes

ENTRANCE REQUIREMENTS

- Pre-Requisite Chart Update
  - Date pre-reqs must be completed: Prior to matriculation.
  - Pre-requisite required grade: C or better
- VMCAS application: Yes
- Transcript Requirements
  - AP Policy
  - International Transcripts
  - WES Report Required: Yes
- Experiences
  - Requirements statement
    - 240 hours minimum
- Letters of Recommendation (eLOR)
  - Letters Guidance Statement
    - Minimum number required: 3
    - Veterinarian Required: Yes
- Bachelor's degree required: No
- Academic Statement
  - Required minimum cumulative GPA 2.75
  - Required minimum science GPA 2.75
- Interview Required: Yes
  - Type of interview Panel

ADMISSIONS PROCESS & DEADLINES

- Admissions Process Statement
  - Deadlines:
    - Application Open Date: May 9, 2019
    - Application Deadline Date: September 17, 2019
  - Interviews held: Sept-Feb
    - Interview format statement Panel
  - Offers released: Rolling Admissions
  - Orientation held: August 24-26, 2020
  - Deposit required: Yes
    - If YES, amount: $200
  - Defers granted: Yes
  - Transfers accepted: Yes

EVALUATION CRITERIA
*If applicable, please enter percentage weighted
- Academic History
- Science GPA
- Cumulative GPA
- eLORS
- Experiences
- Leadership Skills
- Personal Essays
- Contribution to diversity
- Non-cognitive skills
- Readiness to matriculate
- Employment history
- Interview
- Other (please list)

ACCEPTANCE DATA (PRIOR YEAR)
- GPA Average: 3.45
- Number of applications: 986
- Number interviewed: 405
- Number selected: 318
- Number matriculated: 120

TUITION / COST OF ATTENDANCE
*For current year (2019 matriculation)
- Resident (in-State)
  - $61,921
- Non-Resident (out-of-state)
  - $61,921

EDUCATION / RESEARCH
- Clinicals begin 3rd year

PREREQUISITES FOR ADMISSION

Course Description	Number of Hours/Credits	Necessity
Biology	8	Required
Biochemistry	3	Required
General Chemistry	8	Required
Organic Chemistry with Lab	8	Required
Mathematics	6	Required
Physics with Lab	4	Required
English Composition	6	Required
Science Electives	8	Required

A minimum of 64 total semester hours/96 quarter hours is required.

UNIVERSITY OF MINNESOTA

Email: dvminfo@umn.edu
Website: z.umn.edu/prospective

UNIVERSITY OF MINNESOTA
College of Veterinary Medicine

SCHOOL DESCRIPTION

The University of Minnesota College of Veterinary Medicine prepares future leaders in companion animal, food animal, and public health practice, as well as research and education. University of Minnesota students benefit from one of the largest teaching hospitals in the country, as well as world renowned faculty in zoonotic diseases, comparative medicine, and population systems. The College offers state-of-the-art facilities, including the Veterinary Medical Center, Leatherdale Equine Center, and the Raptor Center, which in 1988 became the world's first facility designed specifically for birds of prey. Off-site facilities include farms throughout Minnesota and around the world.

The College of Veterinary Medicine is located on the 540-acre St. Paul campus. Students enjoy a small, intimate campus atmosphere of approximately 3,000 students while benefiting from the numerous amenities available within one of the nation's largest university systems.

The Twin Cities of Minneapolis and St. Paul have a combined population of approximately 2.5 million people and represents one of the largest metropolitan areas where a veterinary college is located. The Twin Cities is the cultural center for the region, abundant with outdoor recreational opportunities, and is repeatedly cited as one of the most livable metropolitan areas in the nation.

In 2013-14, the DVM program underwent a complete curriculum revision. During the first three years of the DVM program, students focus on the study of the normal animal, the pathogenesis of diseases and the prevention, alleviation and clinical therapy of diseases. Students gain hands-on experience throughout the entire program in clinical and professional skills courses.

The program concludes with thirteen months of clinical rotations in the Veterinary Medical Center, during which time students learn methods of veteri-

nary care and develop skills needed for professional practice. Students can choose from over 60 rotation offerings. The fourth year includes up to ten weeks of externship experiences at off-campus sites of the student's choice.

PROGRAM DESCRIPTION

Health & Wellness: We offer a variety of health and wellness related programs, including access to mental health counseling services, wellness initiatives coordinated within each class, student life clubs focused on wellness, on-campus fitness centers, and more.

Diversity & Disadvantaged: We offer a variety of initiatives to promote diversity and inclusion within the student body, starting with the selection of students who contribute and/or support diversity and inclusion. Special scholarships and early admission pathway programs (VetLEAD) support diverse students within the student body. Students can engage in community outreach programs which provide basic veterinary care to low-income or no-income residents in Minnesota or participate on the College-wide diversity and inclusion committee.

Accommodations: Students with documented disabilities will find support from the College's Academic and Student Affairs office in conjunction with the University Disability Resource Center.

- Class Size
  - o Resident #: 53
  - o Non-Resident #: 52
- Applicant Pool (prior year)
  - o Resident #: 190
  - o Non-Resident #: 760
- International School: No
- Accepts International Applicants: Yes
- VMCAS Participant: Yes

ENTRANCE REQUIREMENTS

- Pre-Requisite Chart Update
  - Date pre-reqs must be completed: prerequisite courses must be completed by the end of the spring term of the academic year in which application is made. No more than five prerequisite science and math courses may be pending completion during the fall and spring semesters of the application cycle. A science course and accompanying laboratory are considered as one towards the count of five, even if they are separate classes with independent course numbers.
  - Pre-requisite required grade: C- or better
- VMCAS application: Yes
- Supplemental application: No supplemental application. We do assess an application processing fee of $85. Application fee is payable through our website.
- Transcript Requirements
  - AP Policy: must appear on official college transcripts and be equivalent to the appropriate college-level coursework.
  - International Transcripts: Must be assessed through an evaluation service, such as WES.
  - WES Report Required: Yes
- Test Requirements
  - GRE Test Deadline: Same as application deadline.
- Experiences
  - Requirements statement: Applicants are encourages to have a wide variety of veterinary and animal care experiences. Extracurricular activities, research experience, and other general employment are also highly valued. Experience can be paid, volunteer, or observational.
    - Minimum hours requirements: No minimum requirement
- Letters of Recommendation (eLOR)
  - Letters Guidance Statement: Highly recommend at least one from a veterinarian. Select individuals who know you well through a professional, extracurricular, or educational setting. Committee letters are OK as long as they are routed through the eLOR system.
    - Minimum number required: 3
    - Veterinarian Required: Strongly recommended
- Bachelor's degree required: No
- Academic Statement
  - Required Grades: C- or better
  - Required minimum of last 45: 2.75
  - Required minimum GRE score: 35th percentile
  - Other GPA requirements: Required minimum prerequisite course GPA: 2.75
- Interview Required: Yes
  - Type of interview: Behavioral

ADMISSIONS PROCESS & DEADLINES

- Admissions Process Statement
  - Deadlines:
    - Application Open Date: May 9
    - Application Deadline Date: September 17
    - Transcripts Received Date: September 17
    - eLOR Received Date: September 16
    - GRE Scores Received Date: September 17
  - Interviews held: Late January / early February
    - Interview format statement: Behavioral interview format. One applicant with two interviewers. Approximately 1 hour in length. Learn more about our interview format at our web site: https://z.umn.edu/DVMInterview
  - Offers released: mid to late February
  - Orientation held: Late August
  - Deposit required: Yes
    - If YES, amount: $500
  - Defers granted: Yes
  - Transfers accepted: Yes, on a space available basis

EVALUATION CRITERIA
*If applicable, please enter percentage weighted

- GPA in prerequisite coursework
- GPA in most recent 45-semester credits
- GRE Test scores
- Behavioral interview
- Subjective measures of personal experience
- Employment record
- Extracurricular and/or community service activities
- Leadership abilities
- References
- Maturity/reliability
- Animal/veterinary knowledge, experience, and interest
- Contribution to and support of diversity and inclusion

ACCEPTANCE DATA (PRIOR YEAR)

- GRE Average and Range Verbal: 156 (142-168), Quantitative: 155 (145-167)
- GPA Average and Range: Prerequisite course GPA: 3.67 (2.99-4.0), Last 45-semester credit GPA: 3.74 (3.21-4.0)
- Number of applications: We received 950 applications in 2018-2019
- Number accepted into class: 105
- Number matriculated: 105

TUITION / COST OF ATTENDANCE

*For current year (2020 matriculation)

Expenses include all tuition, fees, and two semesters of health insurance costs (approximately $2,232). Health insurance is mandatory; students can petition out of insurance costs if proof of personal coverage is provided.

Students from Minnesota and South Dakota pay resident tuition rates. Students from North Dakota can apply to the state of North Dakota for tuition support through the Professional Student Exchange Program (PSEP). Approved North Dakota students pay resident tuition rates. North Dakota students not approved pay non-resident tuition rates. Students from all other states or international locations pay non-resident tuition rates.

Students may apply for residency after one year of enrollment.

- Resident (in-State)
  - Tuition & Fees: $31,984
- Non-Resident (out-of-state)
  - Tuition & Fees: $57,490

EDUCATION / RESEARCH

- Special programs / entrance pathways statement
  - VetLEAD: Veterinary Leadership through Early Admissions for Diversity (VetLEAD): VetLEAD creates a pathway into the DVM program for students at under-represented serving partner schools, including Florida Agricultural and Mechanical University (FAMU). High achieving students with relevant experience enrolled at FAMU may apply for an early admissions decision after they have completed at least two semesters at FAMU. Read more about the program at our web site: z.umn.edu/vetlead.
- Combined Programs statement: DVM/PhD:
  - Two options available for formal DVM/PhD study: DVM/PhD in Comparative and Molecular Biosciences or DVM/PhD in Veterinary Medicine. Under the concurrent option, students complete the first two years of the DVM curriculum, then transfer to the PhD program. Following defense of an original PhD thesis, students return to the DVM program to complete clinical training and degree requirements. Alternatively, students may complete all DVM requirements before entering the PhD program full time. Learn more about this program at our web site: z.umn.edu/DVMDual
  - DVM/MPH: In this program veterinary students can simultaneously earn a DVM and a master of public health (MPH) degree in as little as four years. Students obtain the credentials to work in government or industry on issues relating to food safety, emerging infectious diseases, biosecurity, and public health. MPH students complete veterinary and human public health field experience and a "culminating experience" project under the guidance of a faculty adviser. Learn more about this program at our web site: z.umn.edu/dvmmph
- Other Academic Programs statement
  - Summer Scholars: The Summer Scholars program offers first and second year veterinary students the opportunity to participate in research projects related to veterinary, animal, and human health initiatives. Through this experiential learning, students will gain an appreciation of biomedical and veterinary research careers and see firsthand how research contributes to advances in health care and veterinary practice.
- Curriculum Statement
  - The University of Minnesota curriculum is based on progression from normal to abnormal and from the cellular level to the whole animal. The curriculum includes purposeful integration of topics across courses within and between semesters and early introduction to hands-on opportunities with animals in clinical skills courses. Tracking begins in the third year and includes opportunities in small animals, horses, food animals, research, and a mixed track. Clinical training is 13 months in length, with access to over 60 choices of clinical rotations at our Veterinary Medical Center, Equine Center, Dairy Education Center, West

Metro Equine service, and the Golden Valley Humane Society, as well as extensive externship opportunities.
- ○ Clinical skills courses begins the first semester of the first year and continue through each semester of the program. Clinical rotations span the last 13 months of the program.
- • Highlights
  - ○ We offer one of the largest teaching hospitals in the country with over 40,000 cases treated per year. Our unique geographic location in an urban setting, yet close to rural agricultural farmland, provides a well-balanced caseload among multiple species. Students benefit from flexible track options, starting in their third year.

Q&A

- • Top 10 FAQs
  - ○ What is the campus like? We are located on the St. Paul campus of the University of Minnesota Twin Cities. It's a small, scenic campus situated in a friendly suburban setting. It takes about 15 minutes to walk across campus, though the majority of our buildings are connected or just a short walk outside.
    Will you waive prerequisite courses? No, we are unable to waive prerequisite courses.
  - ○ Will you consider online / community college courses towards prerequisite course requirements? Yes, many of our applicants take courses online or through community colleges.
  - ○ Do you have an application processing fee? Yes, we have a separate $85 application processing fee, payable online with credit card.
  - ○ How are "Gap Years" considered? Gap years are viewed neutrally; applicants should feel empowered to take one if needed and supported if they choose not to.
  - ○ Will you accept prerequisite course substitutions? We will only accept substitutions for like courses. For example, we may accept biology II in place of zoology. Applicants should contact the admissions office in advance for guidance.
  - ○ Do I need to submit a transcript if I attended the UMN for undergraduate education? Yes, all transcripts need to be submitted through VMCAS.
  - ○ Do you consider an overall GPA? No, we consider a prerequisite course GPA and a last 45-semester credit GPA.
  - ○ Are video conference interviews permitted? For extenuating circumstances, such as travel complications due to weather, medical conditions, applicants abroad to study, etc.
  - ○ Is the analytical writing section of the GRE considered? No. General writing skill is considered throughout the written application instead.

PREREQUISITES FOR ADMISSION

Course Description	Number of Hours/Credits
English (2 courses)	6
Algebra, Pre-Calculus, or Calculus	3
General Chemistry w/ Labs (2 courses, plus 2 labs)	6
Organic Chemistry	3
Biochemistry	3
General Biology w/ Lab	3
Zoology w/ Lab	3
Genetics	3
Microbiology w/ Lab	3
Physics (2 courses)	6
Liberal Education (3 courses)	9
Statistics	3

PRE-VETERINARY PROFILE: LYDIA SMITH

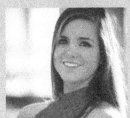

Current School Name
Virginia Tech

What type of veterinary medicine are you interested in pursuing, and why?

Veterinary medicine encompasses so many different routes, it is difficult to choose only one. However, I originally wanted to be a small animal veterinarian with my own private practice. As time went on and I shadowed with more vets, gaining more experience, I saw another path that interested me: shelter medicine. I have always frequented animal shelters, having rescued a total of five dogs across three different facilities. When I started working at a small animal private practice most recently, one of my coworkers was the volunteer and education coordinator for the nearby Animal Care and Adoption Center. She brought in anything from an orphaned less-than-two-pound kitten named Bean to a three-legged dog named Larry, who would always rest his chin on my leg while working. She even had a pig arrive once! A community volunteer accompanies every new shelter patient to aid the animal towards adoption and in some cases, survival. This sense of community, between both animals and humans, through a shelter attracts me as a potential veterinarian because of the 'pack' mindset. A shelter veterinarian treats each animal like an individual of a pack, keeping in mind the whole pack's health and wellbeing. Caring for animals without a paying owner, and ones that can quite literally can be dumped on the doorstep that morning sparks new and unique challenges everyday that you might not find in a typical small animal private practice.

What is/was your major during undergraduate school?

I am currently an Animal and Poultry Sciences major, graduating this May, 2018.

What are your short-term and long-term goals?

My main short term goal, like any other pre-veterinary student, is obtaining that acceptance letter from my dream veterinary school along with graduating my current undergraduate program this spring. One long term goal I have includes someday becoming a board certified veterinary surgeon. Other non-veterinary related long term goals are keeping a healthy mind and lifestyle as well as successfully balancing family, work, and time to recharge myself.

What are you doing as an applicant/pre-vet to prepare for veterinary school?

I started preparing as a veterinary school applicant as early as freshman year in high school, shadowing a local veterinarian on Saturday mornings. Once I came to college, I immersed myself in every animal experience I could as well as chose the major that I believed would give me the most hands-on experience. As time went on, I zeroed in on extracurriculars such as Pre-Veterinary Club, which I am now the President, and worked for over two years in a local small animal clinic, which doubled as both veterinary experience and earning money for future financial commitments. Last year, I ended up being an undergraduate teaching assistant for a class I originally took to only fulfill a requirement. Little did I know, that experience eventually opened a door to other animal research with which I completed my senior capstone project. Every connection I could possibly make, every opportunity that I was presented, I grabbed it by the horns and ran with it.

What extracurricular activities are you involved in currently?

Currently I am the President of the Pre-Veterinary Medical Association (also known as Pre-Vet Club) at my university, Virginia Tech. This takes most of my time and involves extensive planning and attending activities such as our biannual "Puppy Palooza" to alleviate stress for college students, deworming llamas, herding cattle, volunteering at local shelters and a horse rescue, spending time in a clinicals skills lab as well as a necropsy lab, fundraising by making custom pet stockings and filling them with pet treats and toys, and attending the National APVMA Symposium every year. We also have a mentor system which I am involved in that connects pre-vet students to actual veterinary students at the Virginia-Maryland College of Veterinary Medicine. Aside from all things Pre-Vet Club, I am also a member of Dairy Club and the Gamma Phi Beta Sorority. Previously, as I mentioned before, I also served as an undergrad TA for a fungal and mycotoxin course. I also began college residing in a "Living-Learning Community" program, which emphasized strong leadership and professional development.

How old were you when you first became interested in being a veterinarian?

It was at my "future career day" in my kindergarten class where I put on a plastic stethoscope and a white lab coat that I knew I wanted to be a veterinarian. I was five.

MISSISSIPPI STATE UNIVERSITY

Email: MSU-CVMAdmissions@cvm.msstate.edu
Website: www.cvm.msstate.edu

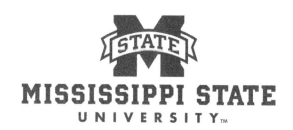

COLLEGE OF VETERINARY MEDICINE

SCHOOL DESCRIPTION
Starkville is home to 22,000 MSU students and their Bulldogs. Starkville is located in northeast central Mississippi and has a population of 24,000. Being a land-grant university, MSU is green and beautifully landscaped. The university includes 9 farms scattered throughout the state. The College of Veterinary Medicine (the Wise Center) was completed in 1982. The college includes 620 rooms on 8 acres, or 360,000 square feet, under one roof.

PROGRAM DESCRIPTION
- Class Size
  - Resident #: 40
  - Non-Resident #: 43
  - Contract 5 South Carolina, 7 West Virginia
- Applicant Pool (prior year)
  - Resident #: 90
  - Non-Resident #: 747
  - Contract: 63 SC applicants and and 25 WV applicants
- International School: No
- Accepts International Applicants: Yes
- VMCAS Participant: Yes

ENTRANCE REQUIREMENTS
- Pre-Requisite Chart Update (See on last page)
  - Date pre-reqs must be completed
    - Prerequisites must be completed by the spring semester prior to matriculation.
  - Pre-requisite required grade
    - C- or better
- VMCAS application: Yes
- Supplemental application: Yes
  - Through VMCAS: Yes
  - External: No

- Transcript Requirements
  - AP Policy: must appear on official college transcripts and be equivalent to the appropriate college-level coursework.
  - International Transcripts
  - WES Report Required: Yes
- Test Requirements
  - TOEFL Test Deadline: same as VMCAS deadline
- Experiences
  - Mississippi State CVM does not require a specified number of hours of experience. The quality of the experience is more important as this allows applicants to make an informed decision on a career in veterinary medicine.
- Letters of Recommendation (eLOR)
  - Mississippi State CVM requires three letters of recommendation, with one being from a DVM. Applicants should choose references that can attest to their passion for veterinary medicine and traits that the applicant possesses that increases their potential for success.
    - Minimum number required: 3
    - Veterinarian Required: Yes
- Bachelor's degree required: No
- Academic Statement
  - Required minimum cumulative GPA 2.8
  - Required Grades C- or better
  - Remediated and repeated courses must be completed before application is submitted.
  - Interview Required: Yes
  - Type of interview
    - Traditional interview consisting of a 3-4 person panel

ADMISSIONS PROCESS & DEADLINES
- Admissions Process Statement
  - Deadlines:
    - Application Open Date: Thursday, May 9, 2019
    - Application Deadline Date Tuesday, September 17, 2019 at 12 Midnight Eastern Time
    - Supplemental Open Date: Thursday, May 9, 2019
    - Supplemental Deadline Date: Tuesday, September 17, 2019
    - Transcripts Received Date: Tuesday, September 17, 2019
    - eLOR Received Date: September 17, 2019
  - Interviews held: Tuesday, September 17, 2019
    - Interview invitations are based on academic and non-academic components. A traditional 3-4 person panel interview is conducted for ~30 minutes.
  - Offers released: February
  - Orientation held: mid June
  - Deposit required: Yes
    - If YES, amount: $500 nonrefundable deposit
  - Defers granted: On an individual basis
  - Transfers accepted: Yes

EVALUATION CRITERIA
*If applicable, please enter percentage weighted
- Academic (40%)
  - Required Math and Science courses GPA
  - Upper Level Math and Science prerequisite GPA
  - Last 45 GPA
- Non-academics (40%)
  - eLORS
  - Experiences
  - Leadership Skills
  - Personal Essays
  - Contribution to diversity
  - Non-cognitive skills
  - Readiness to matriculate
  - Employment history
- Interview (20%)

ACCEPTANCE DATA (PRIOR YEAR)
- GPA Average: 3.7
- Number of applications: 1109
- Number interviewed: 337
- Number selected: 78
  - EEP: 17
- Number accepted into class: 95
- Number matriculated: 95

TUITION / COST OF ATTENDANCE
*For current year (2020 matriculation)
- Resident (in-State)
  - $26,200
- Non-Resident (out-of-state)
  - $47,400

EDUCATION / RESEARCH
- Special programs / entrance pathways statement
- Combined Programs statement

DVM-PhD Program
The mission of the MSU-CVM DVM-PhD program is to prepare exceptional students for careers as veterinary scientists to meet the nation's critical needs in animal and human health research. It is the intent of the MSU-CVM DVM-PhD program to provide the full rigor of training from the DVM and PhD degrees as if they were pursued separately. The program is designed to integrate the research and clinical training programs so that students will experience a logical progression and level of responsibility throughout the program. It is also the intent of the program to provide a system of moral and financial support for the students who have committed to it.

Please contact Dr. Mark Lawrence, Director of Feed the Future Innovation Lab on Fish (FIL), at lawrence@cvm.msstate.edu for more information.
- Other Academic Programs statement

MSU-CVM EARLY ENTRY PROGRAM

The Early Entry Program is a unique program of the College of Veterinary Medicine (CVM) that allows high-achieving high school seniors to earn pre-acceptance (early, pre-approved acceptance) into the CVM.

Students who have an interest in veterinary medicine and meet application requirements during high school may apply for the Early Entry Program. If a student is accepted into this program, he/she begins undergraduate work at MSU after high school graduation, and completes the first three to four years of prerequisite courses, while also working toward completion of a bachelor's degree. After the student has completed all course requirements for the College of Veterinary Medicine and has remained in good standing, he/she matriculates into the CVM as a pre-accepted student. The student does not make further application to the CVM.

Students applying for this program must have the following qualifications:
1. ACT composite score of 27 or SAT score of 1280; and
2. High school grade average of 90 (3.6 on a 4.0 scale)

In addition, the Early Entry Program Admissions Committee considers animal and veterinary experience, work experience, leadership qualities, and non-technical skills and aptitudes (character, community service, etc.) as described in the applicant's written application to the Early Entry Program, and in the applicant's Letters of Recommendation (provided in the application).

Thirty positions are available each year. We normally receive 100-120 applications. Both Mississippi and out-of-state students are eligible for the program.

Applications for the Early Entry Program are available by October 1 each year, and are due for return by January 5 (if January 5 falls on a weekend or holiday, the deadline will moved to the next business following the weekend or holiday). Applicants are notified of acceptance status by early February.

Applications are available online from October 1 through December 31.

CURRICULUM STATEMENT

The curriculum of the MSU-CVM is divided into 2 phases: Phase 1 or Pre-clinical (freshman and sophomore years) and Phase 2 or Clinical (junior and senior years).

Year 1 uses foundation courses to expose the student to important medical concepts and address multidisciplinary problems.

Year 2 is devoted to the study of clinical diseases and abnormalities of animal species. Surgery labs begin in the second year.

- Clinicals begin during Year 3.

Year 3 is comprised of clinical rotations in the College's Animal Health Center, and elective courses.

Year 4 includes core rotations in internal medicine and ICU, large animal ambulatory, neurology, ophthalmology, and the Jackson Emergency/Referral Clinic.

The remainder of the fourth year is largely experiential and offers the student the opportunity to select among approved experiences in advanced clinical rotations, elective courses, and/or externships. The first 3 years of the curriculum are 9-10 months in length, while the fourth year is 12 months.

Q&A

- Top 10 FAQs

Do I have to send transcripts from every college I've attended?
Yes. You must submit an original, official transcript from every college or university you have attended. Transcripts must be submitted directly to VMCAS.

What if the transcripts from my current school contain the grades from my previous schools?
Even if grades from one college or university are reported on a later transcript, you must submit an official transcript from every college or university attended.

If I'm at school at MSU, do I still have to send my MSU transcripts?
Yes. Official transcripts can be requested through the Office of the Registrar.

Does MSU-CVM accept Advanced Placement (AP) credit?
Yes. Course requirements met by AP credit must be listed on your transcript(s).

Where do I send my transcripts?
Transcripts should be sent to:
VMCAS – Transcripts
P.O. Box 9126
Watertown, MA 02471

When do I have to send transcripts showing my fall classes and grades?
We must have your fall transcripts no later than January 15. If your school is unable to meet this deadline, you should contact us to make special arrangements.

Does MSU-CVM require a supplemental processing fee?
MSU-CVM requires payment of a $60 fee. It may be paid by check, money order, or credit card. Please visit our website for information on paying online.

How will MSU-CVM communicate with me after I have applied?
MSU-CVM communicates almost exclusively through email. Please be sure that you are receiving email correspondence from MSU-CVM after the September 17th application date, and please alert the MSU-CVM admissions staff to any changes in your email address.

When and how are interview notifications sent?
Notifications are sent via email in late December. Interviews are typically conducted in January and February. Please note that these dates are subject to change. For the most up to date information, please contact MSU-CVM Admissions.

If I am accepted to MSU-CVM as a non-resident, can I change my residency or lower my fees after I am in school?
No. At the time of application, a candidate's residency is determined based on information provided in the VMCAS application, as well as by any other documents requested by the

Assistant Dean for Admissions, as well as by the college. Each successful applicant must enter a contract with the MSU-CVM prior to final acceptance for admission in which the applicant agrees and obligates himself/herself to pay the tuition, fees and expenses applicable to the applicant's Mississippi resident or Mississippi non-resident status, as determined by the MSU-CVM, that exists on the date the applicant will matriculate; further, the applicant must agree and obligate himself/herself in the contract to continue to pay the tuition, fees and expenses during the applicant's entire MSU-CVM DVM educational experience that are applicable to that same initial status determination, thereby waiving any right to petition for a change in residency status.

PREREQUISITES FOR ADMISSION

Course Description	Number of Hours/Credits	Necessity
English Composition and/or Academic Writing	6	Required
Speech or Technical Writing	3	Required
Mathematics (College Algebra or higher)	6	Required
General Biology and accompanying labs	8	Required
Microbiology with laboratory	4	Required
General Chemistry and accompanying labs	8	Required
Organic Chemistry and accompanying labs	8	Required
Biochemistry	3	Required
Physics (may be Trig-based)	6	Required
Advanced (upper-level) science electives	12	Required
Humanities, fine arts, social sciences and behavioral electives	15	Required

*Upper level science electives are courses 300 and above.

UNIVERSITY OF MISSOURI

Email: seayk@missouri.edu
Website: http://cvm.missouri.edu/prospective-students/

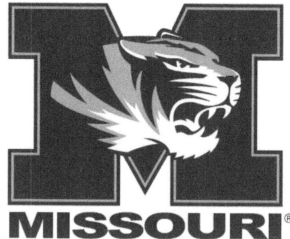

SCHOOL DESCRIPTION

The University of Missouri is located in Columbia, a city renowned for its high quality of life and low cost of living. Located midway between two major metropolises, Kansas City and St. Louis, Columbia abounds with walking trails, state park lands, wildlife refuges, art galleries, boutiques, music clubs and eclectic dining. Mizzou offers SEC football, basketball, baseball, wrestling, soccer, gymnastic and other sports. MU, a major research university with more than 30,000 students, consists of 18 schools and colleges located on a 1,262-acre campus. The College of Veterinary Medicine is noted for its unique curriculum that gives students nearly two years of clinical experience before graduation. Students benefit from exposure to specialty medical areas such as pathology, clinical cardiology, neurology, orthopedics, ophthalmology, and oncology. Students also gain experience with advanced equipment such as a linear accelerator for treatment of cancer, MRI, PET-CT, ultrasonography, extensive endoscopy equipment, cold lasers, a surgery room C-arm for radiography during surgical procedures, and others. Students who attend the MU CVM have the option of applying for Missouri residency after completing their first year. Columbia's proximity to both rural communities and major cities results in exceptional food animal, equine and small animal caseloads. MU is unique in having a medical school, nursing school, engineering college, school of health-related professions, state cancer research center, nuclear research reactor, life sciences center, and department of animal science on the same campus, thus enhancing teaching, research, and clinical services.

PROGRAM DESCRIPTION

- Health & Wellness: A licensed PhD psychologist joint appointed with the MU counseling center provides confidential treatment for students, interns and residents. They also provide seminars for groups on wellness issues.
- Diversity & Disadvantaged / Accommodations: MU has a strong commitment to supporting our diverse student community and have active VOICE and Broad-spectrum clubs. The Associate Dean for Student Affairs is the liaison with the MU office of disabilities and facilitates all ADA accommodations.
- Class Size
  o Resident #: 60
  o Non-Resident #: 60
  o International Seats #: TBD 2019-2020 will be the first year international students are accepted into the MU DVM program. All prerequisites for admission must be taken at a US accredited college.
- Applicant Pool (prior year)
  o Resident #: 157
  o Non-Resident #: 1081
  o Contract # and where: N/A
- International School: No
- Accepts International Applicants: Yes
- VMCAS Participant: Yes

ENTRANCE REQUIREMENTS

- Pre-Requisite Chart Update
  o Date pre-reqs must be completed July 1
  o Pre-requisite required grade C- or higher
- VMCAS application: Yes
- Supplemental application: Yes
  o Through VMCAS: Yes
  o External: No
- Transcript Requirements
  o AP Policy: must appear on official college transcript and be equivalent to the appropriate college-level coursework.

- o International Transcripts No
- o WES Report Required: No
- Test Requirements
  - o GRE Test Deadline: August 31
  - o TOEFL Test Deadline: Date TBD
- Experiences
  - o Requirements statement
    - ▪ Minimum hours requirements 40
- Letters of Recommendation (eLOR)
  - o Letters Guidance Statement
    - ▪ Minimum number required: 3
    - ▪ Veterinarian Required: Yes
- Bachelor's degree required: No
- Academic Statement
  - o Required minimum cumulative GPA: 3.0
  - o Required Grades: C- or higher
  - o Required minimum GRE score: A score of 285 (verbal and quantitative added together) and a 1.5 on the analytical is required.
  - o Other GPA requirements: No
- Interview Required: Yes
  - o Type of interview In person panel interview

ADMISSIONS PROCESS & DEADLINES
- Admissions Process Statement
  - o Deadlines:
    - ▪ Application Open Date: May 9, 2019
    - ▪ Application Deadline Date: September 17, 2019
    - ▪ Supplemental Open Date May 2019
    - ▪ Supplemental Deadline Date: September 17, 2019
    - ▪ Transcripts Received Date: September 17, 2019
    - ▪ eLOR Received Date: September 17, 2019
    - ▪ GRE Scores Received Date: September 17, 2019
  - o Interviews held: Early January through March
    - ▪ Interview format statement In person panel Interview
  - o Offers released: February through April
  - o Orientation held: Mid-August
  - o Deposit required: Yes
    - ▪ If YES, amount: $500
  - o Defers granted: Yes
  - o Transfers accepted: Yes

EVALUATION CRITERIA
*If applicable, please enter percentage weighted
Academic History
Cumulative GPA 20%
Last 45 GPA (last 3 full time undergraduate semesters) 10%
GRE Scores 4%
Undergraduate course load 6%
Experiences 10%
Leadership Skills 5%
Personal Essays 2.5%
Contribution to diversity 5%
Readiness to matriculate 5%
Employment history 5%
Interview 2.5%
Other (please list)
Extracurricular activities 5%
Overall impression 20%

ACCEPTANCE DATA (PRIOR YEAR)
- GRE Average and Range 306
- GPA Average and Range 3.70
- Number of applications 1240
- Number interviewed (or N/A) 339
- Number matriculated 120

TUITION / COST OF ATTENDANCE
*For current year (2020 matriculation)
- Resident (in-State)
  - o Tuition: $ $26,692
  - o Fees: 0
  - o Total COA: $49,724
- Non-Resident (out-of-state)
  - o Tuition: $62,516
  - o Fees: 0
  - o Total COA: $85,548

EDUCATION / RESEARCH
- Combined Programs statement
  - o Students who have earned a bachelor's degree may enroll in graduated classes to earn a Masters of Public Health degree concurrent with the DVM degree. The MPH program required 19 additional credit hours.
  - o Masters of Science and PhD programs are custom designed based on the needs of the faculty advisors and the student. They typically entail and additional year or more of study.
- Other Academic Programs statement
  - o MU CVM has two early admission programs for students who do their undergraduates studies at MU. Students enter as a high school senior or college freshman and must maintain a high academic standard and meet

program requirements to be guaranteed admission.

- Curriculum Statement
  - At MU, the first two years are spent in classrooms and laboratories with the second two years devoted primarily to clinical study in the Veterinary Health Center hospitals.
- Clinicals begin
  - Clinical studies begins October of the third year.
- Research opportunities
  - Approximately 30 percent of the graduating class has actively participated in research projects through either our Veterinary Research Scholars Program (VRSP) or as part of a Laboratory Animal Medicine elective rotation. Additional research activities have occurred on an ad hoc basis.
- Highlights
  - Out-of-state students can easily attain in-state status by the second year.

Q&A

How common is it to obtain Missouri residency for tuition purposes?
It is very common and the majority of out-of-state students obtain Missouri residency by the second year. This greatly reduces the tuition they will pay over the four years. Ninety-nine percent of our students graduate as Missouri residents.

Do Missouri students track?
No. MU provides a mixed animal curriculum for all students. However, the extended time in clinics provides over 25 weeks of self-directed studies in chosen on-campus electives or off campus experiences.

Does attending the University of Missouri for undergraduate coursework provide any more advantage to attending another in–state institution?
No. MU provides an excellent undergraduate education to prepare for the veterinary curriculum, however prospective students should choose an academic institution they feel meets their educational needs and provides sufficient exposure and the necessary preparation pursuant to that profession.

Is community college a viable route into a veterinary curriculum?
Yes. Community college programs are often an economical way to obtain basic general education requirements however upper-level prerequisite requirements are often completed through a four-year program.

Is a veterinary technical program a good path or preparatory field for veterinary medicine?
Sometimes. Students obtain valuable technical skills however many of the programs have courses that do not transfer towards a bachelor's degree and therefore cannot be used to meet admissions requirements.

Does the University of Missouri College Veterinary Medicine have an application fee?
Yes, there is an application processing fee of $100 (charge determined year to year) in addition to the application fee paid to the Veterinary Medical College Application Service (VMCAS) application fee.

Where should transcripts be sent?
All materials including eLORS, GRE scores and official transcripts from the originating institution are sent to VMCAS by their published deadline.

Is a bachelor's degree required to be admitted into a veterinary program?
No. Completion of an undergraduate degree is not required in order to apply or to be admitted into the MU CVM. A bachelor's degree is needed to complete dual DVM/MS/MPH programs.

How much emphasis is placed on shadowing and experience?
Shadowing and veterinary experiences allow a student to decide if the veterinary profession is the correct path for them. The admissions committee values quality of experiences over quantity.

PREREQUISITES FOR ADMISSION

Course Description	Number of Hours/Credits	Necessity
English or Communication	6	Required
College algebra or higher	3	Required
Physics (complete sequence)	5	Required
Biological Science - not AS courses	10	Required
Humanities/Social Sciences	10	Required
Biochemistry with organic pre-req	3	Required
Electives	23	Required

NORTH CAROLINA STATE UNIVERSITY

Email: dvminformation@ncsu.edu
Website: www.cvm.ncsu.edu

NC STATE UNIVERSITY College of Veterinary Medicine

SCHOOL DESCRIPTION

The North Carolina State University College of Veterinary Medicine consistently ranks as one of the leading veterinary educational programs in North America. Located in the state capital of Raleigh, the campus resides in one of the most desirable areas to live and work. The region is home to one of the nation's leading research parks and provides students with opportunities for collaborations in biotechnology, biomedicine, and environmental health with industry and government researchers, clinical trial companies, and other academic colleagues. Featuring 160 faculty members and a capacity for 400 veterinary medical students, the college also offers training for interns, residents, and graduate students. The campus includes a state-of-the-art teaching hospital, classrooms, a working farm, research and teaching laboratories, and a variety of additional amenities. The Randall B. Terry, Jr., Companion Animal Veterinary Medical Center offers cutting-edge technologies for imaging, cardiac care, cancer treatment, and internal medicine and surgery, and handles more than 34,000 referral cases a year. In addition, the educational model has been fully revamped with an eye on the future, equipping students for success in private practice, industry, government, and academia, with emphasis on teamwork, client interactions, and communication skills. The NC State Veterinary Medicine community enhances animal and human health and well-being through the education and advanced training of veterinarians and comparative biomedical scientists. The community is dedicated to providing leadership in veterinary care, biomedical discovery, and societal engagement that addresses complex global issues facing animal, human, and environmental health. It raises the bar for teaching, healing, and scientific discovery in the 21st century.

PROGRAM DESCRIPTION
- Class Size
  - Resident #: 80
  - Non-Resident #: 20
- Applicant Pool (prior year) – 2018 Cycle
  - Resident #: 233
  - Non-Resident #: 835
- International School: No
- Accepts International Applicants: Yes
- VMCAS Participant: Yes

ENTRANCE REQUIREMENTS
- Pre-Requisite Chart Update
  - Date pre-reqs must be completed: Have no more than two (2) pre-requisites outstanding in the spring semester of the application cycle (Spring 2020).
  - Pre-requisite required grade – C-
- VMCAS application: Yes
- Supplemental application: Yes
  - Through VMCAS: No
  - External: Yes
- Transcript Requirements
  - AP Policy: must appear on official college transcripts with course name and credit hours and be equivalent to the appropriate college-level coursework.
  - International Transcripts: all international academic transcripts evaluated by a credential evaluation service.
  - WES Report Required: Yes
- Test Requirements
  - GRE Test Deadline: August 15
  - TOEFL Test Deadline: August 15
  - OTHER Test Deadlines

- Experiences
  - Requirements statement
    - Minimum hours requirements: 200
- Letters of Recommendation (eLOR)
  - Letters Guidance Statement
    - Minimum number required: 3
    - Veterinarian Required: No – 2 are recommended to come from a veterinarian
- Bachelor's degree required: No
- Academic Statement
  - Required minimum cumulative GPA 3.0 Resident, 3.4 Nonresident
  - Required Grades 3.0 Resident, 3.4 Nonresident
  - Required minimum of last 45: 3.0 Resident, 3.4 Nonresident
  - Required minimum science GPA
  - Required minimum GRE score
  - Other GPA requirements
- Interview Required: No

ADMISSIONS PROCESS & DEADLINES
- Admissions Process Statement
  - Deadlines:
    - Application Open Date: May 9, 2019
    - Application Deadline Date September 17
    - Supplemental Open Date: June
    - Supplemental Deadline Date: Wednesday, September 18, 2019, at 1 pm
    - eLOR Received Date: September 17
    - GRE Scores Received Date: September 17
  - Offers released: by March 1
  - Orientation held: August
  - Deposit required: Yes
    - If YES, amount: $300
  - Defers granted: Yes
  - Transfers accepted: No

EVALUATION CRITERIA
*If applicable, please enter percentage weighted
- Academic History
- Science GPA
- Science pre-requisite GPA
- Cumulative GPA
- Last 45 GPA
- GRE Scores
- eLORS
- Veterinary Experience
- Animal Experience
- Educational Experience
- Evaluation Forms/Recommendations
- Personal Statement
- Diversity
- Extracurricular and Community Activities
- Other (please list)

ACCEPTANCE DATA (PRIOR YEAR) 2018 Cycle
- GRE Average and Range
  - Avg – Analytical 65%
    - Range: 8% – 98%
  - Avg - Quantitative – 58%
    - Range – 12% – 97%
  - Avg – Verbal – 69%
    - Range – 24% – 99%
- GPA Average and Range
  - Avg – Overall – 3.72
    - Range – 3.06 – 4.00
  - Avg – Last 45 – 3.75
    - Range – 3.13 – 4.00
  - Avg – Required Course – 3.67
    - Range – 2.95 – 4.00
- Number of applications – 1068
- Number matriculated – 100

TUITION / COST OF ATTENDANCE
*For current year (2020 matriculation)
- Resident (in-State)
  - $19,616
  - $39,686
- Non-Resident (out-of-state)
  - $47,657
  - $67,727

EDUCATION / RESEARCH
- Special programs / entrance pathways statement
- Combined Programs statement
  - DVM/PhD - The Combined DVM/PhD accepts students to the Comparative Biomedical Sciences where they study with faculty who are employing state-of-the-art techniques to address a number of interesting scientific problems in the basic and applied biomedical sciences.
  - Combined DVM/MBA - Applicants interested in the combined degree program must be accepted by both the College of Veterinary Medicine and the Jenkins MBA Program.
- Other Academic Programs statement
  - Food Animal Scholars
  - Fisheries and Aquaculture Scholar Program
  - Laboratory Animal Scholar Program
  - The University of North Carolina (UNC) System Veterinary Education Access (UNC-SVEA) Program

- Curriculum Statement
    - The academic professional program calls for two phases of education. A preclinical three-year phase is followed by a clinical phase in the fourth year of training. The first through the third year of the professional program are concerned with a gradual progression from a basic science presentation to a more clinical application of veterinary science. Two summer vacation periods are allowed in the first three years of the professional program.
- Clinicals begin
    - Fourth-year students must complete required and elective rotations that vary depending on the students' selected focus area. Students must complete 43 credits in the senior year: 40 credits of clinical rotations and three credits in Clinical Conference. The clinic year consists of 24 blocks, two-to-three weeks in length, with up to four vacation blocks and three extramural experiences (Clinician Scientist, Epidemiology, & Food Animal Focus Areas have different extramural requirements). A total of 168 credit hours are required for graduation. Clinical Conference presentations are required of each senior.
    - (Brief description of Summer (or other) research programs)) - Summer Research Internship Program for First- and Second-year Veterinary Medicine Students
        - The objective of the Veterinary Scholars Program is to provide veterinary students with mentored research experiences in biomedical laboratories located within our College of Veterinary Medicine. Students are expected to complete 10 weeks of full time research over the course of the summer. In addition to working in research laboratories, there will be several joint events held during the summer for all participating students.
- Highlights
    - Certificate in Global Health
        - The Certificate in Global Health is a formal academic certificate for veterinary students that examines the complexities inherent in improving health on a global scale.
        - During the program, students will be introduced to global health issues and challenges, and develop an understanding of key concepts, tools and frameworks essential for continued study in global health. Students will learn about the importance of understanding and addressing global health through multidisciplinary frameworks and collaborations, and complete an experiential International Research Project.
    - Teaching Animal Unit
        - The Teaching Animal Unit (TAU) is located just east of the College of Veterinary Medicine on approximately 80 of the campus' 180 acres. The staff and PHP residents are actively involved in training the veterinary students who participate in laboratory training during Years 1-3 of the professional DVM curriculum. The TAU is a dynamic teaching lab for veterinary students to learn husbandry, production management, and routine procedures used in livestock production. Students are able to observe and work with normal animals in a real farm setting.
        - The TAU is consistently one of the most popular activities in which veterinary students engage at NC State. They have regularly scheduled labs during Years 1-3, and make visits as part of their senior rotations during Year 4. The Unit consists of six sub units that reflect the principal food animal groups.
    - House System
        - Students are sorted into four houses as part of a college-wide wellness initiative. Throughout the academic

year, the houses, which boast groups of students reflecting differences in backgrounds and areas of study, compete to earn points by participating in various campus events.

- The house model focuses on promoting intellectual growth, mental and emotional health, social development, cultural competence and physical health.

Q&A

- Top 10 FAQs

What makes an applicant competitive for admissions?

You should meet or exceed our minimum grade requirements for cumulative, required, and last 45 credit hour grade point averages. In addition to academic criteria, you will be evaluated on various non-academic criteria. The Admissions Committee will be looking for students who are academically curious, well-rounded and mature. Students who are interested in veterinary medicine should pursue jobs, clubs and other activities that expose them to the profession and to different species of animals. A diverse amount of veterinary and animal experience is highly recommended.

Do you require an admissions interview?

No. We do not require an interview.

What do I have to submit?

The Veterinary Medical College Application Service (VMCAS) application; the NC State Supplemental Application; official transcripts of completed coursework; Graduate Record Exam (GRE) scores.

Do applications from NC State alumni get preference?

We evaluate all applicants on the same criteria no matter what college they have attended. Each cycle we receive more applications from NC State than any other school. There-fore, we admit and deny more applicants from NC State than any other school.

How many applications do you receive and how many are accepted?

We receive more than 1,000 applications each year and that number continues to increase. We admit an incoming class of 100 students each year – approximately 80 North Carolina residents and 20 non-residents.

Do I have to have a Bachelor's degree to get in?

A bachelor's degree is not required for admission into the DVM program. An applicant just needs to satisfy the prerequisites. However, most admitted students do have their bachelor's degree by matriculation.

Why do you accept so many North Carolina residents?

North Carolina State University is a land-grant university designed to serve the citizens of North Carolina in subject areas including, but not limited to, the practical teaching of agriculture, science, military science, engineering and education. The state of North Carolina funds higher education in an effort to offer strong educational opportunities to its citizenry. Therefore, slot allocation priority is given to North Carolina residents.

Are there majors you prefer?

Students can be any major they choose, and the required pre-professional courses can be obtained through the curricula of a number of fields of study. A majority of applicants are science majors, such as: Biology, Animal Science, Zoology, and Chemistry.

Where should I take the prerequisite courses?

You can take the prerequisite courses at any accredited two-year or four-year college or university. This includes courses taken via distance education at those institutions.

Do you accept online courses?

Yes, prerequisite courses may be completed either online or in a classroom setting. The courses must be completed at an accredited two-year or four-year college or university.

PREREQUISITES FOR ADMISSION

Course Description	Number of Hours/Credits	Necessity
Animal Nutrition	3	Required
Biochemistry	3	Required
Biology	4	Required
Chemistry, General	8	Required
Chemistry, Organic	8	Required
Composition, Public Speaking or Communications	6	Required
Humanities and Social Sciences	6	Required
Microbiology	4	Required
Physics	8	Required
Statistics	3	Required
Genetics	4	Required

THE OHIO STATE UNIVERSITY

Email Address: dvmprospective@osu.edu
Website: www.vet.osu.edu/admissions

THE OHIO STATE UNIVERSITY

COLLEGE OF VETERINARY MEDICINE

SCHOOL DESCRIPTION

The Ohio State University was founded in 1870 and is one of the nation's leading academic centers, consistently ranks as Ohio's best, and one of the nation's top-20 public universities. The campus consists of thousands of acres, hundreds of buildings, more than 15,000 faculty and staff, and more than 56,000 students. The College of Veterinary Medicine offers a robust systems-based curriculum augmented with a variety of elective course offerings and opportunities through local partnerships.

The Veterinary Medical Center includes the Hummel and Trueman Hospital for Companion Animals, Hospital for Food Animals, the Galbreath Equine Center, Veterinary Medical Center in Dublin (24 hour emergency clinic), and Large Animal Services at Marysville (an ambulatory clinic). The patient load is one of the highest in the country and farmlands can be accessed 10 miles from campus. The Veterinary Medicine Academic Building has nearly 10,000 square feet of space and includes research labs, classrooms, a library, computer lab, and academic offices. The Ohio State University College of Veterinary Medicine is ranked fifth in the nation among veterinary schools according to U.S. News & World Report's "Best Graduate Schools."

PROGRAM DESCRIPTION

- Health & Wellness: Office of Counseling & Consultation - The Mission of the CVM Office of Counseling and Consultation is to promote a culture of wellbeing and inclusivity through counseling, consultation, and education that supports College of Veterinary Medicine students in their pursuit of academic and personal development, empowering them to become successful members of the veterinary community and beyond.

- Diversity & Disadvantaged / Accommodations: To best serve the needs of our community, our profession must embrace the broadest definition and fullest spectrum of diversity including race, ethnicity, physical and mental abilities, gender, sexual orientation, gender identity or expression, parental, marital, or pregnancy status, religious or political beliefs, military or veteran status, and geographic, socioeconomic, and educational backgrounds, and challenges that have been overcome. At Ohio State, we understand that diversity promotes a culture of inclusion that understands and appreciates the world beyond our own individual perspective. For the College of Veterinary Medicine, diversity is a fundamental component of excellence and, as such, is not optional, but rather is both necessary and desired.
- Class Size
  - Resident #: 50% of the Class
  - Non-Resident #: 50% of the Class
  - Contract # and where: 0
  - International Seats: Included in Non-Resident seats
- Applicant Pool (prior year)
  - Resident #: 246 applicants
  - Non-Resident #: 1142 applicants
  - Contract # and where: No Contract Seats
- International School: No
- Accepts International Applicants: Yes
- VMCAS Participant: Yes

ENTRANCE REQUIREMENTS

- Pre-Requisite Chart Update
  - Date pre-reqs must be completed: All of the prerequisite courses must be completed by the end of the summer term preceding the autumn term

when you would start vet school. You do not have to have all the prerequisites completed before applying.
- Pre-requisite required grade
- VMCAS application: Yes
- Supplemental application: Yes
  - Through VMCAS: No
  - External: Yes
- Transcript Requirements
  - AP Policy: AP credit given if course is listed on official transcript.
  - International Transcripts
  - WES Report Required: Yes
- Test Requirements
  - GRE Test Deadline: Not Required
  - TOEFL Test Deadline: September 15
- Experiences
  - Requirements statement
    - No minimum hour requirement. We look for diversity and depth of experiences
- Letters of Recommendation (eLOR)
  - The letters of recommendation should include specific information regarding the applicant. It should focus on the skills and attributes the applicant possesses and their ability to be not only a successful veterinary student but a successful veterinarian.
    - Minimum number required: 3
    - Veterinarian Required: Yes
- Bachelor's degree required: No
- Academic Statement
  - Required minimum cumulative GPA: 3.0
  - Required minimum of last 30: 3.0
  - Required minimum science GPA: 3.0
  - Required minimum GRE score: Not Required
- Interview Required: Yes
  - Type of interview: In person interview - traditional interview style with at least two people.

ADMISSIONS PROCESS & DEADLINES
- Admissions Process Statement
  - Deadlines:
    - Application Open Date: May 9, 2019
    - Application Deadline Date: September 17
    - Supplemental Open Date: After submitting the VMCAS application.
    - Supplemental Deadline Date: 10 days after receiving the application.
    - Transcripts Received Date

- eLOR Received Date: September 15
- GRE Scores Received Date
  - Interviews held: January-February
    - In-person interview with two people
  - Offers released: February-March
  - Orientation held: Late August
  - Deposit required: Yes
    - If YES, amount: $25.00 for residents; $300.00 (non-refundable fee) for non-resident applicants
  - Defers granted: No
  - Transfers accepted: No

EVALUATION CRITERIA
*If applicable, please enter percentage weighted
- Academic History
- Science GPA
- Cumulative GPA
- Last 30 GPA
- eLORS
- Experiences
- Leadership Skills
- Personal Essays
- Contribution to diversity
- Non-cognitive skills
- Readiness to matriculate
- Employment history
- Interview

ACCEPTANCE DATA (PRIOR YEAR)
- GPA Average: 3.6 Range 3.0-4.0
- Number of applications: 1388
- Number interviewed (or N/A): 508
- Number selected: 162
- Number accepted into class: 162
- Number matriculated: 162

TUITION / COST OF ATTENDANCE
*For current year (2020 matriculation)
- Resident (in-State)
  - $32,350 (tuition and fees)
  - COA: 54,220
- Non-Resident (out-of-state)
  - $71,494 (tuition and fees first year)
  - COA: 93,364 (first year)

EDUCATION / RESEARCH
Special programs / entrance pathways statement - Full range of specialty services, including veterinary behavior, internal medicine, dermatology, neurology, cardiology, opthomology, oncology, surgery and theriogeniology
- The Veterinary Scholar Summer Research Program Includes:
- A robust summer research program

including grant support for summer research opportunities

- International learning research in Spain, Ethiopia, Brazil, Thailand and other countries.
- Rainier Scholars Program
- The program is designed to engage professional degree/graduate students in veterinary medicine with academic, laboratory and hands-on projects and experiential opportunities to better position them for opportunities in industry.
- Selected students participate in a 12-week research program, a graduate business minor program in health sciences, several specific online electives, and concludes with an industry or translation focused internship for up to six weeks.

- Combined Programs statement
  - Accredited veterinary public health master's degree program (MPH) – concurrent with DVM option.
  - Business Minor

- Curriculum Statement
  - The systems-based curriculum includes enough flexibility to allow students to pursue interests through a variety of elective course offerings and off-site elective rotations. In preparation for their clinical year, students will select a "Career Area of Emphasis" (CAE) to enhance their foundational veterinary education.
- Clinical rotations begin the summer after your 3rd year in Veterinary School.
- Highlights
  - The Galbreath Equine Center offers an equine treadmill and sports medicine expertise, as well as a robust equine field service practice.
  - More than 40,000 animal patients per year and an animal blood bank that provides blood products to veterinary hospitals across America.

PREREQUISITES FOR ADMISSION

Course Description	Semester Hours (hours may vary)	Notes
Biochemistry*	4	If Biochemistry is taught as a 2-part sequence, both parts are required. Lab is not required.
Microbiology*	4	Lab is required.
Physiology**	5	
Public Speaking (Communication)	3	Basics of public speaking & critical thinking. This should be a public speaking course.
Science Electives	35	Includes, but not limited to: Biology, chemistry, anatomy, immunology, cell biology, molecular genetics, animal science, ecology, environmental science or other science courses.
Humanities/Social Science Electives	16	Includes, but not limited to: History, economics, anthropology, psychology, art, music, literature, languages, writing, and ethics.

* = Capstone Courses
**Physiology course work must be a comprehensive, intermediate systems physiology series. Required systems include musculoskeletal, neurology, urinary/renal, endocrine, reproductive, digestive, cardiovascular, and respiratory. Science electives can include courses that are prerequisites for the capstone courses (e.g. biology, general and organic chemistry, etc.).

The number of hours provided is a guideline. In assessing course content for equivalency, actual hours may vary for your institution. In some cases a multiple course series may be needed to fulfill prerequisite coursework. If you are unsure of whether or not a course will be accepted to fulfill a prerequisite, please contact us at dvmprospective@osu.edu.

Capstone courses - Biochemistry, Microbiology, Physiology, and Communication - must be completed with (1) a grade of C or better in each course, (2) a 3.0 (B) average among the courses, and (3) no more than one C between any of the four courses.

•If any of the capstone courses are taken as a multiple-part series, this rule will apply to each part as an individual course.

There may be additional courses that your school requires as prerequisites to the above courses. These additional courses can be used toward the elective requirements.

ADVANCED PLACEMENT
To receive credit for AP courses, they must be listed on official transcripts from a college or university you have attended.

VETERINARIAN PROFILE: DANIEL LOPEZ

YEAR OF GRADUATION
2016

PLACE OF EMPLOYMENT
Cornell University

What is your favorite aspect of being a veterinarian?
My favorite part of veterinary medicine is the diversity in my daily schedule; every day is a surprise. It amazes me to work with veterinarians who have practiced for decades, and with great regularity we see a variation on a case that they have never seen before. It is both humbling and inspiring.

What type of veterinary medicine do you practice?
I am currently a 1st year surgery resident at the Cornell University Hospital for Animals, where I focus on small animal surgery (soft tissue and orthopedics). Occasionally, we will help perform procedures on exotic or wildlife species.

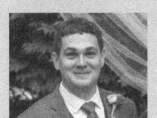

Where did you attend veterinary school?
Cornell University

How long have you been practicing as a veterinarian?
I am currently in my second year of veterinary medicine.

What advice do you have for those considering a career in veterinary medicine?
My advice to those considering a career in veterinary medicine is to keep an open mind; the veterinary profession is so diverse with so many different amazing and unique opportunities. Originally, I was stubbornly adamant that I was going to be a dairy veterinarian. However, after spending time on a small animal surgery rotation outside of my comfort zone, I realized how much I loved surgery. I have never regretted switching, and enjoy going to work every single day.

What challenges have you faced while practicing veterinary medicine?
I have found allowing time to pass to be one of the most important and challenging aspects of veterinary medicine, whether it is monitoring a response to a treatment, allowing a patient to recover from a surgery, or allowing a disease to declare itself if initial diagnostics return inconclusive. Time has definitely tested my patient, however has been so crucial in my practice of medicine.

OKLAHOMA STATE UNIVERSITY

Email Address: dvm@okstate.edu
Website: www.cvhs.okstate.edu

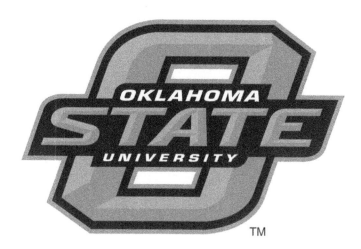

SCHOOL DESCRIPTION

Oklahoma State University is located in Stillwater, which has a population of about 50,000. Stillwater is in north central Oklahoma about 65 miles from Oklahoma City and 69 miles from Tulsa. The campus is exceptionally beautiful, with modified Georgian-style architecture in the new buildings. It encompasses 840 acres and more than 60 major academic buildings.

Three major buildings form the veterinary medicine complex. The oldest, McElroy Hall, houses the William E. Brock Memorial Library and Learning Center, as well as classrooms and laboratories. The Boren Veterinary Medical Teaching Hospital provides modern facilities for both academic and clinical instruction. Completing the triad is the Oklahoma Animal Disease Diagnostic Laboratory, which provides teaching resources for students in the professional curriculum and diagnostic services to Oklahoma agriculture and industry. The College of Veterinary Medicine is fully accredited by the American Veterinary Medical Association. Faculty members in the three academic departments share responsibility for the curriculum. These departments are Veterinary Clinical Sciences, Veterinary Pathobiology, and Physiological Sciences.

PROGRAM DESCRIPTION

- Health & Wellness: The Center for Veterinary Health Sciences Wellness Initiative was launched in 2017 to create awareness and implement strategies to better the wellbeing of students, staff and faculty. Goals include promoting self-care and wellness, creating a culture of camaraderie, inclusion and wellbeing, and providing a curriculum that gives students the necessary tools to enjoy a healthy, productive and rewarding veterinary career. For more information about CVHS Health and & Wellness, visit www.cvhs.okstate.edu/wellness.

- Diversity & Disadvantaged / Accommodations: Oklahoma State University is a land-grant institution committed to excellence in diversity and inclusion. We strive to maintain a welcoming and inclusive environment that appreciates and values all members of the University community.
- Class Size
    - Resident #: 58
    - Non-Resident #: 48
    - Contract 2 and where 1 – Arkansas, 2 - Delaware
    - International Seats #: 2
- Applicant Pool (prior year)
    - Resident #: 129
    - Non-Resident #: 695
- International School: No
- Accepts International Applicants: Yes
- VMCAS Participant: Yes

ENTRANCE REQUIREMENTS

- Pre-Requisite Chart Update
    - Date pre-reqs must be completed: June 1 following application submission
    - Pre-requisite required grade: minimum C in all required courses
- VMCAS application: Yes
- Supplemental application: No
- Transcript Requirements
    - AP Policy: AP credit accepted if documented on college transcript.
    - International Transcripts
    - WES Report Required: Yes
- Test Requirements
    - GRE Test Deadline: September 17
    - TOEFL Test Deadline: September 17
    - OTHER Test Deadlines

- Experiences
  - Requirements statement
- Letters of Recommendation (eLOR)
  - Letters Guidance Statement
    - Minimum number required: #3
    - Veterinarian Required: Yes
- Bachelor's degree required: No
- Academic Statement
  - Required minimum cumulative GPA 2.8
- Interview Required: Yes – OK applicants only
  - Type of interview: standard

ADMISSIONS PROCESS & DEADLINES
- Admissions Process Statement
  - Deadlines:
    - Application Open Date: May
    - Application Deadline Date: September 17
    - Transcripts Received Date: September 17
    - eLOR Received Date: September 17
    - GRE Scores Received Date September 17
  - Interviews held: February
  - Offers released: February
  - Orientation held: Mid August
  - Deposit required: Yes
    - If YES, amount: resident, $100.00; non-resident, $500.00
  - Defers granted: Each request is considered on a case-by-case basis.
  - Transfers accepted: Yes

EVALUATION CRITERIA
*If applicable, please enter percentage weighted
- Total Academic History: 40%
- Pre-requisite GPA: 20%
- Cumulative GPA: 20%
- GRE Scores: 30%

ACCEPTANCE DATA (PRIOR YEAR)
- GRE Average and Range: The class of 2022 had mean scores of 151 verbal, 150 quantitative, and analytical of 4.0.
- Number of applications: 824
- Number interviewed (or N/A): 80
- Number matriculated: 106

TUITION / COST OF ATTENDANCE
*For current year (2020 matriculation)
- Resident (in-State)
  - $24,050 (includes fees)
- Non-Resident (out-of-state)
  - $50,900 (includes fees)

EDUCATION / RESEARCH
- Special programs / entrance pathways statement
- Combined Programs statement
  - The Veterinary Biomedical Sciences Graduate Program provides a multidisciplinary graduate program of excellence in the Oklahoma State University Center for Veterinary Health Sciences, providing a broad base to address individual student interests. Their goal for the future includes continued development of a nationally renowned program of animal health and biomedical research. They offer the following dual degrees: DVM/MPH, DVM/MBA, DVM/MS. For more information on those dual degrees, visit their website: https://cvhs.okstate.edu/students/veterinary-biomedical-sciences/dual-degree.html
- Other Academic Programs statement
- Early Admission Program: The Early Admission Program offers an opportunity for students with superior academic performance to commit to their veterinary medical career goals early in the educational process. Students accepted to the program agree to complete their bachelor's degree with the pre-veterinary required courses and maintain a GPA of 3.5 each semester of their undergraduate education. https://cvhs.okstate.edu/students/early-admission.htmlCurriculum Statement
  - For information regarding the OSU-CVHS curriculum for DVM students, please visit our website: https://cvhs.okstate.edu/students/dvm-curriculum.html
- Clinicals begin: 4th year of the program
- The Summer Research Training Program offers mentored training for veterinary students in biomedical research through a 12-week paid summer immersion experience. The goal of the Summer Research Training Program is to foster the development of the next generation of veterinary research scientists. For more information regading the summer research program, visit our website: https://cvhs.okstate.edu/research/summer-research-training/index.htmlHighlights

Q&A
- For common FAQs, please visit the FAQ portion of our website: https://cvhs.okstate.edu/students/faq.html

PREREQUISITES FOR ADMISSION

Course Description	Minimum Number of Hours/Credits	Necessity
Animal Nutrition	3	Required
Biochemistry	3	Required
Biology/Zoology	8	Required
English, Speech, or Composition	9	Required
Genetics	3	Required
Humanities/Social Science	6	Required
Inorganic Chemistry	8	Required
Statistics	3	Required
Microbiology	4	Required
Organic Chemistry (5-hour survey accepted)	8	Required
Physics 1 & 2	8	Required

OREGON STATE UNIVERSITY

Email: cvmadmissions@oregonstate.edu
Website: www.oregonstate.edu/vetmed

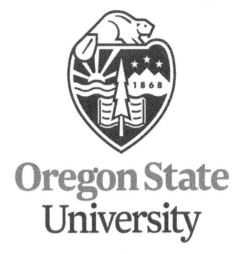

Oregon State University

SCHOOL DESCRIPTION

Oregon State University is located in Corvallis, the heart of the Willamette Valley. Our climate is mild year-round, with ocean beaches less than an hour drive to the west and some of the best snow skiing in the Cascade Range a little over two hours to the east. Corvallis has a population of approximately 55,000 and is a beautiful and friendly place to live and pursue your education. The Oregon State University Carlson College of Veterinary Medicine has one of the smallest class sizes of the DVM programs in the U.S., admitting just 72 students per year. Hands-on education is an important aspect to how our students learn and develop their knowledge of the profession. Our partnership with the Oregon Humane Society provides an opportunity for students to continue acquiring skills and confidence in their ability to perform as professionals. Students at OSU work in state-of-the-art facilities alongside our world-class faculty, including specialists in cardiology, oncology, imaging, and rehabilitation. The individual attention our students get from faculty and hospital staff is, in part, why year after year at least 98% percent of our students pass their board exams.

PROGRAM DESCRIPTION

Health & Wellness: OSU CCVM has a strong commitment to the health and wellness of our students. We have a full-time psychologist on staff to meet with our students individually as well as provide wellness promotion activities and trainings. The SAVMA wellness committee is also very active and regularly plans exercise classes, healthy breakfasts, and visits from therapy dogs.

Diversity & Disadvantaged / Accommodations: The OSU CCVM community recognizes the value of a

diverse student body. Applicants from diverse backgrounds may bring unique perspectives and enrich the veterinary educational experience as well as the profession. Therefore, the Admissions Committee seeks to accept applicants from a variety of ethnic, educational or social backgrounds that may be underrepresented in the veterinary profession. Each applicant is evaluated in terms of their stated background and professional goals in light of current and projected future needs of the veterinary profession.

Accommodations for DVM students are available through the OSU Disability Access Services office. Disability Access Services (DAS) provides accommodations, education, consultation and advocacy for qualified students with disabilities at Oregon State University.

- Class Size
  - o Resident #: 40
  - o Non-Resident #: 32
  - o Contract # and where: WICHE (Arizona, Hawaii, Montana, Nevada, New Mexico, North Dakota, or Wyoming). WICHE seats are included in our 32 non-resident positions.
  - o International Seats. International seats are included in our 32 non-resident positions.
- Applicant Pool (prior year)
  - o Resident #: 98
  - o Non-Resident #: 977
  - o Contract # and where: 98 (Arizona, Hawaii, Montana, Nevada, New Mexico, North Dakota, or Wyoming)
- International School: Yes
- Accepts International Applicants: Yes
- VMCAS Participant: Yes

ENTRANCE REQUIREMENTS

- Pre-Requisite Chart Update
  - Date pre-reqs must be completed-August 1 of year starting the DVM program
  - Pre-requisite required grade: C- or better
- VMCAS application: Yes
- Supplemental application: Yes
  - Through VMCAS: No
  - External: Yes
- Transcript Requirements
  - AP Policy: Test credits for AP must be documented by either an official transcript indicating AP college credit submitted to VMCAS or an official College Board score report submitted to OSU CCVM.
  - International Transcripts: Accepted
  - WES Report Required: Yes
- Test Requirements
  - GRE Test Deadline: Within the past five years.
  - TOEFL Test Deadline: September 17, 2019
- Experiences
  - Requirements statement
    - Minimum hours requirements-N/A
- Letters of Recommendation (eLOR)
  - Letters Guidance Statement
    - Minimum number required: 3
    - Veterinarian Required: Yes, we require at least one letter from a DVM.
- Bachelor's degree required: No
- Academic Statement
- Interview Required: Yes, for selected Oregon residents
  - Type of interview-Multiple Mini Interview

ADMISSIONS PROCESS & DEADLINES

- Admissions Process Statement
  - Deadlines:
    - Application Open Date: May 9, 2019
    - Application Deadline Date: September 17, 2019
    - Supplemental Open Date: May 9, 2019
    - Supplemental Deadline Date: September 17, 2019
    - Transcripts Received Date: September 17, 2019
    - eLOR Received Date: September 17, 2019
    - GRE Scores Received Date: September 17, 2019

- Interviews held: Dates- mid-January
  - Interview format statement: Multiple Mini Interviews
- Offers released: December-February
- Orientation held: September
- Deposit required: No
- Defers granted: Yes
- Transfers accepted: Yes

EVALUATION CRITERIA

*If applicable, please enter percentage weighted: N/A. We use a holistic application review so do not weight any particular part of the application.

- Academic History
- Science GPA
- Science pre-requisite GPA
- Cumulative GPA
- Last 45 GPA
- GRE Scores
- eLORS
- Experiences
- Leadership Skills
- Personal Essays
- Contribution to diversity
- Non-cognitive skills
- Readiness to matriculate
- Employment history
- Interview
- Other (please list)

ACCEPTANCE DATA (PRIOR YEAR)

- GRE Average and Range: Mean GRE Scores: Quantitative- 153 or 52%, Verbal-155 or 68%, Analytical- 4 or 63%
- GPA Average and Range: Mean Cumulative GPA: 3.64
- Number of applications: 986
- Number interviewed (or N/A): 57 Oregon residents
- Number selected: 40
- Number accepted into class: 179
- Number matriculated: 72

TUITION / COST OF ATTENDANCE

*For current year (2020 matriculation) We do not have 2020 rates yet, so am listing estimated costs for Fall 2019.

- Resident (in-State)
  - Tuition & fees: $25,540
  - COA: $43,415
- Non-Resident (out-of-state)
  - Tuition & fees: $48,790
  - COA: $66,665

EDUCATION / RESEARCH

- Combined Programs statement
  - We offer DVM/MS, DVM/MPH, and DVM/PhD options.

- Other Academic Programs statement
  - The Pre-Veterinary Scholars Program is a collaboration between the Honors College (HC) and the OSU Carlson College of Veterinary Medicine (CCVM). This program is designed for incoming HC students who have strong academic abilities and an interest in pursuing veterinary medicine as a career. Pre-Veterinary Scholars will obtain experience, knowledge, and mentorship that will help solidify their career goals and strengthen their application to a professional veterinary program.
- Curriculum Statement
  - The curriculum is essentially traditional with a variety of lecture and lab courses through the third year. These may include flipped classrooms, problem-based learning and other teaching modalities. The fourth year consists entirely of clinical rotations, electives, and preceptorships.
- Clinicals begin: Training in the clinics officially starts with junior clinics in spring quarter of the third year and continues through the entire fourth year.
- Summer research experiences are offered, on a competitive basis, to about 20-25 students per year. These are paid and mentored research experiences that can include laboratory, clinical, and off-site research.
- Highlights
  We have a very successful collaborative program with the Oregon Humane Society (OHS) in Portland, Oregon. We jointly built the Animal Medical Center there in 2005 and our students all participate in a three week on-site rotation at the OHS where they get excellent surgical experience and medical, dentistry and behavior training by providing these services to all of the animals that go through the OHS. Dorms are provided for students. Elective courses include opportunities at Wildlife Safari, the Oregon Coast Aquarium, and an international veterinary service trip.

Q&A

Q: What should I major in at college?
A: No preference is given for any particular major. All prospective applicants are encouraged to develop plans for an alternate career. It is recommended that applicants pursue a bachelor's degree in a desired field in the event they are not accepted into the DVM program, rather than concentrating solely on a pre-veterinary program.

Q: Do all of the prerequisite courses have to be completed before I submit an application?
A: No. While we prefer that applicants have the majority of all required coursework completed at the time of application, pending coursework may be completed throughout the application process. However, all required coursework must be completed prior to August 1 of the year of matriculation, if admitted. (Year of matriculation is the year you enter the DVM program).

Q: Am I required to have a Bachelor's Degree in order to apply?
A: No. As long as you can complete all required prerequisite courses by August 1 of the year of matriculation, you may apply without a Bachelor's Degree.

Q: Are my chances of getting into the OSU CCVM DVM Program better if I attend OSU as an undergraduate student?
A: No. Students may complete their prerequisite coursework at any accredited college or university. The admissions committee does not have a preference for any undergraduate institution over another.

Q: Is there a minimum GPA requirement for applications to be considered?
A: No. We utilize a holistic application review process and do not require a minimum GPA to be considered. However, we require a minimum grade of C- or better in all prerequisite courses.

Q: Can I re-take the GRE multiple times to improve my score?
A: Yes. You can take the General GRE once a month as many times as you would like. The highest set of scores on a particular test date will be used when the GRE has been taken more than once.

Q: What is the GRE institution code for OSU CCVM?
A: The GRE institution code for OSU CCVM is 4565.

Q: What is the class size?
A: We have a maximum of 72 seats available to first year students. The class is comprised of 40 Oregon residents and 32 non-residents.

Q. Do I have to take a public speaking course?
A. Only if you have not yet completed a bachelor's degree and do not intend to before starting our DVM program. If you do plan to complete a bachelor's degree, we will waive all of the General Education prerequisites (English, public speaking, & humanities).

Q: I have questions about becoming an Oregon resident. Who should I contact?
A: For information regarding residency, the regulations regarding this issue can be found at OSU Admissions

page. If you prefer to speak with someone about your specific situation, you may call the residency officer at 541-737-4411 or toll free at 1-800-291-4192.

SUMMARY OF ADMISSION PROCEDURES

- Steps to apply for admission to Oregon State University Carlson College of Veterinary Medicine:
- Begin the VMCAS application process
- Request all transcripts be sent direct to VMCAS, they must be received by September 17, 2019.
  > VMCAS Transcripts
  > P O Box 9126
  > Watertown, MA 02471

- Submit GRE scores directly to VMCAS using ETS code 4565.
- Complete VMCAS with electronic letters of recommendation
- Complete Oregon State University supplemental application by September 17, 2019 at 12 Midnight Eastern Time.
- Pay online supplemental application fee of $50.00

PREREQUISITES FOR ADMISSION

Course Description	Semester/quarter credits	Necessity
General Biology	Two semesters (3 quarters)	Required
Upper Division Biology w/ Lab	One semester (2 quarters) w/ lab	Required
Physics	Eight semester credits (10 quarter credits)	Required
General Chemistry w/ Lab	Two semesters (3 quarters) w/ lab	Required
Organic Chemistry	One semester (2 quarters)	Required
Biochemistry	One semester (2 quarters)	Required
Genetics	One semester (1 quarter)	Required
Calculus or Algebra & Trig	One calculus course or College Algebra & trigonometry courses	Required
Statistics	One semester (1 quarter)	Required
Physiology (Human or Animal)	One semester (1 quarter)	Required
*English	One semester (1 quarter)	Required
*Humanities or Social Sciences	Two semesters (3 quarters)	Required
*Public Speaking	One semester (1 quarter)	Required

*Please note that the General Education Requirements (English, Humanities, & Public Speaking) will be considered met if the applicant has earned a bachelor's degree prior to beginning the DVM program.

UNIVERSITY OF PENNSYLVANIA

Email: admissions@vet.upenn.edu

Website: www.vet.upenn.edu

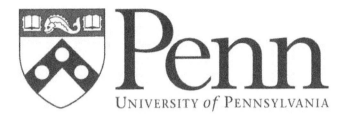

SCHOOL DESCRIPTION

The School of Veterinary Medicine of the University of Pennsylvania, known as Penn Vet, exists to improve the health and welfare of both animals and humans. We are leaders in innovation, committed to raising veterinary medicine to a new level of cutting-edge research and clinical care. We train veterinarians and biomedical scientists to work in a world characterized by globalization, population growth, and rapid technological advances. Our curriculum encompasses both traditional clinical practice and emerging career pathways. We are committed to the principle of One Health as a critical tool for tackling such daunting global challenges as disease, biosecurity, food security, biodiversity, climate change, and antimicrobial stewardship.

PROGRAM DESCRIPTION

- Class Size
  - o Resident #: 40
  - o Non-Resident #: 85
- Applicant Pool (prior year)
  - o Resident #: 219
  - o Non-Resident #: 1019
- International School: No
- Accepts International Applicants: Yes
- VMCAS Participant: Yes

ENTRANCE REQUIREMENTS

- Pre-Requisite Chart Update
  - o Date pre-reqs must be completed: Mid July prior to matriculation in August.
  - o Pre-requisite required grade = C
- VMCAS application: Yes
- Supplemental application: Yes
  - o Through VMCAS: No
  - o External: Yes

- Transcript Requirements
  - o AP Policy: must appear on official college transcripts and count toward degree.
  - o International Transcripts
  - o WES Report Required: Yes
- Test Requirements
  - o GRE Test Deadline: Scores Arrive by Oct 15
  - o TOEFL Test Deadline: If required, arrive by Oct 15
- Experiences
  - o Requirements statement
    - Experience working with animals, direct veterinary work, or research experience is desired. At least 500-600 hours working directly with veterinarians is recommended. Experience should allow applicant to convey to the admissions committee of their motivation, interest, and understanding.
- Letters of Recommendation (eLOR)
  - o Letters Guidance Statement
    - Minimum number required: 3
    - Veterinarian Required: Yes
    - Science Faculty Required: Yes
- Bachelor's degree required: No
- Academic Statement
  - o Required minimum cumulative GPA: no required GPA (incoming average is typically 3.6)
  - o Required Grades: Matriculation requirement C or above
  - o Required minimum GRE score: N/A (incoming average percentile is usually 65+ Quant and 73+ Verbal)
  - o Other GPA requirements

- Interview Required: Yes
  - A formal interview with 2 faculty members or PennVet alum members of the Admissions Committee; Interviewees will also tour Penn Vet and interact with current students.

ADMISSIONS PROCESS & DEADLINES
- Admissions Process Statement
  - Deadlines:
    - Application Open Date: May 9, 2019
    - Application Deadline Date: September 17, 2019
    - Supplemental Open Date: mid-May
    - Supplemental Deadline Date: September 17, 2019
    - Transcripts Received Date: Date as determined by VMCAS (sent directly to VMCAS)
    - eLOR Received Date: Date as determined by VMCAS (sent directly to VMCAS)
    - GRE Scores Received Date: October 15
  - Interviews held: Fridays from early January until completion
    - Interview format statement Invited applicants will have a formal 30 minute interview with 2 faculty members OR alumni members of the Admissions Committee. Interviewees will also tour Penn Vet and interact with current students during the interview day. Interviews are held Jan – Feb and invites are sent from mid-December right up until the final interview date.
  - Offers released: within 14 days after interview
  - Orientation held: late August/early September
  - Deposit required: Yes
    - If YES, amount: $500
  - Defers granted: Yes
  - Transfers accepted: Yes. Entry in second year of VMD if space allows and current institution 1st year curriculum matches closely with Penn Vet 1st year curriculum. Information found at www.vet.upenn.edu/education

EVALUATION CRITERIA
Penn Vet does not place a certain percentage or weight on specific items of an application. In taking a holistic approach, we consider some of the following:
- Your academic record
  - GRE Score
  - Includes cumulative undergraduate grade-point average, achievement in required preprofessional courses, advanced degrees and academic honors.
- Veterinary, animal and/or health science experience
  - This may include the care, knowledge, and experience gained working in a veterinary, agricultural, research, human health and or biomedical setting. Such experience should be of appropriate breadth and depth and should entail more than having provided routine care and feeding of companion animals or family pets.
- Is the applicant a well-rounded and exceptional individual
  - Extracurricular activities, community engagement, leadership roles, employment not related to animals
  - Potential for contribution to, and advancement of, the profession.

ACCEPTANCE DATA (PRIOR YEAR)
- GRE Verbal 74%, Quant 66.2%
- GPA 3.6
- Number of applications 1146
- Number interviewed 280
- Number accepted into class 191
- Number matriculated 126

TUITION / COST OF ATTENDANCE
*For current year (2020 matriculation)
- Resident (in-State)
  - Tuition: $44,910
  - Fees$4,918
- Non-Resident (out-of-state)
  - Tuition: $54,910
  - Fees: $4,918

EDUCATION / RESEARCH
- Special programs
  - Summer VETS Program is offered to current college students each summer. Student will spend 1 week in lectures, labs and clinics at Penn Vet. https://www.vet.upenn.edu/education/vmd-admissions/summer-vets

- Combined Programs statement
  - VMD/PhD, VMD/MBA, VMD/MPH. Please visit https://www.vet.upenn.edu/education/vmd-admissions/life-as-a-penn-vet-student/dual-degree-programs
- Curriculum Statement
  - Penn Vet's curriculum is designed to prepare our students for new career pathways, as well as traditional clinical practice. Its cross-disciplinary approach encourages collaboration among peer practitioners and researchers. Its allegiance to the principle of One Health fosters a perspective that links the wellbeing of humans, animals, and the environment.

FAQs
- Penn Vets Course Requirements are Matriculation Requirements. Completion of course requirements is not necessary in order to apply. All coursework must be completed in mid-July prior to matriculation if accepted.
- Penn Vet reviews all applications after the VMCAS deadline. Time of application submission plays no part in when an application is reviewed. Our full review process begins in Nov.
- Interviews are held in January and February of the application cycle. Invites are sent in December and up through our last interview day in February.
- Penn Vet does not look at fall coursework as part of the review process and therefore, fall transcripts are not required.

PREREQUISITES FOR MATRICULATION

Course Description	Number of Hours/Credits
English (must include at least 3 Credits of Composition)	6
Physics (with lab)	8
Chemistry - General	8
Chemistry - Organic	4
*(Chemistry requires at least 1 lab in General or Organic Chemistry)	
Biology (one course should cover the basics of genetics)	9
Biochem	3
Microbiology	3
Social sciences or humanities	6
Calculus & Statistics (Any Introductory Stats course)	6
Electives	37

PURDUE UNIVERSITY

Email Address: vetadmissions@purdue.edu
Website: www.vet.purdue.edu
Phone: 765-494-7893

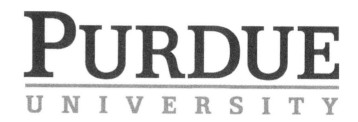

SCHOOL DESCRIPTION

Purdue University is located in one of the largest metropolitan centers in northwestern Indiana. Greater Lafayette occupies a site on the Wabash River 65 miles northwest of Indianapolis and 126 miles southeast of Chicago. The combined population of the twin cities, Lafayette and West Lafayette, exceeds 100,000. The community offers an art museum, historical museum, 1,600 acres of public parks, and more than 60 churches of all major denominations.

Purdue ranks among the 25 largest colleges and universities in the nation. Students represent all 50 states and many foreign countries. Purdue University has the fourth highest enrollment of international students of any college in the United States. Purdue also ranks fourth best in the nation for Best Value institutions in the United States, based on a survey released Wednesday (Sept. 5) by *The Wall Street Journal* and *Times Higher Education*. The Purdue University College of Veterinary Medicine strives to become the leading veterinary school for comprehensive education of the veterinary team and for discovery and engagement in selected areas of veterinary and comparative biomedical sciences. To better prepare individuals for veterinary medical careers in the twenty-first century, our curriculum emphasizes the veterinary team approach, problem-solving, and hands-on experiences.

PROGRAM DESCRIPTION

- Health & Wellness
  - Counseling & Wellness Services: Onsite academic, relationship, and group counseling available Wellness Committee
- Diversity & Disadvantaged / Accommodations
  - Purdue University Disability Resource Center collaborates with students, faculty, and staff to create usable, equitable, inclusive, and sustainable learning environments
  - Veterinary Student Resource Center (VSRC): student-led tutoring
  - Office of Diversity and Inclusion
  - VOICE (Veterinarians as One Inclusive Community for Empowerment) is a student run organization that seeks to increase awareness, respect, and sensitivity to differences among all individuals and communities in the field of veterinary medicine
  - Certificate Program for Pre-Vet Students and Students at Colleges/Schools of Veterinary Medicine: This program is designed for veterinary medical, veterinary technology, and pre-vet students who want to foster inclusive learning environments at their educational institutions and develop the skills to succeed as veterinary professionals.
- Class Size
  - Resident #: 42
  - Non-Resident #: 42
  - Contract # and where: 0
  - International Seats #: Included in the Non-Resident
- International School: No
- Accepts International Applicants: Yes
- VMCAS Participant: Yes

ENTRANCE REQUIREMENTS

- Pre-Requisite Chart Update
  - Date pre-reqs must be completed: All pre-requisites must be completed by the end of the spring semester prior

to matriculation into the veterinary medical program.
- o Pre-requisite required grade
- VMCAS application: Yes
- Supplemental application: No
- Transcript Requirements
  - o AP Policy: will be accepted if it appears on official college transcripts by subject area and is equivalent to the appropriate college-level coursework. Should your institution's official transcript not list the subject area, then you may submit an unofficial transcript with a letter explaining this and indicating which prerequisite courses are met by these credits.
  - o International Transcripts
  - o WES Report Required: Yes
- Test Requirements
  - o GRE Test Deadline: None
  - o TOEFL Test Deadline: September 17, 2019
- Experiences
  - o Requirements statement
    - ▪ Minimum hours requirements No minimum requirements
- Letters of Recommendation (eLOR)
  - o Letters Guidance Statement
    - ▪ Minimum number required: 3
    - ▪ Veterinarian Required: Yes
- Bachelor's degree required: No
- Academic Statement
  - o Required minimum cumulative GPA: 3.0
  - o Required Grades: C- or better
- Interview Required: Yes

ADMISSIONS PROCESS & DEADLINES
- Admissions Process Statement
  - o Deadlines:
    - ▪ Application Open Date: May 9, 2019
    - ▪ Application Deadline Date: September 17, 2019
    - ▪ Transcripts Received Date: September 17, 2019
    - ▪ eLOR Received Date: September 17, 2019
  - o Interviews held: January
    - ▪ Interview format statement Semi-structured Interviews
  - o Offers released: February
  - o Orientation held: Late August
  - o Deposit required: Yes
    - ▪ If YES, amount: $400.00 for residents and $1,000.00 deposit for nonresidents. De-

posit applied to tuition after matriculation. Deposit are not refundable.
- o Defers granted: Yes, with committee approval
- o Transfers accepted: Yes, based on availability

EVALUATION CRITERIA
*If applicable, please enter percentage weighted **Academic Performance 55% (Factors Considered*)**
- Cumulative grade point average
- PVM Core grade point average**
  - **Core GPA includes only the math and science prerequisite courses
- Overall academic performance

Non-Academic Activities 45% (Factors Considered*)
- Veterinary, animal, and/or research experience
- Demonstrated leadership ability
- Communication skills
- Honors & Awards
- Professionalism
- Knowledge of veterinary medicine
- Motivation towards the veterinary profession
- Extracurricular activities
- Paid employment experience
- References
- Interview

ACCEPTANCE DATA (PRIOR YEAR)
- GRE Average and Range: N/A
- GPA Average and Range: Mean GPA
  - o Residents: 3.78; Range: 3.43-4.00
  - o Non-Residents: 3.65; Range: 3.21-4.00
- Number of applications 1468
- Number accepted into class 84
- Number matriculated 84

TUITION / COST OF ATTENDANCE
*For current year (2020 matriculation)
- Resident (in-State)
  - o Tuition: $19,918
  - o COA: $36,796
- Non-Resident (out-of-state)
  - o Tuition: $44,746
  - o COA: $61,774

EDUCATION / RESEARCH
- Special programs / entrance pathways statement
- Combined Programs statement
  - o **DVM MS or PhD Combined Degree Option**
    - ▪ The Purdue University College of Veterinary Medicine offers the option to simultaneously

- pursue a veterinary degree and graduate training leading to a MS or PhD degree.
- Other Academic Programs statement
  - Veterinary Scholar Program: The Purdue University College of Veterinary Medicine offers a Veterinary Scholars Program. This program is designed to recruit highly qualified high school students to our **DVM Program** by offering the opportunity for early admission. Students who are accepted into the Veterinary Scholars Program are guaranteed a position in the DVM program if they successfully complete the required pre-veterinary courses and maintain the academic standards of the Veterinary Scholars Program.
  - VetUp! The Vet Up! College program is a six-week-long residential summer program at the Purdue University College of Veterinary Medicine for 26 educationally or economically disadvantaged undergraduate students each year that will prepare students to be competitive in the DVM applicant pool. Vet Up! College is geared towards rising college juniors and seniors.
  - Vet Up! College participants with a minimum cumulative grade point average of 3.25/4.00 by the start of Vet Up! College, who have not yet applied to another DVM degree program will be invited to apply to Purdue University College of Veterinary Medicine through a highly competitive early admissions process.
- Curriculum Statement
  - The DVM curriculum consists of four years of courses. Success in these courses is dependent upon a strong knowledge base gained from the pre-veterinary course requirements. The first two years of the curriculum focus on the basic sciences while the third and fourth years focus on clinical sciences. A minimum of 18 credits per semester is required in years 1-3. Additional elective courses may be taken.
- Clinicals begin during the 4th year.
- Veterinary Scholars Summer Research Program: Purdue University's College of Veterinary Medicine (PVM) is pleased to announce the availability of summer research fellowships for veterinary and undergraduate students. These fellowships offer veterinary and

undergraduate students the opportunity to work on independent research projects with a faculty mentor and explore non-practice careers.
- Highlights
  - ***The Purdue Advantage:***
    - Educating the entire veterinary team
    - Small class size
    - One-on-one interaction with faculty
    - Hands-on animal learning sessions from day one
    - National award winning educators
    - Emphasis on international learning experiences
    - Diverse and inclusive environment
    - Access to faculty-led research experiences
    - Focus on developing student leadership skills
    - Opportunities for community engagement

Q&A

- Top 10 FAQs

IN ORDER TO APPLY TO YOUR PROGRAM, WHAT INFORMATION AM I TO SEND TO THE SCHOOL DIRECTLY AND TO WHOM DO I SEND IT?
All application materials should be submitted directly to VMCAS. Failure to submit all transcripts from all institutions attended will result in an incomplete application. Transcripts sent directly to Purdue University College of Veterinary Medicine will not be evaluated as part of your application.

DOES PURDUE REQUIRE THE GRE?
No. Purdue does not require the GRE as part of their admissions process. GRE scores submitted will not be evaluated as part of the admissions process, therefore, you do not need to submit your GRE scores to Purdue.

CAN I SUBSTITUTE COURSES (E.G. AN ANIMAL SCIENCE COURSE FOR A BIOLOGY COURSE)?
No. The faculty of our college has approved the courses they believe to be the basic foundation courses needed in order for a student to be successful in our curriculum.
NOTE: Completion of required courses for one veterinary school/college does not guarantee compliance for another. You must complete the prerequisite courses for each veterinary college to which you wish to apply.

CAN I DOUBLE COUNT A COURSE TO MEET TWO DIFFERENT REQUIREMENTS (I.E. GENETICS FOR GENERAL BIOLOGY)?

No. You cannot double count a course to meet two different requirements. A course devoted to the study of genetics will be more in-depth than a general biology course would include.

DO ONLINE/DISTANT LEARNING LABS OR LECTURES MEET THE PRE-REQUISITE COURSE REQUIREMENTS?

Online/distant learning lecture-only courses are accepted by the Admissions Committee. Online/distant learning labs do not meet our pre-requisite course requirements. Labs must be completed onsite at an institution.

DO YOU ACCEPT COURSES TAKEN AT A COMMUNITY COLLEGE?

You can take the prerequisite courses from any two-year or four-year accredited college or university. We recommend attending an undergraduate institution with a rigorous academic program that will prepare you for the academic rigors of the veterinary program.

CAN I HAVE REQUIRED COURSEWORK IN PROGRESS WHEN I APPLY TO YOUR PROGRAM?

Yes. You may have the last of your required coursework in progress when you apply. In other words, your required coursework must be completed by the end of the spring semester prior to fall matriculation. Courses may not be taken during the summer. Our Admissions Committee has determined that summer session is too late for course completion and receipt of summer grades for finalization of admission for fall semester.

IS THERE AN ABSOLUTE MINIMUM AMOUNT OF VETERINARY, ANIMAL AND RESEARCH EXPERIENCE REQUIRED FOR APPLICANTS?

No. We are seeking students from a wide variety of backgrounds and with interests in a diverse range of veterinary careers including private practice, academic, government, industry and research. Your focus should be on the quality of the experience; not quantity.

WHAT ARE SOME EXAMPLES THAT WOULD MEET THE ANIMAL EXPERIENCE REQUIREMENT?

Animal experience can include work on a livestock farm, with a humane society, zoo or kennel, showing animals as 4-H projects, wildlife rehabilitation, and working with animals in other kinds of competitions or businesses. Personal pets are not included.

WHAT ARE SOME EXAMPLES THAT WOULD MEET THE VETERINARY EXPERIENCE REQUIREMENT?

Veterinary experience is gained while working directly with a veterinarian. This can range from on the job shadowing to working with a veterinarian as an assistant in a clinical, research or regulatory setting.

PREREQUISITES FOR ADMISSION

Course Description	Semester(s)	Necessity
General (Inorganic) Chemistry with Lab I	1	Required
General (Inorganic) Chemistry with Lab II	1	Required
Organic Chemistry with Lab I	1	Required
Organic Chemistry with Lab II	1	Required
Biochemistry ((upper-level)	1	Required
General Biology with Lab I	1	Required
General Biology with Lab II	1	Required
Genetics	1	Required
Microbiology with Lab	1	Required
Physics with Lab I	1	Required
Physics with Lab II	1	Required
Statistics	1	Required
English Composition	1	Required
Communication	1	Required
Humanities	3	Required

PRE-VETERINARY PROFILE: KIERRA WALSH

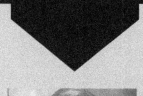

Current School Name
UMass Lowell

What type of veterinary medicine are you interested in pursuing, and why?
I have always found zoo medicine to be especially intriguing as you get to see such a broad range of species and ailments. Every single day offers a new and unique challenge which I find super exciting!

What is/was your major during undergraduate school?
I am studying general biology on a preveterinary track so I take the general biology courses but will also take more focused courses such as animal behavior.

What are your short-term and long-term goals?
My short-term goal is obviously getting into veterinary school! I am looking for a summer internship currently to expand my experience as well as beginning research for my senior thesis at UML focusing on biomaterials. I also hope to being volunteering at a shelter near my school spring semester. My long term goal is to attend veterinary school and get an externship at a zoo and eventually work at one. I would also love to do some travelling working with animals internationally such as in Africa!

What are you doing as an applicant/pre-vet to prepare for veterinary school?
I have worked very hard to balance academics, by maintaining a high GPA, and extracurriculars that will get me a wide range of animal experience. From doing a co-op at Zoo New England over the summer, and continuing to volunteer at their animal hospital, working in a research lab that has animal subjects, to even just dog sitting, I have tried to expand the types of animals and the settings I work with them in. I even started a live animal learning lab at my high school in order to introduce fellow students to exotic pets such as birds, lizards, and snakes as well as teach them animal care as my Girl Scout Gold Award project, which then led to the altering of my high schools biology curriculum to include a zoology course.

What extracurricular activities are you involved in currently?
Currently I volunteer at Zoo New England's Animal Hospital at the Franklin Park Zoo as well as as a research assistant in Dr. Gulden Camci-Unal's biomaterial lab at UMass Lowell. I am also an athlete as President of UMass Lowell's swim and dive team and a lead coach of the Sea Wolves Swim team, and am involved in other school run organizations such as UMass Lowell's difference maker program where I am a team leader for a project to introduce green roof study spaces to campus.

How old were you when you first became interested in being a veterinarian?
I have always wanted to go into veterinary medicine, it was my answer the first time my parents asked when I was little and it still is today. Although back then I could only say vet, veterinarian was a bit hard for a toddler busy conducting "operations" on her very patient golden retriever!

Please describe your various experiences in preparation for applying to veterinary school.
I am involved in the pre-health club at UMass Lowell which has played a large role in preparing me for the application process as well as information I gained from attending the middle school and high school adventures in veterinary medicine programs Tufts offers. I also have a previous year's copy of the *Veterinary Medical School Admissions Requirements* publication to provide some rough guidelines for me.

What characteristics are you looking for in a veterinary school?
I hope to go to a veterinary school that provides a very hands on experience for their students and that allows you to try a bit of everything so that I feel confident in deciding that I do actually want to specialize in zoo medicine. I also am looking for a very collaborative environment with students that are excited to learn and work together, preferably on a more rural campus after completing undergraduate at an urban university! Finally, attending a veterinary school that has a strong support system for their students looking for externships and planning for after graduation would be a huge benefit.

What advice do you have for other pre-veterinary students?
My biggest piece of advice is to never be afraid to ask for something you want. There is no harm in talking to a professor about a research position, or applying to an internship or volunteer position, or reaching out to local clinics or shelters to see if there is anything available.

UNIVERSITY OF TENNESSEE

Email: cvmadm@utk.edu
Website: http://www.vet.utk.edu

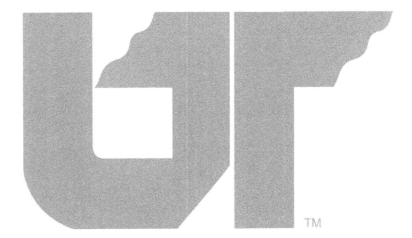

UNIVERSITY OF TENNESSEE
PROFESSIONAL PROGRAM

The University of Tennessee's College of Veterinary Medicine is located in Knoxville, a city of 185,000 situated in the Appalachian foothills of East Tennessee. The surrounding area offers exceptional recreational, cultural and sporting opportunities to enrich the student's educational experience. The modern Clyde M. York Veterinary Medicine Building includes the teaching and research facilities, the W.W. Armistead Veterinary Teaching Hospital, and the Pendergrass Library all contained within the Veterinary Medical Center complex. The curriculum of the College of Veterinary Medicine is a 9-semester, 4-year program. Development of a strong basic science education is emphasized in the first year. The second and third years emphasize the study of diseases, their causes, diagnosis, treatment, and prevention. Innovative features of the first three years of the curriculum include 4 weeks of student-centered small-group applied-learning exercises in semesters 1-4; 3 weeks of dedicated clinical experiences in the Veterinary Medical Center in semesters 1-4; and elective course opportunities in semesters 2-9 that allow students to focus on specific educational and career goals. The UT Veterinary Social Work team is a leader within the veterinary profession. Our staff and licensed counselors provide personal and professional education in health and wellness, communication, and professionalism, through individual counseling and the oversight of a professional course series, One Health and Wellness 1-IV (semesters 1-4). In the final 4 semesters (6-9), students participate exclusively in experiential learning through clinical clerkships. The 68-week clinical program (36 weeks of core rotations and 26 weeks of elective rotations, and 6 weeks of vacation) is conducted in the Veterinary Medical Center, satellite centers, and up to 16 weeks of required off-campus externships. The clinical program does not include a specific tracking curriculum, but allows students to develop individual areas of focus based on their interest and career aspirations. The college has unique programs in zoo, avian, and exotic animal medicine and surgery, cancer diagnosis and therapy, minimally invasive surgery (laser lithotripsy endoscopy, otoscopy), and rehabilitation/physical therapy. Students requiring accommodations to assure optimal learning and achievement are provided support though all 4 years of the professional program. The Student Disability Services Center works closely with the Associate Dean of Academic in providing student accommodations or designing specialized accommodations plans as needed. The College of Veterinary Medicine provides a warm and welcoming atmosphere to all students, faculty and staff and strongly supports diversity within the college and the profession.

PROGRAM DESCRIPTION
- Class Size
  - Resident #: 60
  - Non-Resident #: 25
- Applicant Pool (prior year)
  - Resident # 173
  - Non-Resident # 844
- International School: No
- Accepts International Applicants: Yes
- VMCAS Participant: Yes

ENTRANCE REQUIREMENTS
- Pre-Requisite Chart Update
  - Date pre-reqs must be completed: by the end of the spring term prior to entry.
  - Pre-requisite required grade: C or above
- VMCAS application: Yes
- Supplemental application: Yes
  - Through VMCAS: No
  - External: Yes

- Transcript Requirements
  - AP Policy: must appear on official college transcripts and be equivalent to the appropriate college-level coursework.
  - International Transcripts
  - WES Report Required: Yes
- Test Requirements
  - GRE Test Deadline: August 31, 2019
  - TOEFL Test Deadline: January 25, 2020
- Experiences
  - The College of Veterinary Medicine seeks candidates that are committed to the profession; well- rounded and have clearly demonstrated the thoughtful exploration of careers in veterinary medicine. Meaningful experiences will include a breadth of career areas and animal species, a progression of responsibilities from shadowing into hands-on, and a sufficient duration of experience develop insight into the challenges and rewards of the profession. Students are encouraged to explore 3 or more areas of veterinary medical fields, acquire some variety of small animal, large animal, and alternatives species or career environment, along with hands-on experience as may be legally allowed. No minimum level of experience is required for application to the program. High-quality experiences of 400 hours or more are recommended to attain a maximum score in the evaluation process.
    - Minimum hours requirements – 400 Recommended
- Letters of Recommendation (eLOR)
  - Letters Guidance Statement
    - Minimum number required: 3
    - Veterinarian Required: Yes, at least 2
- Bachelor's degree required: No
- Academic Statement
  - Required minimum cumulative GPA: 3.2 for Out of State Applicants
  - Required Grades: C or above
  - Required minimum of last 45: No Minimum
  - Required minimum science GPA: No Minimum
  - Required minimum GRE score: No Minimum
- Interview Required: Yes
  - Type of interview: Structured and Tentative MMI

ADMISSIONS PROCESS & DEADLINES
- Admissions Process Statement
  - Deadlines:
    - Application Open Date: May 9, 2019
    - Application Deadline Date: September 17, 2019
    - Supplemental Open Date: May 9, 2019
    - Supplemental Deadline Date: September 17, 2019
    - Transcripts Received Date: September 17
    - eLOR Received Date: September 17, 2019
    - GRE Scores Received Date: September 17, 2019
  - Interviews held: October through January
  - Offers released: Late February – Early March
  - Orientation held: Mid-August
  - Deposit required: No
  - Defers granted: Yes, case by case
  - Transfers accepted: No

EVALUATION CRITERIA
*If applicable, please enter percentage weighted
- *Initial academic file review includes:*
  - Academic performance and grade point average
  - GRE Test scores
  - Prerequisite completion
  - VMCAS and Supplemental Application information
  - VMCAS Disadvantaged/Hardship statement (optional)
- *Holistic packet review:*
  - Rigor of educational program and potential for success
  - Personal Statement
  - References (3-5 required – 3 veterinarian letters preferred)
  - Evidence of logical preparation for this career
  - Veterinary and Animal Experience
  - Extracurricular activities/community service
  - Leadership and diversity
  - Disadvantaged/Hardship factors
  - TN: Essay or Personal Statement
- *Interview:*
  - TN: Personal Statement
  - Animal/veterinary experience
  - Communication skills
  - Motivation
  - Understanding of the profession

- o Personal interests and qualities
- o Professionalism
- Other (please list)

ACCEPTANCE DATA (PRIOR YEAR)
- GRE Average and Range Average 309, Range 280 - 333
- GPA Average and Range Average, 3.67, Range 2.83 – 4.00
- Number of applications 1068
- Number interviewed (or N/A) 393
- Number selected 170
- Number accepted into class 85
- Number matriculated 85

TUITION / COST OF ATTENDANCE
*For current year (2018 matriculation)
- Resident (in-State)
  - o $28,734 29, 310
  - o COA 22, 834
- Non-Resident (out-of-state)
  - o $56,540 56,576
  - o COA 22,834

EDUCATION / RESEARCH
- **Combined Programs**
- Dual Master of Public Health – Doctor of Veterinary Medicine
- Dual Master of Science (Animal Science) – Doctor of Veterinary Medicine
- Dual Doctor of Philosophy (PHD) – Doctor of Veterinary Medicine
- Other Academic Programs statement

Special Programs/Entrance Pathways
- **Summer Veterinary Experience**
  - o The Veterinary Summer Experience Program seeks to provide opportunities for current high school students interested in veterinary medicine. To this end, the program is designed to provide valuable educational experiences and acquaint students with all facets of our exciting profession. Students will be assigned paid observational opportunities in their local veterinary practices for five weeks, followed by one week at the University of Tennessee College of Veterinary Medicine. While at the veterinary college, students will participate in various educational and leadership programs including lectures, laboratories, and clinical rotations.
- **Three-plus-one Entry**
  - o The College of Veterinary Medicine participates in three-plus-1 programs that award a Bachelor's Degree to stu-

dents who have met the requirements of their program and attained sufficient credits for graduation when considering the first-year professional curriculum. A contract between individual colleges is required for participation.
- Curriculum Statement
  - o The primary objective of the college is to enable students to attain essential knowledge, skills, attitudes, and behaviors to meet the varied needs of society and the veterinary profession. The professional curriculum provides an excellent basic science education in addition to comprehensive training in diagnosis, disease prevention, medical treatment, and surgery. Development of a strong basic science foundation is emphasized in the first two semesters. Courses consist mostly of pre-clinical subjects of anatomy (gross and microscopic), physiology, immunology, bacteriology, virology, and parasitology. Also included in the first year are clinical subjects of physical diagnosis and normal radiology, along with beginning professional skills that include finance, business, ethics, and communication skills. Considerable integration of subject matter is incorporated during this year. The third through fifth semesters include the study of diseases, their causes, diagnosis, treatment and prevention, and courses are team-taught on an organ system basis. The final four semesters are devoted to intensive education in solving animal disease problems involving extensive clinical experience in the Veterinary Medical Center. Each student will participate in clinical rotations in the Veterinary Medical Center and in required externships (preferably off-campus), with options to participate in research and alternative career studies. The curriculum is a systems-based curriculum that combines different instructional modalities from problem-based learning, standard lecture formats, laboratories, simulations, and clinical training.
- **Clinical Clerkships**
  - o Beginning with the Class of 2022, the final four semesters (6-9) begin immediately following semester five in January of year 3. Students participate exclusively in experiential learn-

ing through clinical clerkships. The 68-week clinical program (36 weeks of core rotations and 26 weeks of elective rotations, and 6 weeks of vacation) is conducted in the Veterinary Medical Center, satellite centers, and in up to 16 weeks of required off-campus externships. The clinical program does not include a specific tracking curriculum, but allows students to develop individual areas of focus based on their interest and career aspirations. The college has unique programs in zoo, avian, and exotic animal medicine and surgery, cancer diagnosis and therapy, minimally invasive surgery (laser lithotripsy endoscopy, otoscopy), and rehabilitation/physical therapy.

- **Highlights**
  - Innovative features of this curriculum include student-centered, small group, applied learning exercises in semesters one through four; dedicated clinical experiences in the Veterinary Medical Center in semesters one through four; and elective course opportunities in semesters two through nine which allow students to focus on individual educational/career goals. Students enrolled in the DVM program may register for up to 10 hours of graduate courses, and these hours will be credited toward the DVM. Elective study offers a unique educational alternative for students in the College of Veterinary Medicine and is intended to enhance professional growth, concentration in an area of interest, and career opportunities.

PREREQUISITES FOR ADMISSION

General inorganic chemistry (with laboratory)	8
Organic chemistry (with laboratory)	8
General biology/zoology (with laboratory)	8
Cellular/Molecular biology*	3
Genetics	3
Biochemistry (exclusive of laboratory)†	4
Physics (with laboratory)	8
English composition	6
Social sciences/humanities	18

* It is expected that this requirement will be fulfilled by a course in cellular or molecular biology. An upper-division cell or molecular biology course is preferred.

† This should be a complete upper-division course in general cellular and comparative biochemistry. Half of a 2-semester sequence will not satisfy this requirement. Applicants are strongly encouraged to complete additional biological and physical science courses, especially comparative anatomy, mammalian physiology, microbiology with laboratory, and statistics.

TEXAS A&M UNIVERSITY

Email: studentadmissions@cvm.tamu.edu
Website: vetmed.tamu.edu

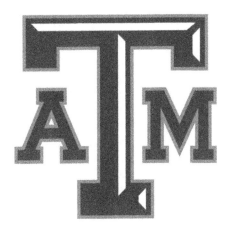

SCHOOL DESCRIPTION

The university is located adjacent to the cities of Bryan and College Station. The two cities have a combined population of approximately 255,500. The student population at Texas A&M is more than 69,000. The College of Veterinary Medicine is one of the 10 original veterinary teaching institutions that existed in the United States prior to World War II.

The College provides an integrated professional curriculum that prepares graduates with a firm foundation in the basic sciences, a broad comparative medicine knowledge base, and the clinical and personal skills to be leaders in the many career fields of veterinary medicine. Professional students are given the opportunity to gain additional education and training in their personal career paths.
Becoming a veterinarian requires much dedication and diligent study. The veterinary medical student is required to meet a high level of performance. The demands on students' time and effort are considerable, but the rewards and career satisfaction are personal achievements that make significant contributions to our society.

PROGRAM DESCRIPTION

- Class Size
  - Resident #: 142
  - Non-Resident #: 10
  - Contract # and where: 0
  - International Seats #: 0
- Applicant Pool (prior year)
  - Resident #: 146
  - Non-Resident #: 6
  - Contract # and where
- International School: No
- Accepts International Applicants: No
  VMCAS Participant: No
  - If "No", how to apply: TMDSAS

ENTRANCE REQUIREMENTS

- Pre-Requisite Chart Update
  - Date pre-reqs must be completed: May 31 of year of application.
  - Pre-requisite required grade
- VMCAS application: No
- Supplemental application: Yes
  - Through VMCAS: No
  - External: Yes
- Transcript Requirements
  - AP Policy: AP credit is accepted as fulfilling selected prerequisites; credit must be reflected on the official undergraduate transcript.
  - International Transcripts
- Test Requirements
  - GRE Test Deadline: September 30
  - TOEFL Test Deadline: Date
  - OTHER Test Deadlines
- Experiences
  - Requirements statement
    - Minimum hours requirements
- Letters of Recommendation (eLOR)
  - Letters Guidance Statement
    - Minimum number required: 3
    - Veterinarian Required: Yes
- Bachelor's degree required: No
- Academic Statement
  - Required minimum cumulative GPA: 2.9
  - Required minimum of last 45: 3.1
  - Required minimum science GPA: 2.9
  - Required minimum GRE score
  - Other GPA requirements
  - Required Grades
- Interview Required: Yes
  - Type of interview: MMI

ADMISSIONS PROCESS & DEADLINES
- Admissions Process Statement
  - Deadlines:
    - Application Open Date: May 1
    - Application Deadline Date: October 1
    - Supplemental Open Date May 1
    - Supplemental Deadline Date: October 1
    - Transcripts Received Date: October 1
    - eLOR Received Date: October 1
    - GRE Scores Received Date: October 1
  - Interviews held: January
    - Interview format statement
  - Offers released: mid-March
  - Orientation held: Late August
  - Deposit required: No
  - Defers granted: Yes
  - Transfers accepted: Yes

EVALUATION CRITERIA
*If applicable, please enter percentage weighted
- Academic History
  34% Cumulative GPA, Last 45 GPA & Science GPA
- Science pre-requisite GPA
- 16% GRE Scores
- 17% eLORS
- 12% Experiences (vet & animal), Leadership Skills, Personal Statement, Contribution to diversity

- Non-cognitive skills
- Readiness to matriculate
- Employment history
- 21% Interview
- Other (please list)

ACCEPTANCE DATA (PRIOR YEAR)
- GRE Average and Range
  Verbal   155
  Quantitative   155
  Analytical   4
- GPA Average and Range
  3.72   2.9 – 4.0
- Number of applications: 601
- Number interviewed (or N/A): 253
- Number selected 152
- Number accepted into class: 152
- Number matriculated 152

TUITION / COST OF ATTENDANCE
*For current year (2020 matriculation)
- Resident (in-State)
  - Tuition: $24,160
  - Fees $320
  - COA $44,710 - $51,840
- Non-Resident (out-of-state)
  - Tuition: $ 37,164
  - Fees $320
  - COA $59,010 – $66,605

PREREQUISITES FOR ADMISSION

Course Description	Number of Hours/Credits	Necessity
General Biology with lab	4	Required
General Microbiology with lab	4	Required
Genetics	3	Required
Animal Nutrition or Feeds & Feeding	3	Required
Inorganic Chemistry I & II with lab	8	Required
Organic Chemistry I & II with lab	8	Required
Biochemistry (lecture hours only)	3	Required
Statistics (upper level)	3	Required
Physics I & II with lab	8	Required
English	6	Required
Public Speaking	3	Required

TUFTS UNIVERSITY

Email Address: vetadmissions@tufts.edu
Website: vet.tufts.edu

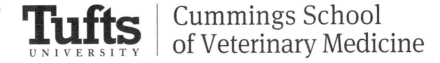

SCHOOL DESCRIPTION

Cummings School of Veterinary Medicine at Tufts University is committed to advancing One Health initiatives that enhance the health and well-being of animals, humans and the environment. Cummings School is well-positioned to apply One Health philosophies, leveraging the collective expertise of Tufts University's constellation of health science schools, including veterinary, medical, dental, and nutrition. The University's leadership in both clinical and research settings reaches across disciplines, into the classroom, and out into the world.

Our faculty advance science, improve patient care and, most importantly, inspire our students to approach their profession with open minds and a desire to make a difference. The relatively small student body ensures close professional relationships and networking opportunities. An array of curricular options, including electives and dual degree programs, allows each student to find and nurture his or her evolving niche within the profession.

Veterinary students play an integral role in the seven hospitals and clinics that comprise Cummings Veterinary Medical Center at Tufts. From their first year onward, students gain valuable expertise and enjoy a rich clinical learning environment at the:

- Foster Hospital for Small Animals, offering one of the largest small animal caseloads in the country, especially in the area of emergency and critical care where we are designated by the American College of Veterinary Emergency and Critical Care as a national Veterinary Trauma Center.
- Lerner Spay and Neuter Clinic, where students hone their surgical skills.
- Hospital for Large Animals, providing active involvement in the diagnosis, treatment and prevention of disease in horses, especially

equine athletes and sport horses, as well as camelids and small ruminants.
- Wildlife Clinic, engaging students in the hands-on practice of wildlife medicine as well as the larger ethical and conservation issues that impact wildlife, people, and the environment.
- Tufts at Tech Community Veterinary Clinic, an innovative, low-cost clinic located within a public technical high school, where students provide primary care to underserved communities in the area.
- Tufts Veterinary Field Service, the largest food animal practice in southern New England, addressing health and production needs of cattle, small ruminants, and horses. The School's farm, just steps away from the classroom, offers additional hands-on experience in agriculture and food supply veterinary medicine.
- Tufts Veterinary Emergency Treatment and Specialties, providing students the opportunity to work in an after-hours urgent care and specialty setting that closely aligns with a private practice business model.

Students engage in a myriad of opportunities, including basic, translational, and clinical research, shelter medicine, comparative oncology, wildlife and conservation medicine, the study of human-animal interactions, regenerative medicine, and more. A major international grant, Emerging Pandemic Threats One Health Workforce and the International Veterinary Medicine certificate program, along with other ongoing projects, allow students to contribute to global One Health. These opportunities create a campus without boundaries, offer unique learning experiences, and ultimately prepare our graduates for exciting and fulfilling careers.

Located just 30 miles west of the city of Boston, students take advantage of the area's internationally renowned teaching hospitals and biomedical research centers, as well as join in the vibrant atmosphere of more than 300,000 college students living, learning, and growing together.

We invite you to explore our website and visit our campus to learn more about Cummings School of Veterinary Medicine at Tufts University: vet.tufts.edu.

PROGRAM DESCRIPTION
- Health & Wellness
  - http://vetsites.tufts.edu/wellness
- Class Size
  - Resident #: 30
  - Non-Resident #: 68
  - Contract # and where: 0
  - International Seats #: included in non-resident #
- Applicant Pool (prior year) Class of 2022: 987
- International School: No
- Accepts International Applicants: Yes
- VMCAS Participant: Yes

ENTRANCE REQUIREMENTS
- Pre-Requisite Chart Update
  - Date pre-reqs must be completed: Prior to enrollment
- VMCAS application: Yes
- Supplemental application: Yes
  - Through VMCAS: Yes
  - External: No
- Transcript Requirements
  - AP Policy: We accept AP credit to fulfill prerequisites courses as long as that credit appears on your undergraduate transcript.
  - International Transcripts: Yes
  - WES Report Required: Yes
- Test Requirements
  - GRE Test Deadline: September 17, 2019
  - TOEFL Test Deadline: September 17, 2019
- Experiences
  - This may include the care, knowledge, and experience gained working in a veterinary, agricultural, research, human health and or biomedical setting. Such experience should be of appropriate breadth and depth and should entail more than having provided routine care and feeding of companion animals or family pets.
- Letters of Recommendation (eLOR)
  - Letters Guidance Statement Tufts requires two academic letters and one veterinary/research letter
    - Minimum number required: 3
    - Veterinarian Required: Yes
- Bachelor's degree required: No

- Interview Required: Yes
  - Type of interview: Meet with two faculty who have reviewed your application

ADMISSIONS PROCESS & DEADLINES
- Admissions Process Statement
  - Deadlines:
    - Application Open Date: May 9, 2019
    - Application Deadline Date: September 17, 2019
    - Supplemental Open Date: May 9, 2019
    - Supplemental Deadline Date September 17, 2019
    - Transcripts Received Date: September 17, 2019
    - eLOR Received Date: September 17, 2019
    - GRE Scores Received Date: October 15, 2019
  - Interviews held: December, January, February
    - Interview format statement Approximately 400 applicants are invited to interview. Applicants are interviewed by a team of two faculty members.
  - Offers released: March
  - Orientation held: Late August
  - Deposit required: Yes
    - If YES, amount: $500
  - Deferments granted: Yes, case by case
  - Transfers accepted: Yes, if spaces exist in second-year class

EVALUATION CRITERIA
*If applicable, please enter percentage weighted (N/A)
- GRE Scores
- eLORS
- Experiences
- Leadership Skills
- Personal Essays
- Contribution to diversity
- Non-cognitive skills
- Readiness to matriculate
- Employment history
- Interview

ACCEPTANCE DATA (PRIOR YEAR) Class of 2022
- GRE Average and Range: The mean GRE scores for the Class of 2022 were: Verbal 159, Quantitative 157, and Analytical Writing 4.5.
- GPA Average and Range: The mean GPA for the class of 2022 was 3.75.
- Number of applications 987
- Number interviewed approximately 400
- Number matriculated 98

TUITION / COST OF ATTENDANCE
*For current year (2018-19)
- Resident (in-State)
  - $51,116
  - Fees $450
- Non-Resident (out-of-state)
  - $56,116
  - Fees $450

EDUCATION / RESEARCH
- Special programs / entrance pathways statement Bachelor's/DVM Early Acceptance Program http://vet.tufts.edu/admissions/dvm-admissions/bachelordvm-program/
- Combined Programs statement
  - DVM/Master of Public Health http://vet.tufts.edu/education/combined-dvm-programs/dvmmaster-of-public-health-program/
  - DVM/MS Laboratory Animal Medicine http://vet.tufts.edu/education/combined-dvm-programs/dvmm-s-in-lab-animal-medicine-2/
  - DVM/MA with the Fletcher School of Law and Diplomacy http://vet.tufts.edu/education/combined-dvm-programs/dvmm-a-with-tufts-university-fletcher-school-of-law-diplomacy/
  - DVM/PhD http://vet.tufts.edu/education/combined-dvm-programs/dvmphd-with-tufts-university-sackler-school-of-graduate-biomedical-sciences/
- Curriculum Statement
  - http://vet.tufts.edu/education/dvm-program/purpose-goals/
- Clinicals begin
  - Students begin hands on opportunities in the first year with Clinical Skills courses and continue building their clinical skills throughout the four years.
- Highlights
  - Selectives, signature opportunities, research options http://vet.tufts.edu/education/dvm-program/special-programs-in-the-dvm-program/

Q&A
- Top 10 FAQs

I'm interested in One Health. What are some examples of ways to get involved in One Health as a Tufts student?
There are too many examples to list! The best answer to your question: if you take the initiative, you can do almost anything. The faculty are here to facilitate and guide your professional growth. Students can choose to work on One Health problems at our Wildlife Clinic, in bench science research labs on campus, and/or on international veterinary projects throughout the world through travel during the summer. Some students pursue a dual DVM/MPH and choose a One Health focus that reflects their areas of interest. There are also many collaborative opportunities with faculty at other Tufts schools and at world-renowned research and clinical facilities in the Boston area. As a first-year student, you can begin to network, discover, and refine your interests in the One Health arena.

What is the annual caseload in Tufts' small animal hospital?
The Foster Hospital for Small Animals is one of the busiest, if not the busiest, hospitals of the 30 U.S. veterinary schools. The school recently completed a multi-million dollar renovation and expansion to accommodate the growing number of cases. Last year, the hospital saw over 32,000 cases, including both primary and referral cases as well as emergency and critical care cases. As a student, you will spend time in each of many specialties throughout the hospital, ranging from emergency and critical care to oncology to diagnostic imaging. Working alongside board-certified specialists on both primary care cases and the more complicated cases, you will develop your diagnostic and clinical skills to become a competent and confident medical professional.

Does Tufts have a "tracking" curriculum for its DVM students?
Students do not choose a specialty track; all students take a core curriculum that provides an education in all aspects of the veterinary profession. This will prepare you for the National Boards and will allow you to sample various aspects of a very diverse profession. In addition to the core curriculum, you will choose from a large variety of selectives and electives which will allow you to focus on topics of your choice.

What percent of Tufts' entering class is from out-of-state?
Seventy percent of each entering class comes from outside of Massachusetts. As a private institution, Tufts University has fewer restrictions with regard to state residency than most other veterinary schools.

Does Tufts have a focus on large animal medicine and surgery?
Yes, as a student you will be required to take many courses in equine and food animal medicine and

surgery. Many selectives and electives are offered as well. Students can choose to work/volunteer on the campus farm, the large animal neonatal team, the colic team, and on various research projects. The veterinary field service provides an opportunity to ride with our faculty to surrounding farms.

Can I pursue and earn another degree while enrolled in the DVM program?

Yes, Tufts veterinary students can choose from a variety of other degree programs. The Master of Public Health and the Master of Science in Laboratory Animal Medicine can be earned within the four years of veterinary school. Students who choose one of these additional programs graduate with both the DVM and a master's degree in four years. Other degrees include the MA at the Fletcher School of Law and Diplomacy, the MS in conservation medicine, the MS in animals and public policy, the MS in infectious disease and global health, and the PhD. Students enrolled in these programs take five years to complete both the DVM and the other degrees (and longer for the PhD).

Do you have a focus on wildlife and conservation medicine?

Built upon the strengths provided by the Tufts Wildlife Medicine Program and the Tufts Center for Conservation Medicine, the school provides a rich learning environment for students who would like to focus on wildlife health and preservation, habitat and species diversity, conservation biology, ecological issues, and natural resources. The school has a busy Wildlife Clinic, which sees indigenous patients from all over New England as well as from the nearby zoos and aquaria. As a student, you can work and/or volunteer at the clinic during the school year/summers, and you will also spend a required clinical rotation there. You can take advantage of the many selectives and electives in wildlife and conservation medicine beginning as early as your first year. The Wildlife, Aquatics, Zoo, Exotics (WAZE) Club is the largest student organization on campus. WAZE promotes education through a variety of lunchtime lectures, workshops, field trips, and rounds throughout the year. At Tufts, you can immerse yourself in wildlife medicine!

Can I do an international project as a veterinary student at Tufts?

Absolutely. Many students choose to enroll at Tufts because of the unique opportunity to participate in international projects. You can work on a mentor's project, work through an NGO, and/or design your own project. All students take the foundation course in international veterinary medicine during their first year and, those who are interested, can delve much deeper as they progress through the curriculum. Read about all of the opportunities available to you here: https://vet.tufts.edu/international-veterinary-medicine-at-cummings-school/

I'm a middle school, high school, or college student. How can I spend time on the Tufts campus?

Tufts offers a popular career exploration program called Adventures in Veterinary Medicine. You can spend one or two weeks immersed in veterinary medicine alongside DVM students and faculty. Learn more: http://vetsites.tufts.edu/avm/

How can I learn more about Tufts?

- Visit our website: https://vet.tufts.edu/
- Make an appointment with an admissions counselor and get a campus tour. Call us at (508) 839-7920.
- Attend our campus-wide Open House in September.
- Call or email us with questions at (508) 839-7920 or vetadmissions@tufts.edu!

PREREQUISITES FOR ADMISSION

Course Description	Number of Hours/Credits	Necessity
Biology with laboratory	8	Required
Chemistry with laboratory	8	Required
Organic Chemistry with laboratory	8	Required
Biochemistry	3	Required
Physics	6	Required
Genetics*	3	Required
Mathematics/Statistics	6	Required
English/Speech	6	Required
Humanities and Fine Arts	6	Required
Social and Behavioral Sciences	6	Required

* unless included in biology

TUSKEGEE UNIVERSITY

Website: https://www.tuskegee.edu/programs-courses/colleges-schools/cvm

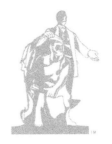

TUSKEGEE
UNIVERSITY

SCHOOL DESCRIPTION

Tuskegee University College of Veterinary Medicine is located in Tuskegee, Alabama, a city of about 13,000. Tuskegee is 40 miles east of the state of Alabama, Capitol City, Montgomery, and twenty miles west of the city of Auburn. It is also within easy driving distance to the cities of Birmingham, Alabama and Atlanta, Georgia. Summers are hot with moderate to mild humidity, and winters are moderate. Its recreational facilities, lakes, and parks can be enjoyed year-round.

Since it was founded by Booker T. Washington in 1881, Tuskegee University (HBCU) has become one of our nation's most outstanding institutions of higher learning. While it focuses on helping to develop human resources primarily within the African-American community, it is open to all.

Tuskegee's mission has always been to provide service to people in addition to education. The University stresses the need to educate the whole person, that is, the hand and the heart as well as the mind. Tuskegee enrolls more than 3,000 students and employs approximately 900 faculty and support personnel. Physical facilities include more than 5,000 acres of forestry and a campus consisting of more than 100 major buildings and structures. Total land, forestry, and facilities are valued in excess of $500 million. The campus has also been declared a historical site by the United States Department of the Interior.

Historically, Tuskegee University College of Veterinary Medicine (TUCVM) was established in 1945 for the training of African-Americans during a time when few had the opportunity to study veterinary medicine because of segregation and other racial impediments.

The Tuskegee University College of Veterinary Medicine (TUCVM) was established in 1945 and is the only veterinary medical professional program located on the campus of a Historically Black College or University (HBCU) in the United States. The TUCVM has educated over 70 percent of the Nation's African American veterinarians, and is recognized as the most diverse of all 30 Schools/Colleges of Veterinary Medicine in the U.S. The primary mission of the TUCVM is to provide an environment that nurtures and promotes a spirit of active, independent and self-directed learning, teaching, research and service in veterinary medicine and related disciplines.

Also, TUCVM's graduates have excelled in private clinical practice, public practice such the government, military, and in corporations such as the pharmaceutical industry. They hold key leadership positions in the government, military, academia, and in the international arena.

PROGRAM DESCRIPTION
- Total class size is 65
- Applicant Pool (prior year)
  - Contract # and where, South Carolina (4) and Kentucky (3)
- VMCAS Participant: Yes

ENTRANCE REQUIREMENTS
- Pre-Requisite Chart Update
  - Date pre-reqs must be completed: Applicants must complete all prerequisites by the end of the spring semester preceding matriculation.
  - Pre-requisite required grade: C or better.
- VMCAS application: Yes
- Supplemental application: Yes
- Transcript Requirements
  - WES Report Required: Yes
- Test Requirements
  - GRE Test Deadline: September 1

- Experiences
  - Requirements statement: Must be with a licensed veterinarian.
    - Minimum hours requirements: 200
- Letters of Recommendation (eLOR)
  - Letters Guidance Statement
    - Minimum number required: 3
    - Veterinarian Required: Yes
- Bachelor's degree required: Yes
- Academic Statement
  - Required minimum cumulative GPA: 3.0
  - Required minimum GRE score
- Interview Required: Yes

ADMISSIONS PROCESS & DEADLINES

- Admissions Process Statement
  - Deadlines:
    - Application Open Date: May 9
    - Application Deadline Date: September 17
    - Supplemental Deadline Date September 17
    - Transcripts Received Date: All final transcripts are required to be submitted to TUCVM, not VMCAS by June 1.
    - eLOR Received Date: September 17
    - GRE Scores Received Date: September 17
  - Interviews held: January-February
    - Interview format statement
  - Offers released: March
  - Orientation held: mid-August
  - Deposit required: Yes
    - If YES, amount: $435.50
  - Defers granted: Yes, One Year, Case by case
  - Transfers accepted: No

ACCEPTANCE DATA (PRIOR YEAR)

- GRE Average and Range   1008
- GPA Average and Range   3.398
- Number of applications   163
- Number interviewed (or N/A)   135
- Number selected   65
- Number accepted into class   N/A
- Number matriculated   N/A

TUITION / COST OF ATTENDANCE

*For current year (2020 matriculation)
- No in-state or out-state fee
- Veterinary Medicine
  - Full-time (12-19 Hours) $20,585.00
  - Each Credit Hour over 19 $1,125.00
- Veterinary Medicine (Part-time)
  - First 2 Credit Hours $4,620.00
  - Each Additional Credit Hour $1,690.00

EDUCATION / RESEARCH

- Special programs / entrance pathways statement
- Combined Programs statement
  - Combined DVM-Graduate Degree Programs are available: PhD in Integrative Biosciences, PhD Interdisciplinary Pathobiology, Master of Science Veterinary Science, Master of Public Health and Master of Science in Public Health.

APPLICATION INFORMATION

Supplemental application fee: TUCVM requires a $100.00 supplemental fee. Send supplemental application fee directly to: Office of Veterinary Admissions and Recruitment, Tuskegee University College of Veterinary Medicine, 1200 West Montgomery Rd, Tuskegee Institute, Al 36088.

For specific application information (availability, deadlines, fees, and VMCAS), please refer to the contact information listed above, or visit the online application process at: https://www.aavmc.org/students-applicants-and-advisors/veterinary-medical-college-application-service.

Residency implications: applications are accepted with special consideration given to Alabama residents and those who have residency in the following contract states, Kentucky, and South Carolina.

Number of resident seats and non-resident seats: none - TUCVM maintains "open access" and selection for seats.

International applications will be considered for admissions into TUCVM.

PREREQUISITES FOR ADMISSION

Academic Courses	Hours
English or Written Composition	6
Humanities and Social Studies (History, Economics, Psychology And Sociology)	6
Liberal Arts (Arts, Any Language, Music and Others)	6
Mathematics	
(Algebra, Calculus, Statistics, or Trigonometry)	6
Medical Terminology	1
Advanced Biology Courses (300 Level & Above)	
(Anatomy, Biology, Immunology, Microbiology, Physiology, or Zoology)	9
Biochemistry with Lab	4
Chemistry with Lab	4
Organic Chemistry with Lab	4
Physics I and Physics II With Labs	8
Electives (Genetics, Marine Biology, or Other Advance Biology Or Science Classes)	8
Introduction to Animal Science	3
Physical Education (If No B.S.)	2
Total Semester Courses	67

** Advanced biology courses, e.g., anatomy, physiology, ecology, immunology, zoology, microbiology , genetics, toxicology, and histology.

All required science courses (Advance biology, biochemistry, chemistry, physics) must have been completed within six (6) calendar years of the time of admission

FIRST-YEAR PROFILE: SHAWN KOZLOV

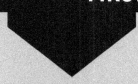

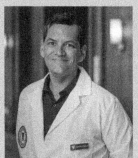

Current School Name
Virginia-Maryland College of Veterinary Medicine

Why do you want to be a veterinarian?
I was initially drawn to the veterinary profession with an interest in biological science and a compassion for animals. This opened my eyes to a profession with a wide-ranging impact on animal lives, human lives, and the environment. There is no shortage of opportunities to make a difference in the world for veterinarians either in small animal practices, biomedical research, or public health. The more I learned about this robust world, the greater my desire became to continue my career in the veterinary field by pursing a degree in veterinary medicine.

What are your short-term and long-term goals?
My short-term goals include being successful and involved in the veterinary program at the Virginia Maryland College of Veterinary Medicine. I am President of the Class of 2021 and want to both succeed and help my classmates succeed in becoming well-qualified, competent members of the field I have come to love. I hope to find a surgery residency where I can put my many years of lab animal surgery experience to good use and learn to be a leader in the animal surgery field.

Long-term, I look forward to contributing to the veterinary field through mentoring, presenting, and maybe one day returning to teach the next generation of veterinary students. I would like to someday be as influential and encouraging to future veterinary students as so many great veterinarians have been to me. I am not sure where my career in veterinary medicine will take me, but I know that one of the great things about being a veterinarian is that you have many diverse and amazing opportunities.

What did you do as an applicant to prepare for applying to veterinary school?
The first piece of advice I would offer to potential applicants is to understand the challenges facing the veterinary field after graduation. It is important to understand the cost of veterinary school both monetarily and emotionally. If the opportunities available as a veterinarian are still appealing—and they certainly are for me—then be prepared for a challenge. The second piece of advice I would give an applicant is to not give up easily. I did not get into a veterinary school my first attempt, and I am very happy I spoke with the admission offices at the schools I was rejected from and tried again.

What advice would you give to applicants or those considering applying to veterinary school?
Be sure—really sure—that it's what you want. Work with, shadow, and talk to vets who are living the career you want; ask them about the difficult, unpleasant, challenging parts of their work. Vet school is just too large an investment of money, time, opportunity-cost, and stress to take on, with anything less than complete confidence in your decision.

What helped make the transition to veterinary school easier for you?
The transition to veterinary school was startling for me at first. I am a nontraditional student who had been working full time for many years. I decided to get involved and make connections with other students and faculty as quickly as possible. This allowed me to feel more like I belonged and less like an imposter. I believe this is good advice for both nontraditional and traditional students. I felt like I was immediately a part of a team working toward my success.

What is your advice on student debt?
Understand it! Understand how loans work, how the repayment plans work, and what veterinarians working in your field of interest typically make. The more you know and understand about the loan and repayment process, the better prepared you can be to make decisions throughout the application and education process. This can help relieve any loan stress you might feel throughout school and when you graduate.

What are you most excited about learning in veterinary school?
As cliché as it might sound, I am excited to learn everything. I have been lucky enough to work in the veterinary field for many years, and I have a good understanding of a lot of concepts. I am excited to learn the details that fill in the blanks and connect concepts of which I had previously only scratched the surface. After my first semester of classes, I have already expanded so much, and I can't wait to expand on everything else.

VIRGINIA-MARYLAND
COLLEGE OF VETERINARY MEDICINE

Email Address: dvmadmit@vt.edu
Website: www.becomeavet.vetmed.vt.edu

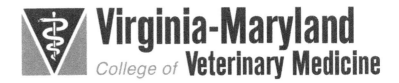

SCHOOL DESCRIPTION

The Virginia-Maryland College of Veterinary Medicine is situated on the campus of Virginia Tech in Blacksburg, Virginia. Blacksburg is located in southwest Virginia between the Blue Ridge and Allegheny Mountains and is a distinct community with a population of about 40,000. Its residents enjoy a wide range of educational, social, recreational, and cultural opportunities. In addition to the main campus in Blacksburg, there are two other campuses, the Equine Medical Center, located in Leesburg, Virginia, and the Gudelsky Center, which is located on the campus of the University of Maryland, College Park.

Our comprehensive four-year curriculum enables students to integrate their knowledge, skills, and professional attributes within diverse learning environments, all while focusing on the major areas of veterinary medicine. Students will gain proficiency while learning in the large classroom, small group integrative sessions, the clinical skills center, and laboratories. After two years of preclinical coursework, students will begin their first clinical experience. The clinical teaching time spans two summer semesters, after which students will immerse themselves in higher level coursework within one of five emphasis areas. At the end of this second teaching time, students will complete their extensive veterinary training within the clinical setting.

PROGRAM DESCRIPTION
- Health & Wellness
    - 2 Full time Mental Health counselors are available to our students.
    - Hokie Wellness: https://hokiewellness.vt.edu/
- Diversity & Disadvantaged / Accommodations
    - http://www.vetmed.vt.edu/about/diversity.asp

- Class Size
    - Resident #: 50 Virginia, 30 Maryland
    - Non-Resident #: 40
    - Contract # and where: 6 West Virginia
- Applicant Pool (prior year)
    - Resident #: 390
    - Non-Resident #: 1266
    - Contract #: 45
- International School: No
- Accepts International Applicants: Yes
- VMCAS Participant: Yes

ENTRANCE REQUIREMENTS
- Pre-Requisite Chart Update
    - Date pre-reqs must be completed: required courses must be completed by the end of the spring term of the year in which matriculation occurs.
    - Pre-requisite required grade: C- or better
- VMCAS application: Yes
- Supplemental application: Yes
    - Through VMCAS: Yes
    - External: No
- Transcript Requirements
    - AP/IB credits will be accepted as long as they appear on the applicants college transcript. We will only accept 1 semester of AP credit for the English requirement.
    - International Transcripts
    - WES Report Required: Yes
- Test Requirements
    - GRE Test Deadline: Not Required
    - TOEFL Test Deadline: September 17, 2019
    - OTHER Test Deadlines
- Experiences
    - Requirements statement
        - Up to 100 hours of veterinary

experience and 100 hours of animal experience. We also consider experience in research, extracurricular activities and volunteer and community services.
- Letters of Recommendation (eLOR)
  - Letters Guidance Statement
    - Minimum number required: 3
    - Veterinarian Required: Yes, 1 of the 3 must come from a veterinarian.
- Bachelor's degree required: No
- Academic Statement
  - Required minimum cumulative GPA: No minimum
  - Required Grades: C- or higher is all prerequisites
  - Required minimum of last 45: No minimum
  - Required minimum science GPA: No minimum
  - Required minimum GRE score: N/A
  - Other GPA requirements
- Interview Required: Yes
  - Multiple Mini Interview

ADMISSIONS PROCESS & DEADLINES
- Admissions Process Statement
  - Deadlines:
    - Application Open Date: May 2019
    - Application Deadline Date: September 17, 2019
    - Supplemental Open Date: May 2019
    - Supplemental Deadline Date: September 17, 2019
    - Transcripts Received Date: September 17, 2019
    - eLOR Received Date: September 17, 2019
    - GRE Scores Received Date: N/A
  - Interviews held: January 18 and 19, 2020
    - Interview format statement
  - Offers released: Mid-February
  - Orientation held: Late August
  - Deposit required: Yes
    - If YES, amount: $100
  - Defers granted: Yes, case by case
  - Transfers accepted: No

EVALUATION CRITERIA
*If applicable, please enter percentage weighted
- 60% Academics: Cumulative GPA, Required Science GPA and Last 45 Credit Hour GPA
- 40% Non-Academics: Related animal experience, veterinary experience, research, letters of recommendation and overall application portfolio review.

ACCEPTANCE DATA (PRIOR YEAR)
- GRE Average and Range
  - N/A
- GPA Average and Range
  - Cumulative: 3.52
  - Required Science: 3.35
  - Last 45 Credit Hour: 3.46
- Number of applications: 1656
- Number interviewed: 325
- Number selected: 126
- Number accepted into class: 126
- Number matriculated: 126

TUITION / COST OF ATTENDANCE
(For 2018-2019 Academic Year)
- Resident (in-State)
  - $24,772
  - COA
- Non-Resident (out-of-state)
  - $53,305
  - COA

EDUCATION / RESEARCH
- Special programs / entrance pathways statement
- Combined Programs statement
  - Dual DVM/PhD
  - Dual DVM/MPH
- Other Academic Programs statement
  - N/A
- Curriculum Statement
  - Our comprehensive four-year curriculum enables students to integrate their knowledge, skills, and professional attributes within diverse learning environments, all while focusing on the major areas of veterinary medicine.
- Clinicals begin
  - Students will complete 15 weeks of clinical rotations the summer between 2nd and 3rd year. They will complete the remainder during Fall and Spring semester of 4th year.

- Highlights
  - During both the third year and clinical rotations, our students are able to select one of the five tracks to focus within. The five tracks are: Small Animal, Food Animal, Equine, Mixed Animal and Public Corporate.

Q&A
- Top 10 FAQs
  - To find these please go to this link: http://becomeaveterinarian.vetmed.vt.edu/inquiryform

PREREQUISITES FOR ADMISSION

Course Description	Number of Semesters	Necessity
General Biology w/lab	2	Required
Organic Chemistry w/lab	1	Required
General or Introductory Physics w/lab	2	Required
Biochemistry	1	Required
Humanities/Social Sciences	2	Required
Math: algebra, geometry, trigonometry, calculus, or statistics	2	Required
English (3 semester hours must be English composition or a writing-intensive designated course)	2	Required
Medical Terminology	1	Required

WASHINGTON STATE UNIVERSITY

Email Address: admissions@vetmed.wsu.edu
Website: www.dvm.vetmed.wsu.edu

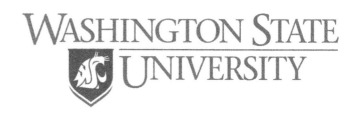

SCHOOL DESCRIPTION

The Washington-Idaho-Montana-Utah (WIMU) Regional Program in Veterinary Medicine is a partnership between the Washington State University College of Veterinary Medicine, University of Idaho Department of Animal and Veterinary Science, Montana State University, and Utah State University School of Veterinary Medicine. Our program accepts students from all of our contract states and seats are available for non-residents on both the WSU and USU campuses. The WSU College of Veterinary Medicine is also a partner with the Western Interstate Commission of Higher Education (WICHE) program and welcomes WICHE-sponsored students from Arizona, Hawaii, Montana, Nevada, New Mexico, North Dakota, and Wyoming. Known for our inclusive and welcoming community of faculty, staff and students, the WIMU Regional program provides a supportive learning environment in state of the art facilities with hands-on experience beginning on day one. In addition to the veterinary curriculum, the WIMU regional program supports an innovative education including courses in ethics, service, and leadership in veterinary medicine. In their second and third years, students take interactive classes to learn skills in clinical communication, diagnostic reasoning, and may elect to take courses on how to manage a veterinary practice as a part of the Veterinary Business Management Association Certificate Program. Students in the WIMU Regional Program have multiple opportunities to engage in dynamic research programs throughout all four years. Opportunities include the Research Scholars Program, Summer Research Program, Research Elective/Supplemental Core Courses, Northwest Bovine Veterinary Experience Program, and combined DVM/graduate studies.

PROGRAM DESCRIPTION

- Two full time counselors provide private counseling, promote student engagement and awareness activities, and conduct workshops and seminars focused on student well-being. A variety of topics include study skills, self-care, stress management, maintaining healthy relationships, time management, compassion fatigue, and wellness
- Provide consultation for diversity/multicultural efforts and outreach within the college
- Actively promotes inclusive language in conversations
- Committed to assisting students who have disabilities with reasonable accommodations through the WSU Access Center
- Class Size
  - Resident #: 55 Washington
  - Non-Resident #: 35
  - Contract # and where: 11 Idaho; 10 Montana; 20 Utah; WICHE
  - International Seats: Included in Non-resident
- Applicant Pool (prior year)
  - Resident: 154
  - Non-Resident: 1014
  - Contract and where: 40 Idaho; 22 Montana; 49 Utah; 155 WICHE
- International School: No
- Accepts International Applicants: Yes
- VMCAS Participant: Yes

ENTRANCE REQUIREMENTS

- Date pre-reqs must be completed: Prerequisite courses must be completed before time of matriculation.

- Pre-requisite required grade: C- or higher
- VMCAS application: Yes
- Supplemental application: Yes
  - Through VMCAS: No
  - External: Yes
- Transcript Requirements
  - Through VMCAS
  - AP Policy: Must meet Washington State University requirements.
  - International Transcripts
  - WES Report Required: Yes
- Test Requirements
  - GRE Test Deadline: VMCAS deadline
  - TOEFL Test Deadline: VMCAS deadline
  - OTHER Test Deadlines: NA
- Experiences
  - Requirements statement
- Applicants are encouraged to include experience in all areas as applicable on the VMCAS application.
- Letters of Recommendation (eLOR)
  - Each applicant must obtain a minimum of three evaluations (the program will accept up to six evaluations) to aid the Admissions Committee in assessing personal traits. The best individuals for these evaluations are those who know the applicant well enough to provide meaningful comments. At a minimum, the application must include the following three evaluations: (1) A veterinarian with whom the applicant has interacted fairly extensively; (2) A current or former academic who can speak to the applicant's academic ability; (3) Individuals who can evaluate the oral and written communication skills as well as the scientific background of the applicant. Graduate students should include an evaluation from their major advisor. Applicants who have been out of school for at least two years do not need to provide an academic reference. Minimum number required: 3
  - Veterinarian Required: Yes
  - Bachelor's degree required: No
  - Academic Statement: When evaluating an applicant, emphasis is placed on physical and biological science preparation. Prerequisite coursework is considered an essential foundation, while excellence in additional upper division science courses further indicates that an applicant is more likely to be able to successfully complete

our program. Applicants can major in any subject area, and are evaluated based on the rigor of the coursework completed as a requirement of that major. The committee strongly recommends completion of the baccalaureate degree prior to matriculation to the DVM program. If a baccalaureate degree has not been earned by the time of application or matriculation, the committee will still base its decisions on the strength and breadth of the applicant's educational background. The Admissions Committee evaluates applicant's academic indices including cumulative GPA, science GPA, math GPA, last 45 semester hour (or last 60 quarter hour) GPA, DVM program science and math prerequisite GPA, grades in upper division science courses, course load per semester, major and academic institution, advanced degrees, Graduate Record Examination (GRE) scores, and record of academic honors, scholarships, etc.
  - No minimum GPA required.
  - Interview Required: Yes. The interview consists of a 30-minute personal interview with two to four members of the Admissions Committee. Designed to ask behavioral and knowledge-based questions.

ADMISSIONS PROCESS & DEADLINES
- Admissions Process Statement
  - Deadlines:
    - Application Open Date: May 9
    - Application Deadline Date: September 17
    - Supplemental Open Date May 17
    - Supplemental Deadline Date: September 24
    - Transcripts Received Date: September 17
    - eLOR Received Date: September 17
    - GRE Scores Received Date: September 17
  - Interviews held: November-February
  - The interview consists of a 30-minute personal interview with two to four members of the Admissions Committee. Designed to ask behavioral and knowledge-based questions, the interview is used to assess the applicant's motivation, communication and teamwork skills, compassion and

empathy, professionalism, integrity and ethics, maturity, experience with a veterinarian in your desired area of interest, and knowledge of the profession. Offers released: November-April
- o Orientation held: Mid-August
- o Deposit required: No
- o Defers granted: Case by case basis
- o Transfers accepted: Yes

EVALUATION CRITERIA
*If applicable, please enter percentage weighted
- Academic History
- Science GPA
- Science and Math Pre-requisite GPA
- Cumulative GPA
- Last 45 GPA
- Math GPA
- Credit Load
- GRE Scores
- eLORS
- Experiences
  - o Veterinary
  - o Animal
  - o Employment
  - o Volunteer
  - o Extracurricular
  - o Research
  - o Achievements
- Leadership Skills
- Work and Family Demands
- Personal Essays
- Non-cognitive skills
- Readiness to matriculate
- Interview
- Other (please list)

ACCEPTANCE DATA (PRIOR YEAR)
- GRE Average and Range
  - o Cumulative average 61%
  - o Verbal average 65%
  - o Verbal range 17%-99%
  - o Quantitative average 55%
  - o Quantitative range 12%-89%
  - o Analytical writing average 63%
  - o Analytical writing range 7%-98%
- GPA Average and Range
  - o Cumulative average 3.670
  - o Cumulative range 2.834-4.000
  - o Total Science average 3.628
  - o Total Science range 2.763-4.000
  - o Pre-Req average 3.595
  - o Pre-Req range 2.912-4.000
  - o Last 45 Semester average 3.707
  - o Last 45 Semester range 2.911-4.000
  - o Math average 3.632
  - o Math range 2.222-4.000

- Number of applications 1434
- Number interviewed Interview Offers 386
- Number offered 222
- Number accepted into class 133
- Number matriculated 133

TUITION / COST OF ATTENDANCE
*For current year (2020 matriculation)
- Resident (in-State)
  - o $25,530
  - o Fees $2026
  - o COA $43,686
- Non-Resident (out-of-state)
  - o $61,086
  - o Fees $2026
  - o COA $79,242

EDUCATION / RESEARCH
- Special programs / entrance pathways statement
- Combined Programs statement (List any combined degree programs with brief statement)
  - o We have no formal combined degree programs within our DVM program. There are opportunities for students to explore combined DVM/PhD or DVM/MS opportunities on an individual basis. Online programs leading toward a Masters in Public Health MPH degree are available for some students participating during their DVM training.
  - o WSU has multiple opportunities to engage in dynamic research programs throughout all four years. Opportunities include the Research Scholars Program, Summer Research Program, Research Elective/Supplemental Core Courses, Northwest Bovine Veterinary Experience Program, and combined DVM/graduate studies.
- Other Academic Programs statement
  - o (List any special admissions pathways such as early entrance, scholars, etc., & brief statement)
  - o Highly motivated and uniquely qualified individuals may gain early acceptance (pre-admission) and early entry (admission) into the professional veterinary medical program. In cooperation with the WSU College of Veterinary Medicine, the WSU Honors College offers the Honors Pre-Admit Veterinary Medicine Program and the Department of Animal Sciences offers the Combined Program in Animal Sciences and Veterinary Medicine

- Curriculum Statement
    - (Brief statement of curriculum (i.e. traditional, PBL, Flipped, etc.))
    - We offer a strong curriculum with the primary goal being to impart the knowledge and skills that our graduates will need to deliver high quality health care to a range of domestic and exotic animal species. A secondary goal is to foster a general curriculum with sufficient flexibility that allows a student to learn the basics while preparing for a specific career path at an entry level. We have a traditional curriculum with the first two years focused on basic science training (with clinical integration), the third year focusing on clinical medicine and the fourth dedicated to hands-on clinical training within multiple rotation experiences through in-house and out-rotations covering a wide range of species and aspects of professional training.
- Clinicals begin
    - (Brief description of Summer (or other) research programs))
    - Veterinary students have opportunities to actively participate in research with CVM faculty through formal programs (Research Scholars Program and/or Summer Research Fellowship Program) or by individually interacting with CVM faculty that are conducting research in an area of mutual interest. The research scholars program is a 3-4 year program that includes two weekly seminar courses, directed readings and completion of an independent research project mentored by CVM faculty. Summer Research fellows receive a stipend while they are actively engaged in research.
- Highlights
    - (Anything you would like to highlight about your DVM program)
    - Cougar Orientation and Leadership Experience (COLE) is a week-long orientation which includes an off-site retreat designed to promote personal leadership, community and wellness.
    - Hands-on Experience begins early in the program through our Veterinary Teaching Hospital (VTH) with caseloads that provide experience in all areas of interest.
    - Students at the Logan and Bozeman get hands-on experiences at primary care veterinary clinics in the greater Logan and Bozeman areas.
    - Clinical Simulation Center in Pullman offers opportunities for students in all four years to practice clinical skills ranging from basic to advanced surgical operations.
    - Innovative Education with a curriculum that exposes students to ethics, service, and leadership in veterinary medicine.
    - Diagnostic Challenges (DC's) are case-based exercises that are conducted collaboratively with faculty in multiple disciplines.
    - Students take classes to learn skills in clinical communication, diagnostic reasoning, and may elect to take courses on how to manage a veterinary practice as a part of the Veterinary Business Management Association Certificate Program.
    - The Northwest Bovine Veterinary Experience Program helps prepare veterinary students for a career working with livestock. Students gain first-hand experience working with veterinarians on commercial dairy or cattle operations.
    - The Humane Society Alliance Education Program is a partnership with regional humane societies to give our students an extraordinary educational opportunity in community-based, wellness-centered, primary care facilities during their final year in school.
    - The Paul G. Allen School for Global Animal Health builds on the college's rich history of research on animal diseases that directly impact human health and offers DVM students the opportunity to participate in that research, in addition to multiple other research opportunities throughout the college.

Q&A

How do I apply to the WIMU Regional Program in Veterinary Medicine to start in Pullman, Logan, or Bozeman?

Students interested in starting the program at any of our campuses will complete the VMCAS application and the WSU/WIMU supplemental application. All applicants apply to Washington State University. Accepted Utah residents attend the Logan campus for their first two years, followed by two years on the Pullman campus. Accepted Montana residents attend the Bozeman campus for their first year, followed by three years on the Pullman campus. Accepted Washington, Idaho, and WICHE-sponsored applicants attend the Pullman campus all four years. Nonresident applicants can apply to the Logan and/or Pullman campus. Nonresidents must indicate on their WSU/WIMU supplemental application for which campuses they would like to be considered.

What should I major in at college?

Veterinary medicine is a rigorous science based field. When evaluating an applicant, emphasis is placed on physical and biological science preparation. Prerequisite coursework is considered an essential foundation, while excellence in additional upper division science courses further indicates that an applicant is more likely to be able to successfully complete our program. Applicants can major in any subject area, and are evaluated based on the rigor of the coursework completed as a requirement of that major. The committee strongly recommends completion of the baccalaureate degree prior to matriculation to the DVM program. If a baccalaureate degree has not been earned by the time of application or matriculation, the committee will still base its decisions on the strength and breadth of the applicant's educational background.

Does it matter where I get my undergraduate degree?

No, what is more important is your success in your academic program. The Committee will review the rigor of the program and its courses, as well as the rigor of an applicant's schedule at a given period of time. Some schools do offer more or less rigorous programs and this should be considered by prospective students.

Is it acceptable to attend a community/junior college?

While some prerequisite courses may be taken at a community college, other coursework may only be available at a four-year institution. If you do attend a community college, be sure to get in touch with a transfer advisor to make sure all credits will be transferable to a four-year institution and a pre-veterinary advisor at your institution to ensure your classes satisfy the prerequisites for the DVM program.

Do all of the prerequisites have to be completed before I submit my application?

No. The Admissions Committee will look for evidence that the physical and biological science prerequisites have been satisfactorily completed or will be completed prior to entry into the DVM program. Applicants are evaluated on the strength of prerequisite coursework completed at the time of application. While some prerequisites may be in progress or planned at the time of application, applicants will be expected to have completed all the prerequisite courses with a C- or higher before entering our program.

How do I know if my college courses satisfy the WSU College of Veterinary Medicine prerequisites?

Prerequisite coursework is checked at the time of application review. We highly recommend speaking with a pre-veterinary or pre-health advisor at your institution if you have questions about prerequisite courses to determine which courses at your institution will fulfill our prerequisites. You can also visit our prerequisite webpage for more information. If you are an academic advisor and need additional assistance please contact us.

Does WSU have a "tracking" curriculum?

A tracking curriculum, in which students are asked to identify species or discipline interests very early in their veterinary medical education, is not practiced at WSU. Our curriculum is designed to provide our graduates with a core knowledge base, meaning that each graduate leaves the DVM program with the knowledge they need to function as an entry-level veterinarian across the full range of domestic species. Students are able to enhance their preparation in specific areas of interest by taking various electives, supplemental core courses, and participating in off-campus experiences.

Where do I send my GRE scores and can I retake the GRE to improve my scores?

Students applying to the WSU/WIMU Regional Program should send their GRE results directly to VMCAS by entering code 4984 on the test form. GRE scores must be received by the deadline set by VMCAS. Please note: test scores that are more than five years old on or before September 17, 2019 will not be accepted. WSU will consider the highest score per section from exams taken within the five year period. Only the general GRE exam is required. Subject tests are not considered.

What if I have a disability?

The WSU/WIMU Regional Program is committed to assisting students who have disabilities with reasonable accommodations. Students with concerns should contact the WSU Access Center.

How are applications from underrepresented groups considered?
The program is committed to recruiting and admitting a highly qualified, diverse student body.

PREREQUISITES FOR ADMISSION

Course requirements and semester hours

Biology (with lab)	8
Inorganic chemistry (with lab)	8
Organic chemistry (with lab)	4
Physics (with lab)	4
Math (algebra or higher)	3
Genetics	3-4
Biochemistry	3
Statistical methods	3
Arts/Humanities/Social Sciences/History*	21
English composition/Communication*	6
TOTAL	64

*General education requirements will be waived if a student has a bachelor's degree.

WESTERN UNIVERSITY OF HEALTH SCIENCES

Email: admissions@westernu.edu
Website: https://prospective.westernu.edu/veterinary/dvm/

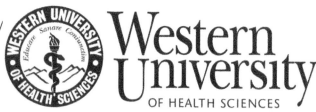

SCHOOL DESCRIPTION

Western University of Health Sciences is an independent, accredited, nonprofit university incorporated in the State of California, dedicated to educating compassionate and competent health professionals who value diversity and a humanistic approach to patient care. The university, located in the San Gabriel Valley of Southern California, about 30 miles east of Los Angeles, grants post baccalaureate professional degrees in nine colleges: the College of Podiatric Medicine, the College of Dental Medicine, the College of Optometry, the Graduate College of Biomedical Sciences, the College of Health Sciences, the College of Graduate Nursing, the College of Osteopathic Medicine of the Pacific, the College of Pharmacy, and the College of Veterinary Medicine. The American Veterinary Medical Association Council on Education granted the College of Veterinary Medicine full accreditation status in May 2013. Western U's CVM admitted its charter class Fall 2003. The founding principles of the College of Veterinary Medicine include:

- Commitment to student-centered, lifelong learning. The curriculum is designed to teach students to find and critically evaluate information, to enhance student cooperative learning, and to provide an environment for professional development.
- Commitment to a Reverence for Life philosophy in teaching veterinary medicine. The College strives to make the educational experience one that enhances moral development of its students and is respectful to all animals and people involved in its programs. Students only practice clinical and surgical skills on live animals when it is medically necessary for that animal.

- Commitment to excellence of student education through strategic partnerships in the public and private veterinary sectors.

This commitment seeks to maximize the learning experience in veterinary clinical practice and to educate practice-ready veterinarians capable of functioning independently upon graduation. In the 3rd and 4th years of the curriculum students are trained primarily off-campus at state of the art facilities.

PROGRAM DESCRIPTION

- Four year program with a Problem-Based Learning curriculum format
- Class Size
    - Resident #: 47
    - Non-Resident #: 53
- Applicant Pool (prior year)
    - Resident #: 306 (in-state)
    - Non-Resident #: 477 (out-of-state)
- International School: No
- Accepts International Applicants: Yes
- VMCAS Participant: Yes

ENTRANCE REQUIREMENTS

- Pre-Requisite Chart Update
    - Date pre-reqs must be completed: Must be completed by the end of the Spring term prior to matriculation (or June 15 at the latest).
    - Pre-requisite required grade: C- or better
- VMCAS application: Yes
- Supplemental application: No
- Transcript Requirements
    - ALL official transcripts are to be submitted directly to VMCAS and received by the deadline.

- o AP Policy – must appear on official college transcripts and be equivalent to the appropriate college level coursework. AP test subject and number of credits must also be specified on the transcript. (e.g. total/sum of credits not accepted)
- o International Transcripts are accepted with an official WES evaluation report submitted and received by VMCAS by the deadline.
  - WES Report Required: Yes
  - Scores must be received by WesternU on or before the application deadline. No exceptions.
- Test Requirements
  - o GRE Test Deadline: August 31
  - o TOEFL Test Deadline: September 1
- Experiences
  - o Requirements statement
    - Minimum hours requirements: Candidates must complete at least 300 hours by the application deadline and 500 hours by June 1, 2020.
- Letters of Recommendation (eLOR)
  - o Letters should come from individuals who can speak to the candidate's anticipated success as a student and/or future veterinarian and should include behavioral examples.
    - Minimum number required: 3
    - Veterinarian Required: Yes
- Bachelor's degree required: No
- Academic Statement
  - o Required minimum cumulative GPA: 2.75
  - o Required Grades C or higher in all prerequisite courses
  - o Other GPA requirements: Minimum GPA requirement must be met the end of the Summer term of the application year.
- Interview Required: Yes
  - o On-campus interview in November. Comprised of two, 15-minute interviews along with other required activities such as Q&A panels, campus tour, and a mock PBL session.

ADMISSIONS PROCESS & DEADLINES
- Admissions Process Statement
  - o Deadlines:
    - Application Open Date: May 9, 2019
    - Application Deadline Date: September 17
    - Transcripts Received Date: September 17
    - eLOR Received Date: September 17
    - GRE Scores Received Date: September 17
  - o Interviews held: November
  - o Offers released: January
  - o Orientation held: August
  - o Deposit required: Yes
    - If YES, amount: $500
  - o Defers granted: Yes, reviewed case by case after offer is accepted and deposit paid.
  - o Transfers accepted: No

EVALUATION CRITERIA
*If applicable, please enter percentage weighted
- Academic History
- Science GPA
- Science pre-requisite GPA
- Cumulative GPA
- Last 45 GPA N/A
- GRE Scores
- eLORS
- Experiences
- Leadership Skills
- Personal Essays
- Contribution to diversity
- Non-cognitive skills
- Readiness to matriculate
- Employment history
- Interview
- Other (please list) N/A

ACCEPTANCE DATA (PRIOR YEAR)
- GRE Average and Range: 153, 4.0
- GPA Average and Range: 3.26
- Number of applications: 772
- Number interviewed: 399
- Number selected: 105
- Number accepted into class: 105
- Number matriculated: 105

TUITION / COST OF ATTENDANCE
*For current year (2020 matriculation)
- Resident (in-State) – First Year
  - o $54,220
  - o Fees: $23,291
  - o COA: $77,511
- Non-Resident (out-of-state) – First Year
  - o $54,220
  - o Fees: $23,291
  - o COA: $77,511

EDUCATION / RESEARCH

- Curriculum Statement
    - The curriculum uses a problem-based learning approach and is guided by a reverence-for-life philosophy. Groups of approximately seven students engage in the learning process while faculty facilitate and provide subject-matter knowledge.
- Clinicals begin
    - Clinical exposure begins in the very first week of class, and more extensive third year clinical experience than is available at most other veterinary schools.
- Highlights
    - WesternU's interprofessional curriculum provides a forum for you to **collaborate and learn from students in eight other health-care programs**. This curriculum provides an opportunity for early networking with other health professionals and ultimately prepares you to better serve your patients through interprofessional collaboration and referrals.
    - Dedicated clinical and basic science faculty with many years of teaching experience are committed to working closely with you to help you succeed in our rigorous program. You will have a faculty advisor who serves as a mentor throughout your academic career by providing advice, referrals, letters of recommendation, and other support.

Q&A

- Top FAQs

What is considered an upper division/advanced course?
This varies from institution to institution. Check with your undergraduate academic advisor for clarification. Upper division/advanced courses are typically taken in your junior and senior year, are not offered at community or junior colleges, and require one or more lower-division courses to be taken prior to enrollment. Please visit the prerequisite database for a listing of approved upper-division courses offered at various institutions. Please note that these are typically not accepted if taken at a community/junior college.

Can I substitute life experience for any of the prerequisites?
No, prerequisite courses are all essential to an applicant's preparation for veterinary school and future career as a veterinarian. Therefore, we require that you take all of these classes without exception.

May I use a single course to satisfy more than one prerequisite?
No, you may not use a single course to satisfy multiple prerequisites. Each prerequisite must be satisfied by a unique course.

How can I see if my course satisfies a prerequisite?
All prerequisite courses you wish to use must appear as approved in our Prerequisite Database. If the course is not listed in the database you must submit a syllabus for review by the Admissions Committee.

When will I learn if I have been selected for an interview? Candidates will be notified by email after the committee has made a decision on the application. Interviews take place in November and require the candidate to appear on our campus for the interview.

Do you accept online laboratories? Online/virtual labs are not accepted to satisfy any of the laboratory requirements for our prerequisites requiring labs.

Do you accept online courses? We will accept online lectures provided that the course you wish to take is listed as approved in our Prerequisite Database.

PREREQUISITES FOR ADMISSION

Course Description	Number of Hours/Credits	Necessity
Organic Chemistry with Lab	3	Required
Biochemistry or Physiological Chemistry	3	Required
Upper-Division Biological and Life Sciences with Lab	9	Required
Microbiology	3	Required
Upper-Division Physiology (Animal, Human, or Comparative Only)	3	Required
Genetics	3	Required
General or College Physics with Labs	6	Required
Statistics (General, Introductory, or Bio-)	3	Required
English Composition	6	Required
Humanities/Social Sciences	9	Required

PRE-VETERINARY PROFILE: BRIANNE GRYSPEERD

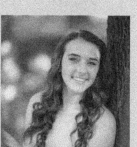

Current School Name
Oakland University

What type of veterinary medicine are you interested in pursuing, and why?
I am interested in pursuing small-animal veterinary medicine (like canine, feline, and other small mammals). This specific area interests me because the majority of veterinarians I have shadowed are in this field. I grew up with dogs and cats (no farm animals of my own), and those are the kinds of animals I would like to work with in the future.

What is/was your major during undergraduate school?
Biological sciences.

What are your short-term and long-term goals?
My short-term goals are to finish my first year of college in good academic standing. I am also looking for an internship, job, or summer-long shadowing experience with a veterinarian clinic in 2018. One of my goals includes completing at least 10 hours of community service with an animal shelter.

Some of my long-term goals include graduating from Oakland University and graduating from Oakland's Honors College. In or after 2018, I plan to get involved with some sort of animal-related research on campus. I then plan to apply for veterinary school and hopefully go to Michigan State or another university after my undergraduate degree. After vet school, I would be very interested in working with sled dogs in Alaska or northern Canada for a few years.

What are you doing as an applicant/pre-vet to prepare for veterinary school?
To prepare for veterinary school, I am researching the different school options and taking the required classes. I am also trying to build hours in work experience (a job at McDonald's), veterinary work experience (job shadowing), undergraduate research, and animal-related community service (volunteering at shelters).

What extracurricular activities are you involved in currently?
My extracurricular activities include being an active member in the Honors College Student Association and the Pre-Veterinary Medicine Association at Oakland. I am also a part of the 4-H club, K-9 and Kompany, where I show animals, complete community service, and educate youth.

How old were you when you first became interested in being a veterinarian?
I have wanted to be a veterinarian all my life. Throughout middle and high school, I showed dogs and discovered my passion for animals. I also love science classes (specifically biology), so the educational aspect of veterinary medicine is also very interesting. After job shadowing for two summers during high school, I was certain veterinary medicine was my dream career.

Please describe your various experiences in preparation for applying to veterinary school.
As a freshman in college, I have been learning more about the application process and trying to build hours that may set me apart from other applicants. I plan to demonstrate that I have a strong academic background with grades in my major, and that I am well rounded with my work and service experiences. I have around fifty hours of job shadowing experience with veterinarians from recent years.

What characteristics are you looking for in a veterinary school?
I am looking for a veterinary school close to Michigan. Within the neighboring states would be ideal; however, I am interested in some colleges on the west side of the country.

What advice do you have for other pre-veterinary students?
My advice to other pre-vet students is to focus on other areas of applying to vet school, not just the grades. Good academic standing is great, but the experiences an individual has endured improve how they view the field more than anything else can.

UNIVERSITY OF WISCONSIN

Email: oaa@vetmed.wisc.edu
Website: www.vetmed.wisc.edu

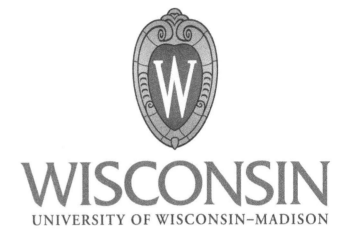

SCHOOL DESCRIPTION
The University of Wisconsin is located in Madison, the state capital, which has a population of about 240,000. The School of Veterinary Medicine facility has a modern veterinary medical teaching hospital, modern equipment, and high-quality lab space for teaching and research. The curriculum provides a broad education in veterinary medicine with learning experiences in food animal medicine and other specialty areas. The school has an outstanding research program and many faculty members have joint appointments with the College of Agricultural and Life Sciences, the School of Medicine and Public Health, the Wisconsin National Primate Research Center, the McArdle Laboratory for Cancer Research, the National Wildlife Health Laboratory, and the North Central Dairy Forage Center. These connections provide educational opportunities for students. The School of Veterinary Medicine is committed to creating an inclusive and diverse learning environment for all students.

PROGRAM DESCRIPTION
- Please see www.vetmed.wisc.edu for more information
- Class Size
  - Resident #: 62
  - Non-Resident #: 34
  - International Seats #: International students are included in non-resident student pool
- Applicant Pool (prior year)
  - Resident #: 155
  - Non-Resident #: 1160
- International School: No
- Accepts International Applicants: Yes
- VMCAS Participant: Yes

ENTRANCE REQUIREMENTS
- Pre-Requisite Chart Update
  - Date pre-reqs must be completed July 1 prior to matriculation
  - Pre-requisite required grade C/2.0
- VMCAS application: Yes
- Supplemental application: Yes
  - Through VMCAS: No
  - External: Yes
- Transcript Requirements
  - AP Policy: must appear on official college transcripts and be equivalent to the appropriate college-level coursework.
  - International Transcripts
  - WES Report Required: Yes
- Test Requirements
  - GRE Test Deadline: October 1
  - TOEFL Test Deadline: October 1
- Experiences
  - Prospective applicants are encouraged to obtain experience with the veterinary medical profession and in the care and handling of a variety of species of animals, including food animals.
- Letters of Recommendation (eLOR)
  - Letters Guidance Statement
    - Minimum number required: 3
    - Veterinarian Required: Yes
- Bachelor's degree required: No
- Academic Statement
  - Required Grades C/2.0 in required coursework
- Interview Required: No

ADMISSIONS PROCESS & DEADLINES

- Admissions Process Statement
  - Deadlines:
    - Application Open Date: May 9, 2019
    - Application Deadline Date: September 17, 2019
    - Supplemental Open Date Mid-November
    - Supplemental Deadline Date Mid-December
    - Transcripts Received Date: September 17, 2019
    - eLOR Received Date: September 17, 2019
    - GRE Scores Received Date: October 15
  - Offers released: late February
  - Orientation held: late August
  - Deposit required: No
  - Defers granted: Yes
  - Transfers accepted: No

EVALUATION CRITERIA

*If applicable, please enter percentage weighted

- Academic History
- Required coursework GPA
- Cumulative GPA
- Last 30 GPA
- GRE Scores
- eLORS
- Experiences
- Leadership Skills
- Personal Essays
- Contribution to diversity

ACCEPTANCE DATA (PRIOR YEAR)

- GRE Average GREV 156, GREQ 156, WA 4.4
- GPA Average 3.69
- Number of applications 1,315
- Number accepted into class 96
- Number matriculated 96

TUITION / COST OF ATTENDANCE

*For current year (2020 matriculation)
These figures are for 2019 matriculation. 2020 matriculation tuition figures have not been set.

- Resident (in-State)
  - Tuition: $30,515
  - Please see our website for current fees and COA information
- Non-Resident (out-of-state)
  - Tuition: $49,203
  - Please see our website for current fees and COA information

EDUCATION / RESEARCH

- Special programs / entrance pathways statement
  - The Food Animal Veterinary Medical Scholars (FAVeMedS) initiative is a highly selective program to identify and mentor academically gifted first-year undergraduate students who are highly motivated toward a lifelong career in food animal veterinary medicine. Students who are accepted into FAVeMedS are, at that time, simultaneously granted admission to the DVM program after three years of undergraduate studies, provided that they successfully complete the academic, research, and mentored clinical experiences required of program participants.
- Combined Programs statement
  - The UW School of Veterinary Medicine offers several dual degree and certificate programs for DVM program students:
    - DVM + MS (Comparative Biomedical Sciences)
    - DVM + PhD (Comparative Biomedical Sciences; other graduate programs)
    - DVM + PhD (Major or Minor in Clinical Investigation)
    - DVM + MPH (Master of Public Health)
    - DVM + Certificate in Global Health
- Curriculum Statement
  - A traditional comprehensive curriculum provides each graduate with a broad veterinary medical education and the skills necessary for the profession.
- Clinicals begin
  - Clinicals begin in May following the completion of the third year of the DVM curriculum; students have a 12-month clinical experience.
- Highlights
  - New Highlight: "The School of Veterinary Medicine is centrally located on the vibrant University of Wisconsin-Madison campus within walking distance of the School of Medicine and Public Health, the School of Pharmacy, and the School of Nursing. Inter-professional research and education opportunities abound including access to a robust dual DVM/MPH degree program and a certificate

program in Global Health in collaboration with the School of Medicine and Public Health.

Q&A
- Top 10 FAQs

Do you offer pre-vet advising?
Yes, please call the Office of Academic Affairs at 608-263-2525 to schedule an appointment.

How many students are accepted into the DVM program each year?
96

Do you give preference to Wisconsin residents?
A minimum of 62 seats in each class are reserved for Wisconsin residents.

Can I establish residency while enrolled in the DVM program?
Typically one cannot establish residency for tuition purposes while enrolled in the DVM program.

Do you require interviews?
No

Can a writing-intensive course in another academic discipline be used to fulfill the English composition requirement?
Yes

Can I apply prior to completing all of the required prerequisite coursework?
Yes, you can apply with up to four outstanding prerequisite courses however no more than two of those courses can be completed in the spring semester prior to matriculation.

Do I need to take a standardized examination?
The GRE General Test is required of all applicants.

May I submit more than one set of GRE scores?
Yes

Is a particular major required or preferred when applying?
One undergraduate major does not have an advantage over another with respect to admission to the DVM program.

Prerequisite Course Description	Number of Hours/Credits	Necessity
Biology or Zoology	4	Required
Genetics or Animal Breeding	3	Required
General Chemistry	8	Required
Organic Chemistry	3	Required
Biochemistry	3	Required
General Physics	6	Required
Statistics	3	Required
English Composition or Journalism	6	Required
Social Science or Humanities	6	Required
Anatomy	3	Recommended
Microbiology	3	Recommended
Physiology	3	Recommended
Cell/Molecular Biology	3	Recommended

INTERNATIONAL
VETERINARY MEDICAL SCHOOLS
COE Accredited

ATLANTIC VETERINARY COLLEGE AT THE UNIVERSITY OF PRINCE EDWARD ISLAND

Email: registrar@upei.ca
Website: www.upei.ca/programsandcourses
/professional-programs/doctor-veterinary-medicine

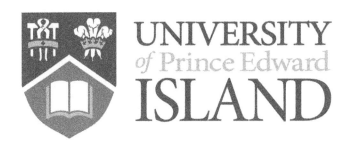

SCHOOL DESCRIPTION

The Atlantic Veterinary College (AVC) opened in 1986 and, since then, has graduated over 1,600 Doctors of Veterinary Medicine. It is fully accredited by the American Veterinary Medical Association and the Canadian Veterinary Medical Association, and is recognized by the Royal College of Veterinary Surgeons (UK).

Located on Canada's eastern seaboard (650 miles northeast of Boston), the Atlantic Veterinary College makes its home in beautiful Charlottetown, Prince Edward Island. With a population of just over 145,000, which jumps to over a million during the summer tourist season, Prince Edward Island is a mixture of rural and urban living, with agriculture, fishing, and tourism the mainstays of its economy. The capital city of Charlottetown (population 35,000) combines a small-town lifestyle with the amenities of larger cities, including dining and theatre. Residents also enjoy outdoor activities, such as golfing, cycling, sailing, and cross-country skiing.

The college is a completely integrated teaching, research, and service facility. The four-story complex contains the veterinary teaching hospital, diagnostic services, fish health unit, farm services, postmortem services, animal barns, laboratories, classrooms, information technology services, offices, cafeteria, and study areas.

The AVC Veterinary Teaching Hospital is the most comprehensive veterinary referral hospital in Atlantic Canada and provides care for over 7,000 animals yearly. Students have the opportunity to work closely with faculty clinicians to manage the care and treatment of dogs, cats, horses, and cattle as well as a variety of other domestic and non-domestic species.

PROGRAM DESCRIPTION
- Class Size
  - Resident #: 10
  - Contract # and where: 16 Nova Scotia, 13 New Brunswick, 3 Newfoundland
  - International Seats #: 26

- Applicant Pool (prior year)
  - Resident #: N/A
  - Non-Resident #: N/A
- International School: Yes
- Accepts International Applicants: Yes
- VMCAS Participant: Yes
  - If "No", how to apply

ENTRANCE REQUIREMENTS
- Pre-Requisite Chart Update
  - Date pre-reqs must be completed: At least 20 prerequisite courses must be completed or in progress at the time of application
  - Pre-requisite required grade
- VMCAS application: Yes
- Supplemental application: No
  - Through VMCAS: No
  - External: No
- Transcript Requirements
  - AP Policy: will only be accepted if credit has been granted from the home post-secondary institution and in situations where the applicant would not otherwise meet the prerequisites for the DVM program.
  - International Transcripts
  - WES Report Required: Yes, for academic institutions outside of North America only.
- Test Requirements
  - GRE Test Deadline: August 31
  - TOEFL Test Deadline: September 17
- Experiences
  - All applicants are required to submit structured descriptions of their veterinary and animal experiences prior to application to the DVM program. The goal of these experiences is to

provide applicants with insight into the breadth of the veterinary profession and assist them in making an informed career choice. For details regarding these experiences, please go to http://www.upei.ca/programsandcourses/professional-programs/doctor-veterinary-medicine/dvm-non-academic-requirements.

- ■ Minimum hours requirements: No
- Letters Guidance Statement
  - o Minimum number required: 3
- Bachelor's degree required: No
- Academic Statement
  - o There is no minimum academic average or GPA required for application or acceptance into the DVM program, however, competition can be intense and significant academic achievement must be demonstrated. Applicants are encouraged to review http://www.upei.ca/programsandcourses/professional-programs/doctor-veterinary-medicine/dvm-academic-requirements for information about the academic achievement of past accepted applicants.
- Interview Required: Yes
  - o Applicants invited to interview meet individually with two members of the Admissions Committee to review their veterinary and animal experience and discuss the applicant's understanding of the profession. Communication skills are also evaluated. In addition to the interview, non-academic aptitude is also assessed via a personality inventory that has been designed, validated and standardized with a population of candidates applying to professional academic programs. Each scale in the test was designed to evaluate critical approaches and behaviours found in daily academic and professional situations.

ADMISSIONS PROCESS & DEADLINES
- Admissions Process Statement
  - o Deadlines:
    - ■ Application Open Date: May 9
    - ■ Application Deadline Date: September 17
    - ■ Transcripts Received Date: September 17
    - ■ eLOR Received Date: September 17

- ■ GRE Scores Received Date: September 17
  - o Interviews held: November
    - ■ Applicants participate in an individual interview with two members of the Admissions Committee focusing on the applicant's understanding of the profession and communication skills.
  - o Offers released: January
  - o Orientation held: Late August
  - o Deposit required: Yes
    - ■ If YES, amount: $500Can
  - o Defers granted: Yes, case by case
  - o Transfers accepted: Yes

EVALUATION CRITERIA
*If applicable, please enter percentage weighted
- Cumulative GPA: 50%
- GRE Scores: 10%
- Interview: 20%
- Other (please list): Work and school approach and Behaviour Test 20%

ACCEPTANCE DATA (PRIOR YEAR)
- GPA Average and Range: Mean GPA 3.7

TUITION / COST OF ATTENDANCE
*For current year (2020 matriculation)
- Resident (in-State)
  - o Tuition: $12,746Can (approx.)
- Non-Resident (out-of-state)
  - o Tuition: $66,500Can

EDUCATION / RESEARCH
- Curriculum Statement
  - o The DVM curriculum is four years in duration consisting of three preclinical years followed by one clinical year. It combines a broad based, multispecies core with elective opportunities that allow students to shape their own career paths in Years 3 and 4.
- Clinicals begin
  - o DVM students are encouraged to actively participate in research beginning in their first year. Summer research employment opportunities as well as research elective course work are available throughout the program.
- Highlights
  - o Our DVM program is fully accredited by the American and Canadian Veterinary Medical Associations, and is recognized by the Royal College of Veteri-

nary Surgeons in the United Kingdom. That means that our graduates are eligible for licensure in Canada, the United States, the United Kingdom, Australia, New Zealand and beyond! We are committed to producing graduates with the knowledge, skills, aptitudes, and attitudes to become proficient entry-level veterinarians in multi-species clinical practice, with the flexibility to pursue a variety of focused opportunities in clinical practice or other career tracks available to the veterinary profession.

PRE-REQUISITE COURSES

Animal Biology 1
Animal Biology 2
Animal Biology 3
Genetics
Mathematics 1
Mathematics 2 (Statistics)
Chemistry 1
Chemistry 2
Chemistry 3 (Organic Chemistry)
English (Composition)
10 Electives

The following prescribed Science courses must have a laboratory component in order to be accepted: Animal Biology 1, Animal Biology 2, Animal Biology 3, Chemistry 1, Chemistry 2, Chemistry 3 (Organic Chemistry).

UNIVERSITY OF CALGARY*

Email: vet.admissions@ucalgary.ca
Website: vet.ucalgary.ca/dvmprogram

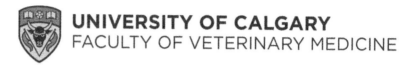

UNIVERSITY OF CALGARY
FACULTY OF VETERINARY MEDICINE

SCHOOL DESCRIPTION
The University of Calgary Faculty of Veterinary Medicine (UCVM) offers a four-year professional degree leading to a Doctor of Veterinary Medicine (DVM). Completion of at least 4 or more semesters of full-time post-secondary instruction at a recognized university or at a college providing university-equivalency in coursework is required prior to application to the DVM program.

PROGRAM DESCRIPTION
- Class Size
  - Resident #: 30-34
- International School: No
- Accepts International Applicants: No
- VMCAS Participant: No
  - If "No", how to apply: Access to the online application form for the Faculty of Veterinary Medicine can be found on the website (https://vet.ucalgary.ca/dvmprogram)

ENTRANCE REQUIREMENTS
- VMCAS application: No
- Supplemental application: No
- Transcript Requirements
- Test Requirements
- Experiences
  - Requirements statement: While no specific animal or veterinary-related experience is required, such experience is an asset.
- Letters of Recommendation (eLOR)
- Bachelor's degree required: No
- Academic Statement
  - Required minimum cumulative GPA
  - Required Grades
  - Required minimum of last 45

- Required minimum science GPA
- Required minimum GRE score
- Other GPA requirements
- Interview Required: Yes
  - Type of interview: non-academic factors are assessed. On interview day, applicants are required to complete an on-site essay and participate in a series of interviews and other activities.

ADMISSIONS PROCESS & DEADLINES
- Admissions Process Statement
  - Deadlines:
    - Application Open Date: October 1
    - Application Deadline Date: November 30
    - Transcripts Received Date: January 18
    - eLOR Received Date: November 30
  - Interviews held: March 9
  - Offers released: June
  - Deposit required: Yes
    - If YES, amount: $500
  - Transfers accepted: Yes, but not for those who have withdrawn or been expelled.

EVALUATION CRITERIA
*If applicable, please enter percentage weighted
- Academic History
- Science GPA
- Science pre-requisite GPA
- Cumulative GPA: 30%
- Last 45 GPA
- GRE Scores
- eLORS: 5%

- Experiences
- Leadership Skills
- Personal Essays
- Contribution to diversity
- Non-cognitive skills
- Readiness to matriculate
- Employment history
- Interview 45%
- Other (please list): On-site essay Performance 20%

ACCEPTANCE DATA (PRIOR YEAR)
- GRE Average and Range
- GPA Average and Range
- Number of applications
- Number interviewed (or N/A)
- Number selected
- Number accepted into class
- Number matriculated

TUITION / COST OF ATTENDANCE
*For current year (2020 matriculation)
- Resident (in-State)
  - Tuition: ~$10,860.00 CDN

EDUCATION / RESEARCH
- Special programs / entrance pathways statement

APPLICATION INFORMATION
Access to the online application form for the Faculty of Veterinary Medicine can be found on the website (https://vet.ucalgary.ca/dvmprogram). Applicants must be Alberta residents at the time of application, as defined by the Province of Alberta. The Alberta Government Guidelines within the Student Financial Assistance Regulations will be used to determine residency status. Details of these requirements can be found on the Alberta Government website at: https://studentaid.alberta.ca/before-you-apply/eligibility.aspx. Proof of Alberta residency will be required with your application.

Completed application forms include the following: complete personal information; a signed statement verifying Alberta residency status and verifying completion of the academic requirements; post-secondary transcripts submitted by the appropriate academic institution; a statement of work experience; and a statement of major extra-curricular activities. Official transcripts should be sent directly from the reporting institution to the UCVM Admissions Office.

English language proficiency must be demonstrated for all applicants for whom English is not their first language.

PREREQUISITE COURSES

Required Undergraduate Course	e.g. University of Calgary Equivalent Course
Two Introductory Biology Courses (*a lab component is required for each course*)	BIOL 241 and BIOL 243
Two Introductory Chemistry Courses (*a lab component is required for each course*)	CHEM 201 and CHEM 203
One Introductory English Course (*must contain a writing component*)	ENGL 201
One Introductory Organic Chemistry Course (*a lab component is required*)	CHEM 351
One Introductory Statistics Course	STAT 205
One Introductory Biochemistry Course (*a lab component is optional*)	BCEM 341 or BCEM 393
One Introductory Genetics Course (*a lab component is optional*)	BIOL 311
One Introductory Ecology Course (*a lab component is optional*)	BIOL 313

UNIVERSITY COLLEGE DUBLIN

Email:vetprogrammes@ucd.ie
Website: www.ucd.ie/vetmed
Phone: +353 1 7166100

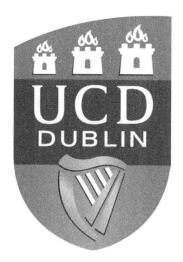

SCHOOL DESCRIPTION

UCD School of Veterinary Medicine is the sole provider of a veterinary medicine degree programme on the island of Ireland, and is accredited by the American Veterinary Medical Association.

Students of the veterinary medicine programme benefit from the outstanding facilities of the purpose-designed UCD Veterinary Sciences Centre and UCD Veterinary Hospital on the main university campus at Belfield, Dublin. Located on a 132 Ha site 5km south of Dublin's City Centre, UCD is Ireland's largest university with over 30,000 students. This is complemented by Lyons Estate Farm where students have practical classes at all stages of the curriculum.

Ireland is a small island with a big reputation – located on the western edge of Europe, it's a strategic gateway to Europe and one of the most globalised countries in the World. Dublin, the capital, is a lively city, built on hundreds of years of history and culture. Today, Dublin is a truly global city, and its multi-cultural population make it a cosmopolitan and vibrant destination.

Dublin frequently ranks highly in the QS Best Student Cities, described as a great location for those whose 'idea of a perfect student city involves combining top-class study facilities and historic surroundings with a cracking social scene and famously friendly locals.'

UCD is Ireland's global university, and its most popular university for international students – 30% of international students coming to Ireland choose UCD. We have 139 nationalities within the student body, with international students accounting for 27% of our overall student numbers, and some 30% of our staff are international. We also have a global network of alumni, with 269,000 alumni across 165 countries.

Our university is one of Europe's leading research-intensive universities; an environment where undergraduate education, masters and PhD training, innovation and community engagement form a dynamic spectrum of activity. UCD has the most engaged student body in Ireland, and with over 140 clubs and societies on campus, there really is something for everyone to get involved in. Your experience as a vet student at UCD will guarantee life-long friendships. You can find further information on attending UCD as an international student at http://www.ucd.ie/international

PROGRAM DESCRIPTION

- Class Size
    - Resident #: 90
    - Non-Resident #: 40
- Applicant Pool (prior year)
    - Non-Resident #: 230
- International School: Yes
- Accepts International Applicants: Yes
- VMCAS Participant: Yes

ENTRANCE REQUIREMENTS

- Pre-Requisite Chart Update
    - Date pre-reqs must be completed: all required courses should be completed prior to August of the year of admission.
- VMCAS application: Yes
- Supplemental application: Yes
    - Through VMCAS: No
    - External: Yes
- Transcript Requirements
    - AP Policy: AP - Combined score of 12 (Across a maximum of 4 subjects). Math Req - AP 2, Chemistry Req - AP 3. For more information Contact UCD team in the US at northamerica2@ucd.ie
    - International Transcripts: Yes
    - WES Report Required: No

- Test Requirements
  - GRE Test Deadline: August 31
- Experiences
  - Requirements statement: Applicants are expected to have gained relevant work experience of handling animals. This should, where possible, include not only seeing veterinary practice, but also spending time on livestock farms and other animal establishments.
    - Minimum hours requirements
- Letters of Recommendation (eLOR)
  - Letters Guidance Statement: A minimum of two references must be provided (one from an academic source, and one from a practicing veterinary surgeon – Signed on Headed Paper).
    - Minimum number required: 2
    - Veterinarian Required: Yes (Signed and on Headed paper).
- Bachelor's degree required: Yes
- Academic Statement
  - Required minimum cumulative GPA: 3.2
  - Required Grades
  - Required minimum of last 45 Required minimum science GPA
  - Required minimum GRE score
  - Other GPA requirements
- Interview Required: No (at the direction of the Admissions Committee)
  - Type of interview

ADMISSIONS PROCESS & DEADLINES
- Admissions Process Statement
  - Deadlines:
    - Application Open Date: May 9
    - Application Deadline Date: September 17
    - Supplemental Open Date
    - Supplemental Deadline Date: November 1
    - Transcripts Received Date: September 17
    - eLOR Received Date: September 17
    - GRE Scores Received Date: September 17
  - Interviews held: January/February
    - Interview format (At the Direction of the Admissions Committee)
  - Offers released: By early April
  - Orientation held: Late August/Early

September
  - Deposit required: Yes
    - If YES, amount: €2,000, required within 2 weeks of acceptance
  - Defers granted: **No**
  - Transfers accepted: **No**

EVALUATION CRITERIA
*If applicable, please enter percentage weighted
- Academic History
- Science GPA
- Science pre-requisite GPA
- Cumulative GPA
- Last 45 GPA
- GRE Scores
- eLORS
- Experiences
- Leadership Skills
- Personal Essays
- Contribution to diversity
- Non-cognitive skills
- Readiness to matriculate
- Employment history
- Interview
- Other (please list)

ACCEPTANCE DATA (PRIOR YEAR)
- GRE Average and Range
- GPA Average and Range
- Number of applications
- Number interviewed (or N/A)
- Number selected
- Number accepted into class
- Number matriculated

TUITION / COST OF ATTENDANCE
*For current year (2020 matriculation)
- Resident (in-State)
  - Tuition: €20,700 EU students that enter Graduate Entry Veterinary Medicine from 2019/20 onwards will be subject to annual increases of between 2-4%
- Non-Resident (out-of-state)
  - Tuition: €37,000 per annum for 4 year. Non-EU students that enter Graduate Entry Veterinary Medicine from 2019/20 onwards will be subject to annual increases of between 2-4%

PROGRAMME/SYLLABUS
Our veterinary programme is accredited by the Veterinary Council of Ireland, the American Veterinary Medical Association, and the European Association of Establishments in Veterinary Education. It is designed to educate you to the best

international standards in veterinary medicine and to prepare you for entry to any branch of the veterinary profession. Veterinary medicine is concerned with the promotion of the health and welfare of animals of special importance to society. This involves the care for healthy and sick animals, the prevention, recognition, control and treatment of their diseases and the welfare and productivity of livestock. Veterinarians also safe-guard human health through prevention and control of diseases transmitted from animals to man, through ensuring the safety of foods of animal origin, and through advancing the science and art of comparative medicine.

Veterinary graduates have a wide spectrum of careers to choose from including private practice (companion animals, food animals, horses, exotics, or a mixture of these), government service (animal health, food safety, public health), research or industry.

US applicants through VMCAS are eligible to apply to enter this programme provided they have the prerequisites as outlined below. Further curricular details are published on our web site, www.ucd.ie/vetmed.

The Graduate-Entry Programme is organised into four stages. In stage 1 of the programme students will build on their knowledge of the basic biological sciences by taking modules designed to demonstrate how this knowledge is applied in the practice of veterinary medicine, and gain a firm grounding in animal welfare, behaviour and handling. A key objective will be to ensure that students have the required knowledge, skills and competences to progress to Stage 2. Starting with stage 2 students will take modules with students of the five-year undergraduate veterinary medicine programme. As the programme progresses students will develop clinical skills and study each of the clinical sciences using a "body systems" approach. All stages of the programme include a "professionalism' module which addresses the professional attributes required to contribute as a productive member of the veterinary profession.

The final year of the programme consists of clinical rotations in the UCD teaching hospital where students study alongside experienced and specialist staff clinicians, and participate in patient care and client communication. Each student has a personalized timetable ensuring that they participate in rotations in Large and Small Animal Surgery, Diagnostic Imaging, Anesthesiology, Small Animal Medicine, Emergency Medicine, Farm Animal Clinical Studies including Herd Health, Diagnostic and Clinical Pathology, as well as a rotation in shelter medicine, which is provided in collaboration with the Dublin Society for the Prevention of Cruelty to Animals (DSPCA). Throughout the programme students are required to participate in extra-mural studies. In the early years, this consists of gaining experience in the handling and management of farm and companion animals, and in later years, of working with veterinarians in practice (clinical extra-mural experience).

Course Requirements	Full Semester
Physics with lab	1
Biochemistry	1
General biology	1
General inorganic chemistry with lab	1
Microbiology	1
Cellular biology	1

Course completion deadline: all required courses should be completed prior to August of the year of admission.

5-Year Undergraduate Programme MVB
Those candidates with a non-science degree or lacking some prerequisites or sufficient relevant experience will be considered entry to the 5-year MVB programme.

Standardized examinations: none required. GRE results will be considered if submitted.

UNIVERSITY OF EDINBURGH

Email: vetug@ed.ac.uk
Website: https://www.ed.ac.uk/vet

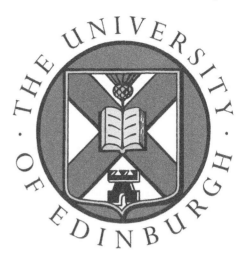

SCHOOL DESCRIPTION

The Royal (Dick) School of Veterinary Studies was founded by William Dick in 1823, and sits within the College of Medicine and Veterinary Medicine at the University of Edinburgh. The School is a recognized world leader in veterinary education, research and clinical practice. The BVM&S degree is accredited by the Royal College of Veterinary Surgeons (RCVS), the American Veterinary Medical Association (AVMA), the Australasian Veterinary Boards Council (AVBC), the South African Veterinary Council (SAVC), and the European Association of Establishments for Veterinary Education (EAEVE), allowing our graduates to practice veterinary medicine throughout the United Kingdom, North America, Europe, Australasia and beyond.

Veterinary Medicine at Edinburgh mixes the best of tradition with award winning, progressive teaching. Clinical and professional skills are taught from the earliest stages. Our approach is to ensure optimum integration of the core subjects throughout the curriculum. While many of our graduates enter and remain within the veterinary profession, many others find that training at Edinburgh enables them to succeed in a wide range of careers in research, government, private enterprise and academia.

The Easter Bush campus houses the Royal (Dick) School of Veterinary Studies which incorporates The Roslin Institute, The Jeanne Marchig International Centre for Animal Welfare Education and the Veterinary Oncology and Imaging Centre. The Roslin Institute (now the research arm of the Veterinary School) is an animal sciences research institute, which won international fame in 1996, when Ian Wilmut, Keith Campbell and their colleagues created Dolly the sheep, the first mammal to be cloned from an adult cell.

Within the University of Edinburgh, there are over 260 student societies – more than any other university in the UK – covering everything from juggling to horse riding to volunteering, which can cater to your interests. Our sports, music and drama facilities are ranked among the best in the UK.

Edinburgh, the inspiring capital of Scotland, is an historic, cosmopolitan and cultured city, which offers a unique living and learning experience. One of the most vibrant cities in Europe, the city of Edinburgh is regularly voted as one of the most desirable places to live in the world and has been rated the "friendliest city in the UK." This cosmopolitan, safe and welcoming atmosphere encourages all students to feel at home very quickly. With a population of around 500,000, Edinburgh is a compact city, which is easy to travel around on foot or by the efficient public transport network. Edinburgh International Airport has an extensive range of national and international services with direct flights to most major cities in Europe and to a number of major cities worldwide. Many students also take the opportunity to travel around Europe during vacation periods, or even for the weekend, as there are many cheap flight options available from Edinburgh.

For more information on our Veterinary Medicine and Surgery degree programs, refer to the following link: www.ed.ac.uk/schools-departments/vet/studying/bvms-degree.

The Graduate Entry Program (GEP) is a four-year program which allows graduates with a relevant first degree in a biological or animal science subject to attain a Bachelor of Veterinary and Surgery (BVM&S) degree and register as a veterinary surgeon. The BVM&S is the equivalent of a DVM. The GEP is tailored to cover key areas of integrated anatomy and physiology in a case-based format with additional courses on introductory pathology, infectious disease, animal husbandry and population medicine. Studying Veterinary Medicine at Edinburgh will give you transferable skills such as effective communication, teambuilding and understanding of business management. Veterinary training also provides an outstanding background for those who wish to pursue a career in biomedical research, including both veterinary and human medicine. Our long-standing combination of tradition and cutting-edge veterinary teaching benefits from a close-knit collegial community of students.

PROGRAM DESCRIPTION
- Class Size
  - Resident #: 40
  - Contract # and where: 32 England, Wales & Northern Ireland
  - International Seats #: 35 (5-year), 63 (4-year)
- Applicant Pool (prior year)
  - Resident #: 962
  - Non-Resident (international) #: 485
- International School: Yes
- Accepts International Applicants: Yes
- VMCAS Participant: Yes
  - Also accepts UCAS applications.

ENTRANCE REQUIREMENTS
- Pre-Requisite Chart Update
  - mid-June
  - Pre-requisite required grade: C or better
- VMCAS application: Yes
- Supplemental application: No
  - Through VMCAS: No
  - External: No
- Transcript Requirements
  - AP Policy
  - International Transcripts
  - WES Report Required: No
- Test Requirements:
  - GRE Test Deadline: September 30
  - TOEFL Test Deadline: June 1
  - OTHER Test Deadlines N/A
  - Note that the following tests are NOT required for candidates applying to the BVM&S programs at the University of Edinburgh:
    - BioMedical Admissions Test (BMAT)
    - UK Clinical Aptitude Test (UKCAT)
    - Medical College Admission Test (MCAT)
    - Veterinary College Admission Test (VCAT)
- Experiences
- Letters of Recommendation (eLOR)
  - Letters Guidance Statement
    - Minimum number required: 2
    - Veterinarian Required: Yes

- Bachelor's degree required: Yes
- Academic Statement
  - Required minimum cumulative GPA: 3.4
- Interview Required: Yes
  - Multiple Mini Interviews

ADMISSIONS PROCESS & DEADLINES
- Admissions Process Statement
  - Deadlines:
    - Application Open Date: May 9, 2019
    - Application Deadline Date: September 17 (VMCAS), October 15 (UCAS)
    - Supplemental Open Date
    - Supplemental Deadline Date
    - Transcripts Received Date: September 17 (VMCAS), October 15 (UCAS)
    - eLOR Received Date: September 17 (VMCAS), October 15 (UCAS)
    - GRE Scores Received Date: October 1
  - Interviews held: early to mid-February (held in the U.S.)
  - https://www.ed.ac.uk/vet/studying/4-year-programme/edinburgh-interview Offers released: early April at the latest
  - Orientation held: early August (4-year Graduate Entry Program), early September (5-year program)
  - Deposit required: Yes
    - If YES, amount: £1500 for non-EU applicants.
  - Defers granted: No
  - Transfers accepted: No

EVALUATION CRITERIA
*If applicable, please enter percentage weighted
- Academic History
- Science GPA
- Science pre-requisite GPA
- Cumulative GPA
- GRE Scores
- eLORS
- Experiences
- Leadership Skills
- Personal Essays
- Contribution to diversity
- Non-cognitive skills
- Readiness to matriculate
- Employment history
- Interview
- Other (please list)

ACCEPTANCE DATA (PRIOR YEAR)
- GPA Average 3.49
- Number of applications 427 (for 4-year program)
- Number interviewed 215
- Number selected 139
- Number accepted into class 74
- Number matriculated 73

TUITION / COST OF ATTENDANCE
*For current year (2020 matriculation)
- Resident (in-state)
  - Tuition: (£1,820 - £9,250)
  - Further information about additional fees is available here: https://www.ed.ac.uk/vet/studying/4-year-programme/fees-and-funding
- Non-Resident (out-of-state)
  - Tuition: £31,450 per annum (2019 matriculation), fixed for the duration of the program
  - Further information about additional fees is available here: https://www.ed.ac.uk/vet/studying/4-year-programme/fees-and-funding

EDUCATION / RESEARCH
- Curriculum Statement
  - The BVM&S curriculum adopts a blended approach with traditional lectures, case based and flipped classroom approaches according to subject area.
- Clinicals begin
  - The Clinical phase comprises the final 3 years of the programme, although clinical skills training begins in the first year.
  - Many students participate in research projects usually conducted during the summer months.

- Highlights
  - The School has an extensive exotics animal practice with significant clinical and research expertise across exotic, wildlife and conservation medicine
  - Students graduate with significant practical experience due to opportunities on course (lecture free final year) and participation in clinical extramural studies
  - The World leading Roslin Institute comprises the research arm of the veterinary school. This research rich environment informs the student environment and the schools clinical practice.

Q&A
- Top 10 FAQs
  - A full list of our FAQs is available in our BVM&S booklet here: https://www.ed.ac.uk/vet/studying/bvms-booklet

PREREQUISITE POLICY
Candidates who want to be considered for the 4 year graduate programme (GEP) must achieve high grades (C or better) in the following subjects:
- Biology/Zoology
- Physics
- Biochemistry
- Organic and Inorganic Chemistry
- Mathematics/Statistics

In addition, gaining high grades (C or better) in the following subjects would strengthen an application for the GEP
- Genetics
- Microbiology
- Cell Biology

UNIVERSITY OF GLASGOW

Email Address: vet-sch-admissions@glasgow.ac.uk
Website: http://www.gla.ac.uk/schools/vet

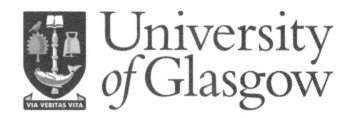

SCHOOL DESCRIPTION

The School of Veterinary Medicine is located on the 80 hectare Garscube campus at the Northwest boundary of the city, four miles from the University's Gilmorehill campus. The School was founded in 1862 and gained independent Faculty status in 1969. In 2010, the Faculty translated from the "Faculty of Veterinary Medicine" to the "School of Veterinary Medicine" within the College of Medical, Veterinary and Life Sciences. The School has a 190 hectare commercial farm and research centre at Cochno, 15 minutes from the Garscube campus (5 miles north).

The city of Glasgow has a population of around 600,000 and is Scotland's largest city. One of Europe's liveliest places with a varied and colorful cultural and social life, it can cater to every taste. Situated on the River Clyde, Glasgow has excellent road and rail links to the rest of the UK and air services to a wide range of destinations, both home and overseas.

Wherever you come from, you can be sure of building friendships that last a lifetime at Glasgow. According to the travel guide *Lonely Planet*, Glasgow is one of the world's top ten cities.

The School has approximately 200 staff (academic, research, and support) with an additional 65 postgraduate research students, 30 postgraduate clinical scholars, and 600 undergraduate students.

The school is pre-eminent in teaching, research, and clinical provision, and attracts students, researchers, and clinicians from around the world. Our internationally accredited school provides an expert referral centre via the Small Animal Hospital, the Weipers Centre for Equine Welfare, and the Scottish Centre for Production Animal Health & Welfare for animal owners and referring practitioners throughout the UK.

Following the first ever international UK accreditation visit to be undertaken conjointly between the American Veterinary Medical Association (AVMA)

Council on Education, the Royal College of Veterinary Surgeons (RCVS), the European Association of Establishments for Veterinary Education (EAEVE), and the Australasian Veterinary Boards Council (AVBC) in April 2013, the University of Glasgow's School of Veterinary Medicine has achieved full accreditation for a further period of seven years.

The BVMS programme is based on integration of clinical and science subject areas and has a spiral course structure, meaning that you will revisit topics as you progress through the programme, each time with increasing clinical focus. In conjunction, there is a vertical theme of professional and clinical skills development to help you acquire the personal qualities and skills you will need in professional environments.

The programme is delivered over five years and is divided into three phases. Years 1 and 2, Foundation Phase, Years 3 and 4, Clinical Phase, Year 5, Professional Phase.

In the recent Research Excellence Framework 2014 (REF2014), the Grade Point Average for Glasgow's veterinary and animal health research activity was ranked top amongst the UK veterinary schools.

PROGRAM DESCRIPTION

- Health & Wellness: The School of Veterinary Medicine is committed to supporting student wellbeing and recognises that a positive approach to the management of physical and mental health is crucial to supporting student learning and academic achievement.
- Diversity & Disadvantaged / Accommodations: The University of Glasgow is committed to equality, diversity and inclusion and to promoting a positive culture in which all can thrive.
    - The School will provide all reasonable support to enable disabled students

or those with health conditions to complete their studies. Appropriate support can be provided for many circumstances even if the effects of disability or ill health are substantial and it is important to know that no health condition in itself would automatically preclude a student from studying veterinary medicine and we consider any disability or health condition on an individual basis. However, because of a requirement to ensure patients, clients and colleagues are not harmed through involvement in veterinary training, if you have a condition which would make it impossible for you to work safely with patients, clients or colleagues, or to acquire the skills necessary to complete training, even with adjustments and support, then you cannot be accepted onto the undergraduate veterinary medicine programme.

- o You should not assume that your disability or health condition will prevent your take-up of a place and we would be pleased to speak with you, in confidence, at the earliest opportunity about any concerns you may have either pre or post-application.
- Class Size
  - o Resident #: 72
  - o Non-Resident #: 65
- Applicant Pool (prior year)
  - o Resident #: 565
  - o Non-Resident #: 408
- International School: Yes
- Accepts International Applicants: Yes
- VMCAS Participant: Yes

ENTRANCE REQUIREMENTS
- Pre-Requisite Chart Update
- Required Courses – Biology/Zoology, Organic chemistry, Inorganic chemistry, Biochemistry, Physics, Maths/Statistics
- Recommended Courses – Genetics, Microbiology, Cellular Biology
  - o Date pre-reqs must be completed: Required courses should be completed prior to admission in the fall.
  - o Pre-requisite required grade B
- VMCAS application: Yes
- Supplemental application: No
- Transcript Requirements
  - o AP Policy: not applicable
  - o International Transcripts: Yes
- Test Requirements

- Experiences
  - o Requirements statement
    - Minimum hours requirements
    - A minimum of 6 weeks work experience with at least 2 weeks with a veterinary surgeon and have had hands on experience with both farm and companion animals where possible.
- Letters of Recommendation (eLOR)
  - o Letters Guidance Statement
    - Minimum number required: 2
    - Veterinarian Required: Yes
- Bachelor's degree required: No
- Academic Statement
  - o Required minimum cumulative GPA: 3.4
  - o Required minimum science GPA: 3.0
- Interview Required: Yes
  - o Type of interview: Face to Face and Situational Judgement Test

ADMISSIONS PROCESS & DEADLINES
- Admissions Process Statement
  - o Deadlines:
    - Application Open Date: May 9
    - Application Deadline Date: September 16
    - Transcripts Received Date: September 16
    - eLOR Received Date: September 16
  - o Interviews held: November-February (In North America)
    - Interview format statement
- The interview consists of a 30-minute meeting and a computer based exercise which explores ethical awareness and critical thinking. The discussion will cover work experience, hobbies and interests and school work. You should have a good knowledge of the profession as a whole and what would be expected of you as a veterinary surgeon. We not only assess the breadth of candidates' experience of working with livestock and companion animals, but we also examine personal attributes which demonstrate responsibility, self-motivation, a caring ethos and resilience. We are interested to hear of candidates' special interests, or hobbies, outside veterinary science. You should be aware of any current topical veterinary issues so it is advisable to keep up to date with Media information.
  - o Offers released: Prior to 15 April
  - o Orientation held: late September
  - o Deposit required: Yes
    - If YES, amount: £1,000
  - o Defers granted: Yes
  - o Transfers accepted: No

EVALUATION CRITERIA

*If applicable, please enter percentage weighted
A holistic approach is taken when evaluating applications taking into account the science GPA, cumulative GPA, experiences and leadership. If the application fulfils these requirements candidates are invited to attend an interview where they are assessed on a level playing field.

- Academic History
- Science GPA
- Science pre-requisite GPA
- Cumulative GPA
- GRE Scores
- eLORS
- Experiences
- Leadership Skills
- Personal Essays
- Contribution to diversity
- Non-cognitive skills
- Readiness to matriculate
- Employment history
- Interview
- Other (please list)

ACCEPTANCE DATA (PRIOR YEAR)

- GPA Average and Range
- Average: 3.52
- Range: 3.1 – 3.96
- Number of applications: 973
- Number interviewed: 469
- Number selected: 313
- Number accepted into class: 140
- Number matriculated: 140

TUITION / COST OF ATTENDANCE

*For current year (2020 matriculation)
- Resident (in-State)
  - £9,250/yr
- Non-Resident (out-of-state)
  - Tuition: Tuition fees are updated annually and can be found here
  - https://www.gla.ac.uk/undergraduate/fees/intlfees/#/tuitionfees2019/20 (fees are fixed in UK pounds stering at the point of entry, but please be aware there can be some fluctuation in the exchange rate).

EDUCATION / RESEARCH

- Curriculum Statement
  - The BVMS programme is based on integration of clinical and science subject areas and has a spiral course structure, meaning that you will revisit topics as you progress through the programme, each time with increasing clinical focus. In conjunction, there is a vertical theme of professional and clinical skills development to help you acquire the personal qualities and skills you will need in professional environments. The programme is delivered over five years and is divided into three phases. Foundation phase years 1 and 2, Clinical Phase years 3 and 4 and the Professional Phase year 5.
- Highlights
- Extra Mural Studies
- In common with all veterinary students in the UK you will be required to undertake an additional 38 weeks of extra-mural studies (EMS) during your vacation time. The first period of 12 weeks is dedicated to gaining further experience of the management and handling of domestic animals. After this initial period is completed you start the clinical period of 26 weeks, which can be used to gain experience in veterinary professional environments. Satisfactory completion of EMS is a requirement for graduation.

Q&A

- Top 10 FAQs

Q. Are the tuition fees fixed for the full term of the programme?
A. Yes, tuition fees are fixed in Pounds Sterling at the point of entry however there will be fluctuations in the exchange rate which you must make allowances for.

Q. Can you outline the structure of the curriculum?
A. Information on the course structure can be found at https://www.gla.ac.uk/undergraduate/degrees/veterinarymedicine/#/

Q. What provisions do you have for supporting students with a disability or have additional needs?
A. Students can register with Disability Services to arrange an assessment, and the School will endevour to make reasonable adjustment where possible Full details can be found at https://www.gla.ac.uk/myglasgow/disability/

Q. How does assessment work on the programme?
A. There is limited continual assessment throughout the year and an end of year examination which determines progression to the following year of the programme.

Q. Are international students guaranteed university accommodation?
A. International students are guaranteed accommodation in the first year provided they apply before the August deadline.

Q. Do I need a visa to study in the UK?
A. International students require a Tier 4 Student Visa to study in the UK. Further information can be found at https://www.gla.ac.uk/international/support/

Q. Is there any assistance to prepare for the NAVLE exam?
A. All final year students are given support with preparing for the NAVLE examination. They are given access to a bank of questions called Vet Prep and further guidance is provided by an academic member of staff.

Q. Are pets allowed in University accommodation and how do I go about bringing them to the UK?
A. If you are bringing a pet to the UK you are unable to stay in university accommodation, but help will be given to find private accommodation which accepts pets. Guidance on bringing your pet to the UK can be found here: https://www.gov.uk/take-pet-abroad

Q. What is the cost of living to study in Glasgow?
A. Further information can be found at https://www.gla.ac.uk/international/support/livinginuk/costofliving/

Q. What is the weather like in Glasgow
A. Glasgow enjoys a very stable climate with relatively warm summers and quite mild winters. The temperature in Glasgow is often milder than the rest of Scotland.

Seasons:

The spring months (March to May) are mild and cool. Many of Glasgow's trees and plants begin to flower at this time of the year and parks and gardens are filled with beautiful spring colours.

The summer months (May to September) can vary considerably between mild and wet weather, or warm and sunny. The winds are generally westerly, due to the warm Gulf Stream. The warmest month is usually July, the daily high averaging no more than 20C. (The highest recorded temperature is 31.2C, on the 4th of August 1975.)

Despite some infrequent clear or dry days, winters in Glasgow are normally damp and cold. (The lowest recorded temperature is -17C on the 29th of December 1995). Winds and rainfall are often fairly chilling and strong, like the rest of western Scotland. Severe snowfalls melt within days and rarely lie in the city centre. December, January and February are the wettest months of the year, but can often be sunny and clear.

Glasgow is known with those who have lived there to be able to produce all 4 seasons in one day. So as a general piece of advice, make sure you are suitably equipped with clothing. And when it rains in Glasgow, there is almost always wind to accompany it – umbrellas frequently break.

Course requirements
Applicants are expected to have completed at least 3 years Pre-Veterinary or science courses at College or University, with a minimum of one year in chemistry (including organic chemistry and organic chemistry lab), biology, or biochemistry, and either physics, maths, or statistics.

UNIVERSITY OF GUELPH

Email: vetmed@uoguelph.ca

Website: www.ovc.uoguelph.ca/ recruitment/en /index.asp

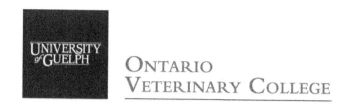

ONTARIO VETERINARY COLLEGE

SCHOOL DESCRIPTION

The Ontario Veterinary College (OVC) at the University of Guelph is a world leader in veterinary health care, learning and research. We work at the intersection of animal, human, and ecosystem health.

Founded in 1862, OVC is the oldest veterinary school in Canada and the United States, and is one of only five veterinary schools across Canada. OVC is located in Ontario, at the University of Guelph, and is a short drive from one of Canada's largest and well-known hubs of activity and culture, Toronto. A drive north takes you to the first of Canada's many popular lakes, known for clear waters and havens of nature.

Academically, OVC is consistently ranked as one of Canada's top universities. In fact, we're renowned worldwide for excellence in teaching, research and service, with graduates of the program practicing veterinary medicine, conducting research or working in related industry across the globe.

With faculty and administration sharing like-minded ideas on furthering animal care, research and innovative teaching methodologies, OVC offers a rich and intense learning environment to students. Our Health Sciences Centre offers both primary care in addition to advanced large and small animal specialty services, intensive care, and oncology. Through the Health Sciences Centre, veterinary student experiential learning can be tailored to meet each person's specific career goals in a student-centered manner.

Researchers at OVC conduct innovative, collaborative research aimed at improving the health and well-being of animals, humans, and ecosystems. This work covers a broad scope of disciplines ranging from basic laboratory investigation, to epidemiological field studies, to applied clinical research on companion and food animals as well as wildlife. More recently, cross-disciplinary research in One Health is a key focus for the College. Research at OVC is performed within a framework of the following guiding principles: Excellence, Uniqueness, Collaboration, Innovation, Communication, and Training.

DVM students can work on summer research projects with OVC faculty and participate in our Summer Career Opportunities and Research Exploration Program.

The OVC is accredited by the American Veterinary Medical Association, giving graduates a broad spectrum of veterinary career opportunities across multiple countries.

PROGRAM DESCRIPTION
- Class Size
  - Canadian Ontario resident #: 105
  - International Seats #: 15
- Applicant Pool (prior year)
  - Resident #: 450
  - International #: 218
- International School: Yes
- Accepts International Applicants: Yes
- VMCAS Participant: Yes

ENTRANCE REQUIREMENTS
- Pre-Requisite Chart Update
  - Date pre-reqs must be completed: August 31st, the year prior to anticipated Fall entry.
  - Pre-requisite required grade: Average 3.2
- VMCAS application: Yes
- Supplemental application: Yes
- Transcript Requirements
  - AP Policy
  - International Transcripts: Yes
- Test Requirements
  - TOEFL Test Deadline: November 1 (for those whose first language is not English)
- Experiences: Veterinary experience may be voluntary or paid, but must be done with a

supervising veterinarian in placements such as clinical practice, research laboratories, animal shelters, animal rehabilitation facilities, public health settings or another related industry where a veterinarian is employed. The aim is to provide the candidate with an understanding of the veterinary profession. It is expected that this category of experience will involve job shadowing/assisting the veterinarian(s) and not just reception or other administrative duties. Although there is no minimum required number of hours needed for application, it is strongly advised that applicants log as many hours as possible.

- Letters of Recommendation (eLOR): It is important that all your referees understand what is required of veterinarians in a Canadian/US context. **Two of your referees must be veterinarians with whom you have obtained veterinary and/or animal experience.** This experience does not have to be clinical. It can include research and working in government or industry sectors. The goal of having the two veterinary references is to allow those already in the profession to assess whether you are a suitable candidate to become a member of the profession. All of your referees have to be qualified to give an unbiased, informed and critical assessment of you as an applicant. They should be individuals who know you in a supervisory or professional context and are able to assess you objectively. None of your referees can be family members, or long standing friends of you or your family, or be employed by you or your family, even if they are veterinarians. Applications from candidates with referee assessments which the Admissions Committee does not consider to be appropriate will not be further considered.
  - Number required: 3
  - Veterinarian Required: Yes, 2.
- Bachelor's degree required: No
- Academic Statement
  - Required minimum average of the last two full time semesters GPA: 3.2 or higher
  - 8 Prerequisite courses average 3.2 or higher
- Interview Required: Yes
  - Type of interview: MMI

ADMISSIONS PROCESS & DEADLINES
- Admissions Process Statement
  - Deadlines:
    - Application Open Date: May
    - Application Deadline Date: September 16
    - Supplemental Open Date: May

- Supplemental Deadline Date: November 1
- Transcripts Received Date: September 16
- eLOR Received Date: September 16
  - Interviews held: February , (International applicants), May (Domestic undergraduate applicants)
    - Interview format: MMI
  - Offers released: By end of February (international)
  - Orientation held: September starting on Labor Day
  - Deposit required: Yes
    - If YES, amount: $500 Canadian Funds
  - Defers granted: With appropriate grounds

EVALUATION CRITERIA
*If applicable, please enter percentage weighted
- Pre-requisite GPA 32.5%
- Last 2 semester GPA 32.5%
- eLors
- Experience
- Leadership
- Personal Essays
- Interview 35%
- Communication Skills

ACCEPTANCE DATA (PRIOR YEAR)
- GPA average was 3.63 and the range was 3.28-4.0
- Number of applications: 218
- Number interviewed: 63
- Number selected: 15
- Number accepted into class: 15
- Number matriculated: 14

TUITION / COST OF ATTENDANCE
*For current year (2020 matriculation)
- Domestic resident (in-Province)
  - Tuition: $10, 271 Canadian Funds per year
  - Fees: $514.35 Canadian Funds per year
- International
  - Tuition: $66,236 Canadian Funds per year
  - Fees: $514.35 Canadian Funds per year

EDUCATION / RESEARCH
- Curriculum Statement
  The Program Learning Outcomes of our DVM curriculum may be found online here and the overview of the four-year program here.

- ○ Phase Learning Outcomes and courses for each year of the program are found online: Phase 1, Phase 2, Phase 3, Phase 4.
- Clinicals begin
  - ○ Student participation in experiential and applied clinical learning starts within the first year, with increasing clinical application as the program progresses. By the end of the third year, all subsequent training is embedded in experiential learning placements or clinical rotations.
  - ○ The Summer Career Opportunities and Research Exploration (CORE) Program is an additional educational program offering summer research placements for students to have the opportunity to experience research, prepare a research poster, visit several research facilities, hear exciting talks, attend round table discussions, and network with DVMs having a variety of career paths.

Q&A

- Top FAQs
- How easy is it to go on to work in the US after graduating from OVC? Since you write the NAVLE and our school is fully accredited, it is quite easy to work in the USA right out of the program.
- Do I need a VISA to study in Canada? Yes, you would need a student VISA. You can apply for this online or apply when crossing the border for your first fall semester.

- To assist you with your transition to living and studying in Canada, we have an International Peer Helper who will connect you with resources and support you as you join the class of 2024.
- Why should I choose the Ontario Veterinary College? The Ontario Veterinary College is a world leader in veterinary health care, learning and research. We are consistently rated highly in world rankings of veterinary programs, have exceptional student retention, and our students' demonstrate a very high success rate in passing the North American Veterinary Licensing Exam (NAVLE). Our international students tell us that they chose OVC because of the warm and supportive atmosphere here. We support our students and maintain a cooperative and caring environment focusing on student wellness and inclusion.
- Where is Guelph, Ontario? The City of Guelph is one of Canada's fastest growing cities, and part of one of Ontario's strongest economic regions, offering easy entry to major Canadian and U.S. markets.
- Surrounded by gently rolling farmland, Guelph is a vibrant, eco-friendly community of 120,000 people and is one of Canada's safest cities. Guelph offers a wonderful lifestyle with quick, 1-hour driving access to Toronto, Canada's biggest and most multicultural city. Guelph is a 90-minute drive to the US border and Buffalo NY, and about 3 hours from Detroit MI.
- http://www.guelph.ca

PREREQUISITES FOR ADMISSION

Course Description	Number of Hours/Credits
Biological Sciences	6
Cell Biology	3
Biochemistry	3
Statistics	3
Genetics	3
Humanities/Social Science*	6

*Consider topics such as ethics, logic, critical thinking, determinants of human behaviour and human social interaction.

PRE-VETERINARY PROFILE: SAMANTHA LARKIN

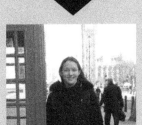

Current School Name
Juniata College

What type of veterinary medicine are you interested in pursuing, and why?
I have a particular interest in wildlife medicine and exotic animals. I have always had a passion for exotics and wildlife, and I think I will enjoy the challenge of working with different animals.

What is/was your major during undergraduate school?
Zoology.

What are your short-term and long-term goals?
I have multiple short-term goals. Since I am a senior in college, the most immediate goals concern the gap year that I plan to take. I am seeking jobs or volunteer opportunities with wildlife for this time. I am also attempting to put together my application for veterinary school. My next goals concern getting into vet school and doing well, and then studying a specialty. My ultimate long-term goal is to dedicate myself to helping endangered species; however, I am very open to the possibility of my goals changing as I learn more and go through veterinary school.

What are you doing as an applicant/pre-vet to prepare for veterinary school?
During college, I have worked to get all the prerequisites, grades, and opportunities to gain hours for my application to be considered. I also researched schools this summer to ensure I had all the prerequisites for the schools to which I may want to apply. I am currently working on putting my application together. I took a class during the fall semester of my senior year that gets the application process started. We are asked to write our personal statement and to outline all of our experiences and explain why they are meaningful to help with our application.

What extracurricular activities are you involved in currently?
I am an officer of the Tri-Beta organization (biology honor society) at my college; a member of concert band; an officer in the equestrian club; a student assistant in Academic Support; and a tutor for chemistry, biostatistics, and vertebrate zoology.

How old were you when you first became interested in being a veterinarian?
I was very young when I found my passion for animals. I love to help people and animals alike, so I have wanted to be a veterinarian for most of my life. I have considered other careers, and during certain times I have been unsure if this was truly the path I wanted to pursue. However, looking into other careers always seemed to solidify my desire to be a veterinarian.

Please describe your various experiences in preparation for applying to veterinary school.
I started working at a horse farm my senior year of high school and I continued to work there the summer I got home from college to gain experience working with animals other than dogs and cats. I also did some limited shadowing over the summer between my freshman and sophomore year of college. My junior year, I shadowed veterinarians one day a week during the fall. I had the opportunity to participate in an EPA program where I worked 20 hours a week in a veterinary practice for four months in London. When I came home, I was able to get a job at a veterinary physical therapy facility for the summer as a veterinary technician.

What characteristics are you looking for in a veterinary school?
I am looking for a school with opportunities to work with various animals in different disciplines. I hope to find one that offers opportunities to work with wildlife and exotic animals in particular. I also hope to attend a school where most of the learning is hands-on.

What advice do you have for other pre-veterinary students?
You should get as much experience as possible, but try to take care of yourself. You should work hard to get the grades and find opportunities to work with animals whenever possible, but also find your interests and follow them. Don't be afraid to try new things. The veterinary field is larger than most people imagine; there are so many specialties to discover and shadow if you look for the opportunities.

MASSEY UNIVERSITY

Email Address: vetschool@massey.ac.nz
Website: www.massey.ac.nz/vetschool

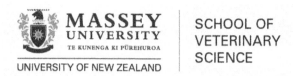

MASSEY UNIVERSITY
TE KUNENGA KI PŪREHUROA
UNIVERSITY OF NEW ZEALAND

SCHOOL OF
VETERINARY
SCIENCE

SCHOOL DESCRIPTION

The Massey University veterinary program was the first veterinary program in the southern hemisphere to gain AVMA accreditation. It has an international reputation for providing an excellent veterinary education with a strong science background, a broad knowledge of companion, equine, and production animal health, and a focus on independent thinking and problem-solving skills. You can be sure that as a Massey graduate you'll be well prepared for your veterinary career. At Massey we believe that veterinary school is a part of your life, not your whole life, and there are a lot of great places to see and experiences to be had while in New Zealand. In a country renowned for an excellent lifestyle, Massey University is a great place to study abroad for your highly ranked, AVMA accredited veterinary degree.

PROGRAM DESCRIPTION

Health & Wellness: All vet students have access to the student health and counselling service as well as staff and senior student mentors. There is also an extensive recreation centre, fitness facilities, sport courts and numerous social and competitive sport leagues.

- Class Size
  - Resident #: 100
  - Non-Resident #: See international
  - International Seats #: 24
- Applicant Pool (prior year)
  - International #: ~100
- International School: Yes
- Accepts International Applicants: Yes
- VMCAS Participant: Yes
  - Applicants may apply through VMCAS or directly to the university online

ENTRANCE REQUIREMENTS

- Pre-Requisite Chart Update
  - Date pre-reqs must be completed: December of year prior to matriculation.
  - Pre-requisite required grade: C
- VMCAS application: Yes (or direct application)
- Supplemental application: Yes
  - Through VMCAS: No
  - External: Yes
- Transcript Requirements
  - AP Policy We do not recognize AP credits directly, but where a US/Canadian tertiary institution has given credit for their courses based on AP courses taken, we will recognize the tertiary institution credit.
  - International Transcripts: from VMCAS (or direct)
  - WES Report Required: Yes
- Test Requirements
  - TOEFL OR IELTS Test Deadline: November 1 (not required of applicants who have completed at least 6 years of secondary or post-secondary education in English. IELTS is our preferred test to TOEFL).
- Experiences
  - Clinical work experience - A minimum of 10 days (80 hours) verified by the veterinarian. eLOR's submitted through VMCAS usually satisfy this requirement.
    - Minimum hours requirements: 80
- Letters of Recommendation (eLOR)
  - Letters Guidance Statement We do not consider letters of recommenda-

tion in our admission process. They will only be considered for verification of clinical work experience hours
- Minimum number required: 0
- Veterinarian Required:
- Bachelor's degree required: No
- Academic Statement
  - Required minimum science GPA: 3.0
- Interview Required: Yes
  - Type of interview: Skype

ADMISSIONS PROCESS & DEADLINES
- Admissions Process Statement
  - Deadlines:
    - Application Open Date
    - Application Deadline Date: September 17 (VMCAS) November 1 (Direct)
    - Supplemental Open Date
    - Supplemental Deadline Date: November 1
    - Transcripts Received Date November 1
    - eLOR Received Date N/A
    - GRE Scores Received Date N/A
  - Interviews held: Dates
    - Applicants will be interviewed online in December of year prior to matriculation.
  - Offers released: After interviews (mid-December to late January)
  - Orientation held: Mid July
  - Deposit required: Yes
    - If YES, amount: $NZ 1,500
  - Defers granted: No
  - Transfers accepted: Yes

EVALUATION CRITERIA
*If applicable, please enter percentage weighted
- Academic History 50%
- Science GPA (Incl. in Academic History)
- eLORS Non-weighted. Used to verify hours only.
- Experiences Non-weighted.
- Non-cognitive skills 50%
- Interview (Incl. in Non-Cognitive skills)
- Other (please list)

ACCEPTANCE DATA (PRIOR YEAR)
- GRE Average and Range N/A
- GPA Average and Range 3.54 (3.20-3.90)
- Number of applications ~100
- Number interviewed (or N/A)
- Number selected 24
- Number accepted into class 24
- Number matriculated 24

TUITION / COST OF ATTENDANCE
*For 2019 (2020 matriculation TBC)
- Resident (New Zealand)
  - Tuition: Subsidized
- Non-Resident (International)
  - Tuition: $NZ 64,040 NZD per year ($NZ 32,020 per semester)*
  - Fees ~ $NZ 1000 per year
  - COA ~ $NZ 15,000 per year (excl. Tuition)

  *Cost in USD will depend on the exchange rate at the time.

EDUCATION / RESEARCH
Special programs / entrance pathways statement
- Combined Programs statement
- Other Academic Programs statement
- Students who aren't selected through the process described above can apply for Group 1 entry (see FAQ on degree structure).
- Curriculum Statement
  - See FAQ section
- Clinicals begin in the final year
  - Students interested in research can apply for summer student research scholarships to complete projects with the vet school staff.
- Highlights
  - Great accreditation and international ranking
  - Safe, first world country
  - Friendly, welcoming faculty and students
  - Federal aid approved institution
  - Convenience of all degree years on the same campus so you don't have to move cities or countries during your degree

Q&A
- Top 10 FAQs

What is your program accreditation? and ranking?
Massey University was the first veterinary program to gain AVMA accreditation in the southern hemisphere, and is also fully accredited by the Australasian Veterinary Board Council (AVBC), the Royal College of Veterinary Surgeons (RCVS) and reciprocally recognized by the South African Veterinary Association (SAVA). So as a Massey veterinary graduate you could work not only in the USA and Canada, but also New Zealand, Australia, the United Kingdom, and many other countries.

What is your program ranking?
The QS ranking is the longest standing ranking system of veterinary programs around the world (including North America). Since it began, Massey has ranked in the top 30 veterinary science programs globally every year, and for the employer ranking has been ranked as high as number 1 in the world.

Where is the Massey University veterinary school?
In Palmerston North, a student-friendly town of ~85,000 in the lower North Island of New Zealand. Palmerston North is a one-hour flight south of Auckland, is close to west coast beaches, and is just under a two-hour drive to the Hawke's Bay wine region, skiing and snowboarding at Mt. Ruapehu and the capital city, Wellington. Nicknamed "student city," Palmerston North offers free bus services for Massey students and has great cafés, restaurants, bars, and outdoor recreational activities.

Will I need a VISA to study in New Zealand?
All non-New Zealand resident students require a student visa to study in New Zealand. As long as you don't have criminal convictions, this is easily obtained following an offer of admission into the vet program. It is a visa requirement that students can demonstrate adequate finances for the duration of their course (e.g. Federal Aid loan approval)

Can I access Federal Aid loans while studying at Massey University?
Yes, Massey University is an approved institution for Federal Aid loan lending.

Why isn't your veterinary degree called a DVM?
In New Zealand, all the professions (Medicine, Law, Dentistry and Vet) are undergraduate programs that can be entered directly out of high school. Our veterinary degree is called a Bachelor of Veterinary Science, but as it is AVMA accredited you can be assured that it is the equivalent of a DVM degree.

What is the structure of the degree?
Our veterinary program is 5 years (10 semesters) in length, split into a one semester "pre-selection" (aka pre-vet) phase, and the "professional" phase (9 semesters). In the pre-vet phase students complete the four pre-requisite classes and develop a GPA for ranking for selection into the professional phase. There are limited places in the professional phase so not everyone who completes the pre-selection phase will be selected. If you're applying through VMCAS you'll be applying for direct entry into the professional phase (we call this Group 2 entry). If you don't meet our minimum requirements for Group 2 or aren't ranked highly enough to be selected, you could attempt the pre-vet semester (called Group 1 entry) to prove your ability for vet school. This is a great option for people who want to get into vet school as soon as possible after high school, or who would like to change careers.

What is the professional phase curriculum like?
You will study core science for veterinarians, normal and then abnormal animal structure and function. Then you'll be taught how to "fix" animals, or return them to normal function through clinical studies, medicine, surgery, and health management of companion and agricultural animal species. The final year is composed almost entirely of clinical rotations.

We aim to increase your learning and understanding by integrating topics within and between years, and introducing problem oriented learning throughout the curriculum. This encourages you to apply the information learned in the various courses to veterinary cases and scenarios designed to develop your problem solving and critical thinking. We also place a substantial emphasis on developing your non-technical skills (e.g. communication) to enhance your future career success.

Does your school do tracking?
Prior to the clinical year, all students complete the same curriculum. In the final year of the degree you would choose a clinical track from the following options: small animal, production animal, equine or mixed animal, or other areas as approved (e.g., wildlife, research). All tracks share a core of 18 weeks of rotations covering multiple species and services. You will then have another ~8-10 weeks prescribed based on your track, and ~8-10 weeks of externships of your choice (within New Zealand or overseas). The semi tracked curriculum allows you to further explore your area of interest while ensuring wide coverage of the main veterinary species.

How do I apply?
You can find more specific information on the Massey University veterinary school website, and can apply directly online from the website, or through VMCAS.

UNIVERSITY OF MELBOURNE

Website: www.fvas.unimelb.edu.au

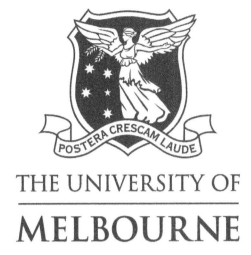

SCHOOL DESCRIPTION

The University of Melbourne has a 150-year history of leadership in research, innovation, teaching and learning. Throughout its history the University of Melbourne has educated some of the world's most eminent scientists and researchers and this tradition continues today. Currently, we are the top ranked university in Australia.

The Melbourne Veterinary School's heritage began in 1886 as the first veterinary college in Australia, and we celebrated our centenary as a Faculty of the University of Melbourne in 2009. In July 2014, through consolidation of university faculties, the new Faculty of Veterinary and Agricultural Sciences was created. The Faculty is now comprised of the Melbourne Veterinary School and the School of Agriculture and Food. Our internationally accredited DVM degree program and our globally respected research and research-training programs are now taught and managed within The Melbourne Veterinary School.

Our veterinary program is delivered across two sites: the city-center Parkville campus and the regional Werribee campus with our clinical teaching facilities. Our veterinary teaching hospital is designed to support top-class veterinary education with modern diagnostic capabilities including endoscopy, CT, MRI, image intensification, scintigraphy, on-site diagnostic pathology laboratories and a 24-hour small animal emergency and critical care unit. The university has recently transformed both campuses by constructing major additions to the veterinary teaching hospital and new state-of-the-art teaching facilities.

The veterinary program provides hands-on experience which includes industry integrated practical learning and clinical externship opportunities. Students gain experience in animal handling, care, and management by undertaking professional work-expe-

rience during and between the academic years. The school has strong programs in specialty disciplines for companion animals, horses, dairy cattle, sheep, and beef cattle. The school also has very strong primary care and emergency practices wherein DVM students gain Day-1 readiness. In addition to their broad-based core training, our students select a track in the third year to supplement their learning in a chosen area of interest. The tracks available are:

- o Production Animals
- o Small Animals
- o Horses

GOVERNMENT, INDUSTRY, AND CONSERVATION HEALTH

Our DVM degree is accredited by the American Veterinary Medical Association (AVMA), by the Royal College of Veterinary Surgeons (UK), and by the Australasian Veterinary Boards Council Inc. These accreditations reflect the high quality and international standing of the course and permits graduates of the course to work as veterinarians in a wide range of countries including North America. Our success has been achieved by insisting on international excellence. Talented people from all over the world come to visit, study and work at the University of Melbourne. At last count, the University's student community of 44,000 included more than 9,800 international students from over 100 countries.

We invite you to join our tradition and discover why staff and students of the highest caliber are attracted to study at the Melbourne Veterinary School.

- Class Size
  - o Resident #: 80
  - o International Seats #: 50
- Applicant Pool (prior year)
  - o Resident #: 373
  - o Non-Resident #: 230

- International School: Yes
- Accepts International Applicants: Yes
- VMCAS Participant: Yes

ENTRANCE REQUIREMENTS
- Pre-Requisite Chart Update
  - Date pre-reqs must be completed
  - Pre-requisite required grade
- VMCAS application: Yes
- Supplemental application: No
- Transcript Requirements
- Test Requirements
  - GRE Test Deadline: N/A
  - TOEFL Test Deadline: According to conditional offer lapse date
  - OTHER Test Deadlines According to conditional offer lapse date
- Experiences
- Bachelor's degree required: Yes
- Academic Statement
  - Required minimum cumulative GPA: 3.2
  - Required Grades
  - Required minimum of last 45
  - Required minimum science GPA
  - Required minimum GRE score
  - Other GPA requirements
- Interview Required: No

ADMISSIONS PROCESS & DEADLINES
- Admissions Process Statement
  - Deadlines:
    - Application Open Date: May 9, 2019
    - Application Deadline Date: September 17
    - Transcripts Received Date: September 17
    - eLOR Received Date: September 17
  - Offers released: On a rolling basis
  - Orientation held: Late February
  - Deposit required: Yes
    - If YES, amount: $10,000
  - Defers granted: No
  - Transfers accepted: No

EVALUATION CRITERIA
*If applicable, please enter percentage weighted
- Science GPA: Yes
- Other: Personal statement score, additional (relevant) study

ACCEPTANCE DATA (PRIOR YEAR)
- GPA Average and Range: 3.2+
- Number of applications: approx. 600
- Number selected: 130

- Number accepted into class: 130
- Number matriculated: 120

TUITION / COST OF ATTENDANCE
*For current year (2020 matriculation)
- Resident (in-State)
  - Tuition: Approx. AU$60,000
  - COA: Free
- Non-Resident (out-of-state)
  - Tuition: Approx. AU$70,000
  - COA: $100

EDUCATION / RESEARCH
- Curriculum Statement
  - Integrated systems-based curriculum in the first 2 years, illustrating the clinical relevance with the use of case-enhanced learning, working through case examples in small groups.
  - DVM3 teaching is based around clinical presentation (e.g. lameness, collapse) and the core curriculum is augmented by the Tracks Program, providing additional practical experience in your area of interest.
  - Lecture-free clinical final year.
- Clinicals begin
  - Research projects are undertaken during the 3rd and 4th years of the DVM.
  - Students are mentored by researchers working in a wide variety of research fields.
- Highlights
  - Extensive brand new state of the art learning and teaching facilities and hospital extension.
  - Veterinary anatomy, physiology, pathology and pharmacology are integrated in a systems-based curriculum in the first 2 years, with the use of case-enhanced learning to illustrate the clinical relevance of each area.
  - The new Tracks program in 3rd year provides additional practical experience in your area of interest.
  - Additional selective clinical rotations also available in final year.

Q&A
- Top 10 FAQs
  - FAQs can be found on our website: https://study.unimelb.edu.au/how-to-apply/dvm-faq

PREREQUISITES FOR ADMISSION
- Entrance to the DVM via the Melbourne Bachelor of Science: North American students

should refer to the University's international prospectus for up to date details about entrance requirements for the Bachelor of Science by visiting www.course search.unimelb.edu.au.

- Entrance to the DVM as a graduate: Applicants will require a science or agricultural science degree from the University of Melbourne or another institution. Examples of appropriate degrees include Bachelor's degrees with majors in: Agriculture, Animal Science, Biochemistry, Biomedicine, Physiology or Zoology. Prerequisites for entry as a graduate are at least one semester of study in each of general or cellular biology and biochemistry as part of a science or agricultural degree.

- Entrance to the DVM as an undergraduate: After completing prerequisite first and second year subjects in the Bachelor of Science, students will be eligible to apply for entry to the Veterinary Bioscience specialization of the Animal Health and Disease major in third year. Students who successfully complete their studies will have guaranteed entry into the DVM, with credit for one year of study, leaving three years of study in the DVM.

- There is no standardized test or interview required.

NATIONAL AUTONOMOUS UNIVERSITY OF MEXICO (UNAM) COLLEGE OF VETERINARY MEDICINE*

Email: lazq@unam.mx
Websites: www.fmvz.unam.mx
escolar.fmvz.unam.mx

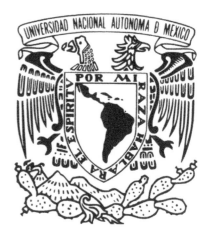

PROGRAM DESCRIPTION
- Accepts International Applicants: Yes
- VMCAS Participant: No
  - If "No", how to apply: Students coming from high schools other than UNAM's own high school system compete for available places through a standardized test administered by UNAM. The test evaluates general abilities and knowledge in all areas, with emphasis on chemistry, biology, mathematics, and Spanish. Students taking the test are assigned to the Veterinary School according to the grade obtained (highest first), until the quota reserved for non-UNAM students is filled.

ENTRANCE REQUIREMENTS
- VMCAS application: No
- Bachelor's degree required: No

ADMISSIONS PROCESS & DEADLINES
- Admissions Process Statement
  - Deadlines:
    - Application Deadline Date: January and April
  - Orientation held: August
  - Deposit required: No
  - Defers granted: Yes

TUITION / COST OF ATTENDANCE
*For current year (2020 matriculation)
- Resident (in-State)
  - Tuition: $500 USD per year
- Non-Resident (out-of-state)
  - Tuition: $500 USD per year

APPLICATION INFORMATION
Undergraduate admission of new students to the National Autonomous University of Mexico (UNAM) is done through the General Administration Scholar Affairs Direction (DGAE).

Students coming from high schools other than UNAM's own high school system compete for available places through a standardized test administered by UNAM. The test evaluates general abilities and knowledge in all areas, with emphasis on chemistry, biology, mathematics, and Spanish. Students taking the test are assigned to the Veterinary School according to the grade obtained (highest first), until the quota reserved for non-UNAM students is filled.

There are two annual applications dates: January and April. Information for specific applications dates can be reviewed at www.escolar.unam.mx (the semester starts in August).

In 2017, a total of 3,281 students applied for 85 places; the score of the accepted students in the standardized test was at least 108 out of 128 points.

VETERINARIAN PROFILE: COREY REGNERUS

YEAR OF GRADUATION
2017

PLACE OF EMPLOYMENT
Ministry for Primary Industries

What is your favorite aspect of being a veterinarian?
The aspect of veterinary science that I love and really thrive on is the license for innovative thinking and problem solving. We are faced every day with a new challenge, or even on old challenge and have the opportunity to really consider it from all angles and develop some life changing opportunities for our patients and their owners. Critical thinking and global assessment are part of the unwritten curriculums at veterinary school, and I personally think they should be very much in the written ones and really driven home.

What type of veterinary medicine do you practice?
I am currently working as a mixed practice veterinarian in New Zealand treating everything from rats and rabbits, cats and dogs, through to dairy cattle, alpacas and llamas!

I will however be leaving clinical practice for the most part and taking a government role at the start of the year. I will be starting at the front line helping with animal welfare and biosecurity at the meat works, but hope to be able to move into management and possibly work towards influencing policy to either help with international trade and the New Zealand economy, or within the animal welfare sphere.

Where did you attend veterinary school?
Massey University in Palmerston North, New Zealand

How long have you been practicing as a veterinarian?
2 months

What advice do you have for those considering a career in veterinary medicine?
Do it! There are a lot of reasons not to do things in the world, and if you think you have a passion for veterinary science and medicine, then do it! You will soon find that there are so many doors that open with a veterinary degree beyond a clinical role that you have probably been imagining since you were just a wee thing. Never close any door or burn any bridges, consider options that at first might not sound appealing as you never know where those paths might lead, and I am sure you will be pleasantly surprised!

What challenges have you faced while practicing veterinary medicine?
While only being a new graduate, I stepped straight into a locum veterinarian at a busy 3 vet practice and have gained a wealth of experience so far. I have had my challenges of missing simple diagnoses, looking for zebras when I should be looking for horses, and being in the position to make the call to euthanise an animal for the first time. They all take their toll, but I have found so much more pleasure than I expected in the client interactions, the relationships that form, and the opportunity to continue to learn every day.

UNIVERSITÉ DE MONTRÉAL*

Email: saefmv@medvet.umontreal.ca
Website: fmv.umontreal.ca/fmv

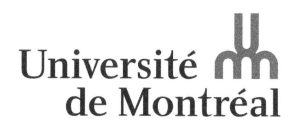

Université
de Montréal

PROGRAM DESCRIPTION
- Class Size
  - Resident #: 45
  - Non-Resident #: 51
- International School: No
- Accepts International Applicants: Yes, only for the second year.
- VMCAS Participant: No
  - If "No", how to apply: Through the Université de Montréal portal.

ENTRANCE REQUIREMENTS
- Pre-Requisite Chart Update
  - Date pre-reqs must be completed: The applicant must have completed all prerequisites at the time of application.
- VMCAS application: No
- Bachelor's degree required: Yes
- Interview Required: Yes

ADMISSIONS PROCESS & DEADLINES
- Admissions Process Statement
  - Deadlines:
    - Application Open Date: November 1
    - Application Deadline Date: January 15
  - Orientation held: Late August
  - Deposit required: Yes
    - If YES, amount: 300$CAN

TUITION / COST OF ATTENDANCE
*For current year (2020 matriculation)
- Resident (in-State)
  - Tuition: $100CAN per Credit
- Non-Resident (out-of-state)
  - Tuition: 300$CAN per credit

APPLICATION INFORMATION
- Applications Available: November 1
- Online: 96,50$CAN
- Application Deadline: January 15
- Residency Implications: Canadian citizenship or permanent residency in Canada is required. A total of 96 students are admitted each year. To be considered for admission, one must: a) meet the above requirements for citizenship, and b) have completed the required studies. Note: All lectures are given in French. Examinations must be written in French.
- The DMV is a 5-year program.
- Condition concerning the knowledge of French: to be admissible, the candidate must demonstrate that he/she has acquired the minimal level of proficiency in French as required by the chosen program, as established by the university. To this end, the candidate must either:
- Succeed the Épreuve Uniforme de Langue et Littérature Française of the ministry of education of Quebec or; obtain a score of at least 785/990 on the international French exam (Test De Français International TFI).
- Performance score: this score is obtained by comparing the student's grade in each course with the class average.
- Course completion deadline: the applicant must have completed all prerequisites at the time of application.
- Additional considerations (in order of importance)
- Academic record
- Admission test

PREREQUISITES FOR ADMISSION

DEC (Diplôme d'Etudes Collégiales) including the following courses:

Course requirements

Physics	101, 201, 301–78
Chemistry	101, 201, 202
Biology	301, 401
Mathematics (including calculus)	103, 203

MURDOCH UNIVERSITY*

Email Address: international@murdoch.edu.au
Website: http://www.murdoch.edu.au/School-of-Veterinary-and
-Life-Sciences

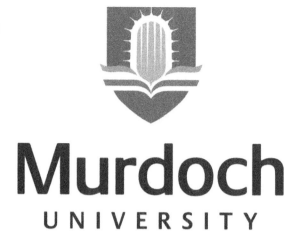

SCHOOL DESCRIPTION

Western Australia is a beautiful part of Australia with a warm, sunny climate. It has some of the world's most precious natural phenomena including Ningaloo Reef and the 350-million-year-old Bungle Bungle Range in the north, and the towering Karri forests of the south west. Perth is a modern, safe cosmopolitan city with a relaxed lifestyle that focuses on the outdoors. There are wineries, beaches, bushland, and unique wildlife within easy reach of the city, and a cosmopolitan mix of cafes, restaurants, pubs and thriving nightlife in the city center.

Murdoch University is a public university based in Perth, with campuses also in Singapore and Dubai. It began operations as the state's second university in 1973, and accepted its first students in 1975. The University is located 15km south of the central business district of Perth, and about 8 kilometers east of the port city of Fremantle. It currently is home to over 22,500 students including approximately 3,000 international students from over 90 countries.

Veterinary students from Murdoch graduate with a double degree (Bachelor of Science [Veterinary Biology] and Doctor of Veterinary Medicine) from a course that takes a total of five years to complete. The course is designed to enable students to acquire the knowledge and skills necessary for the diagnosis, treatment and prevention of disease in pets, farm animals, wildlife and laboratory animals. Veterinary students learn in a practice atmosphere with the final year of study lecture-free and devoted entirely to clinical exposure, including time spent at Perth Zoo.

The Veterinary Biology degree (3 years) encompasses both normal and abnormal aspects of vertebrate structure and function. The first year comprises units which introduce the scientific process, analysis of data and the form and function of the animal body; units in the second year include information on animal development, structure, function and metabolism; and units in the third year cover general aspects of the causes and nature of disease and its control. A further 6 trimesters of study over 2 calendar years leads to a Masters level degree of Doctor of Veterinary Medicine (DVM) which is a registrable veterinary qualification.

Murdoch students have access to excellent facilities, all on the one campus, including a 24-hour emergency clinic, large and small animal practices, an on campus farm and an equine hospital, as well as production animal and equine ambulatory services. The thriving practices have busy caseloads, serviced by many specialist clinicians, so that students can gain extensive experience.

The new BSc/DVM curriculum is designed to keep Murdoch at the forefront of veterinary education. This curriculum allows more time for students to develop areas of special interest through non-core rotations, externships and extramural experience. A Veterinary Professional Life stream is integrated throughout the course to assist students in their transition to future careers in veterinary science and provides a strong focus for developing professional life skills within the veterinary profession.

The veterinary science degree is accredited by the American Veterinary Medical Association (AVMA), the Royal College of Veterinary Surgeons (UK), and the Australian Veterinary Boards Council. Completing your Veterinary Science degree Murdoch saves you years of study, and potentially thousands of dollars; this is because with the correct preparation, the 4 years of veterinary specific tuition can be entered into after only one year of tertiary study in general biological science. Once you have finished your degree at Murdoch, you are eligible to sit your exams with the AVMA just as you would if you completed your studies in North America.

PROGRAM DESCRIPTION

- Class Size
  - Non-Resident #: 45
- International School: Yes
- Accepts International Applicants: Yes
- VMCAS Participant: No
  - If "No", how to apply: Apply directly through Murdoch.

ADMISSIONS PROCESS & DEADLINES

- Admissions Process Statement
  - Deadlines:
    - Application Deadline Date: November 20th
  - Orientation held: Mid-February, late July
  - Deposit required: Yes
    - If YES, amount: $1,000 AUD

TUITION / COST OF ATTENDANCE

- Non-Resident (out-of-state)
  - Tuition: $29,000 AUD progressing to $81,000 AUD

PREREQUISITE COURSE

Currently the prerequisites include units in chemistry, statistics and data analysis, introductory animal anatomy and physiology, cell and molecular biology and vertebrae structure and function, plus a unit that explores the basic building blocks for science students and another that introduces the history and philosophy of science and the interconnected nature of scientific disciplines. A unit covering the principles of livestock science in an Australian context is also a prerequisite. This unit incorporates mandatory components that include animal handling competence of the common farm animals and a farm safety course.

THE UNIVERSITY OF QUEENSLAND

Email Address: enquire@science.uq.edu.au
Website: veterinary-science.uq.edu.au

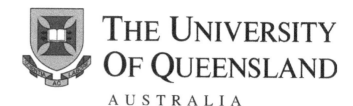

THE UNIVERSITY
OF QUEENSLAND
AUSTRALIA

SCHOOL DESCRIPTION

The veterinary qualification of The University of Queensland (UQ) is accredited with the American Veterinary Medical Association, the Australasian Veterinary Boards Council (Australia and New Zealand), the Royal College of Veterinary Surgeons (United Kingdom), Malaysian Veterinary Council and the South African Veterinary Council.

The School of Veterinary Science's purpose-built facilities are located at UQ's Gatton campus and include Veterinary Teaching Laboratories, the Clinical Studies Centre, and the Veterinary Medical Centre (VMC) with fully equipped Equine and Companion Animal Hospitals, complete with the latest instrumentation for diagnostic imaging and surgical techniques. The VMC has recently commenced an ambulatory service for treatment of production animals on the rural properties surrounding the campus.

The UQ Gatton campus is approximately 40 miles west of Brisbane, the capital city of the state of Queensland in Australia. The campus is easily accessible within one to two hours' drive from the major urban and tourism centres of Brisbane, the Gold Coast and Toowoomba, and has a rural atmosphere with on-campus access to domesticated animals including horses, cattle, pigs, poultry, cats, dogs and wildlife including kangaroos, reptiles and birds.

The School's co-location with the Queensland Animal Science Precinct makes the Gatton campus the most comprehensive animal research and training centre in Australia.

Since its first intake of students in 1936, the UQ School of Veterinary Science has been recognised for a sustained record of excellence in teaching and learning across the veterinary disciplines, and for the quality of its research.

With state-of-the-art facilities, and an ambitious academic recruitment program that has attracted an excellent cohort of staff, the School is at the forefront of veterinary education, supporting UQ's global ranking in the top 100 universities.

The diverse group of academic and clinical staff in the School, including those who have been recognised through nationally accredited awards, have made major contributions to tropical/subtropical animal health and medicine to benefit farm and companion animals, their owners and industry sectors.

The curriculum of the School of Veterinary Sciences is a 10-semester (5-year) program that runs from February to November in the first four years and November to October in the final year. The first year provides core foundational training in biological sciences, with emphases on animal biology, biochemistry, cellular physiology, anatomy and professional studies. In the second and third years, the emphasis becomes the understanding of diseases, and their causation, diagnosis, treatment and prevention. In the fourth year, a strong clinical focus is provided, which is then reinforced in fifth year through 38 weeks of core and elective clinical rotations, both in the Veterinary Medical Centre and off-campus practices.

A strong commitment to research training in veterinary sciences is provided through clinical research electives. The School of Veterinary Science has outstanding teaching and research programs encompassing all aspects of veterinary science, with particular strengths in biosecurity and infectious diseases, genetics, medicine, nutrition, Australian wildlife, farm animal and equine medicine, production and reproduction.

PROGRAM DESCRIPTION

- Class Size
  - Resident #: 90
  - International Seats #: 40
- Applicant Pool (prior year)
  - Resident #: 739
  - Non-Resident #: 212
- International School: Yes

- Accepts International Applicants: Yes
- VMCAS Participant: No
  - If "No", how to apply: Submit your application to the Queensland Tertiary Admissions Centre (QTAC) if you are an international student who is currently:
    - Completing Australian year 12 (either in Australia or offshore), or
    - Studying the International Baccalaureate Diploma in Australia.
  - Apply now to UQ
    - All other international applicants
    - If you're not currently studying Year 12 or the International Baccalaureate (IB) in Australia, submit your application directly to UQ using our online application form or through an approved UQ agent in your country.

ENTRANCE REQUIREMENTS
- Pre-Requisite Chart Update: Queensland Year 12 or equivalent English, Chemistry, and Mathematics B PLUS one of Physics or Biology. Applicants must also complete a situational judgement test. *View the Pre-requisites guide for more information about subject equivalents for interstate high schools, overseas high schools, university subjects and pathways and bridging programs.*
- VMCAS application: No
- Supplemental application: No
- Transcript Requirements
- Test Requirements
  - TOEFL Test Deadline: by application close date
  - OTHER Test Deadlines
    - IELTS
    - Situational Judgement Test (SJT)
- Experiences
- Letters of Recommendation (eLOR)
  - Letters Guidance Statement
    - Veterinarian Required: No
- Bachelor's degree required: No
- Academic Statement
  - Required minimum cumulative GPA
  - Required minimum of last 45
- Interview Required: No

ADMISSIONS PROCESS & DEADLINES
- Admissions Process Statement
  - Deadlines:
    - Application Deadline Date: November 30
  - Orientation held: February
  - Deposit required: Yes
    - If YES, amount: $10,000
  - Defers granted: Yes
  - Transfers accepted: Yes

EVALUATION CRITERIA
*If applicable, please enter percentage weighted
- Academic History
- Science GPA
- Science pre-requisite GPA
- Cumulative GPA
- Last 45 GPA
- GRE Scores
- eLORS
- Experiences
- Leadership Skills
- Personal Essays
- Contribution to diversity
- Non-cognitive skills
- Readiness to matriculate
- Employment history
- Interview
- Other (please list)

ACCEPTANCE DATA (PRIOR YEAR)
- GRE Average and Range
- GPA Average and Range
- Number of applications
- Number interviewed (or N/A)
- Number selected
- Number accepted into class
- Number matriculated

TUITION / COST OF ATTENDANCE
*For current year (2020 matriculation)
- Resident (in-State)
  - $10,581
- Non-Resident (out-of-state)
  - $63,120

EDUCATION / RESEARCH
- Special programs / entrance pathways statement
- Combined Programs statement
- Other Academic Programs statement
  - UQ has introduced a situational judgement test for the Bachelor of Veterinary Science (Honours).
  - The situational judgement test used by UQ is called CASPer, which appli-

cants sit online. You will have to sit the test if you are applying to study the Bachelor of Veterinary Science (Honours) from: 2020 for international students.

○ We recognise that skills and attributes such as resilience, critical thinking and communication are essential for veterinarians, but are not always reflected in academic performance alone.

○ The situational judgement test will be used to select and identify applicants who are best suited to the rigours of veterinary science and the profession.

○ Exact dates are published on the CASPer website, and registration is now open until the day before the scheduled September or October exam date.

○ When taking the CASPer test, you will need access to a computer, internet connection and webcam. Using a tablet to take the test is not recommended.

○ There are no designated testing centres; the test can be completed anywhere that a reliable internet connection is available. System checks and internet connection speed tests are included in the registration process.

○ Find out more about the CASPer test, including:
  ▪ Technical requirements
  ▪ Fees and dates
  ▪ Example questions
  ▪ Results
  ▪ Curriculum Statement
  ▪ Clinicals begin
  ▪ Highlights

PREREQUISITES FOR ADMISSION

To gain entry into The University of Queensland program an international student must have: completed recognised upper secondary or equivalent year 12 studies to the required standard as outlined in the prospectus; satisfied English language requirements and satisfied individual program requirements which include training in English, Mathematics, Chemistry and either Biology or Physics. Applicants must also complete a situational judgement test. Further information about the minimum entry requirements is available on The University of Queensland Future Students website (future-students.uq.edu.au/apply/undergraduate/international/entry-requirements).

Multiple pathways for entry into UQ programs are available for students who do not meet the English language requirements (future-students.uq.edu.au/english-language-pathways).

FOURTH-YEAR PROFILE: MARY RENTFROW

School you are attending
University of Florida

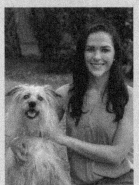

What has been your favorite thing about attending veterinary school so far?
My favorite thing about veterinary school has been collaborating with my peers, residents, and clinicians both in the classroom and on clinics. My class and the faculty are so much like a family that it makes it exciting to be a part of this community. The people have made this experience unforgettable and incredibly rewarding.

What advice do you have for prospective veterinary school applicants?
Get well-rounded experiences with a variety of species and to focus on building meaningful relationships with your mentors during that time. The veterinarians I shadowed or worked with during undergrad wrote my letters of recommendation, presented me with my white coat, and will be part of my graduation. Whenever I have needed any help during school, those doctors have all gone above and beyond to help me succeed. Those relationships may seem like a means to an end now, but the value of solid mentorship throughout your career cannot be understated.

What are your short-term and long-term goals?
My short-term goals are to work in small animal general practice and do relief work with emergency medicine, international wildlife campaigns, and disaster aid when possible. My long-term goals include possibly starting a business within the field or owning a practice.

What extracurricular activities are you involved in during veterinary school?
During veterinary school, I have been a member of a number of clubs and organizations, including SAVMA and the VBMA. I also acted as one of the wet lab coordinators for both surgery club and internal medicine club. Outside of school, I spent a lot of time taking classes at the gym and played intramural beach volleyball.

What was the biggest challenge you faced during veterinary school?
The biggest challenge I faced in veterinary school was trying to prioritize my time. In the beginning, I wanted to be actively involved in every organization on campus while also working part time. I realized I had to prioritize what I was most passionate about to really get the most out of school.

What advice do you have for other students who are currently in veterinary school?
My advice would be to support each other throughout these four years. No one else understands the stress of school better than your classmates. Also, don't spend all of your time studying. It is definitely important and vital to your success, but burnout is a real problem in veterinary medicine. Creating good habits and striving for a healthy work-life balance now will better prepare you to have a sustainable career later in life.

Why do you want to be a veterinarian?
I want to be a veterinarian because I find it both challenging and exciting. Each case requires you to think critically and empathetically. Most importantly, every day you get the chance to save lives and help not only the animals, but also their humans.

What field of veterinary medicine are you interested in pursuing and why?
I am most interested in a career in small animal general practice because I love building lasting relationships with clients and patients. I also enjoy doing a little bit of everything when it comes to medicine, surgery, cardiology, anesthesia, and so forth, and general practice allows me to do that. I have a passion for exotics, as well, and I hope to volunteer abroad in the future.

ROSS UNIVERSITY SCHOOL OF VETERINARY MEDICINE

Email: VetAdmissions@RossU.edu
Website: veterinary.rossu.edu

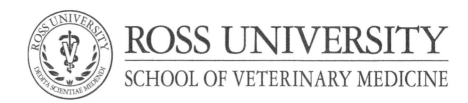

SCHOOL DESCRIPTION

Ross University School of Veterinary Medicine (Ross Vet) prepares its students to become leaders that advance human and animal health through research and learning. Since its founding in 1982, Ross Vet has graduated more than 5,000 veterinarians, many practicing in every US state, in Canada and Puerto Rico, and abroad.

The accelerated Doctor of Veterinary Medicine (DVM) program can be completed in 10 consecutive semesters, which gets you into practice sooner than most other DVM programs. The seven-semester preclinical curriculum takes place on the technologically advanced campus in St. Kitts, where you will be challenged by a broad-based curriculum that integrates unique research opportunities, classroom study and hands-on clinical training. The remaining three semesters, often called your clinical year, is completed with one of our affiliated AVMA-accredited veterinary schools in the US (22 schools) or abroad (9).

Ross Vet operates on rolling admissions and has three semester starts: January, May and September.

Guided by faculty passionate for educating the veterinarians of tomorrow, Ross Vet graduates are eligible to practice veterinary medicine in all 50 states, Canada and Puerto Rico upon completion of their clinical years and passing the requisite licensing requirements. Ross Vet students who are U.S. citizens/permanent residents and meet the Department of Education's qualifying criteria may be eligible for Federal Stafford Loans and Federal Graduate PLUS Loans.

PROGRAM DESCRIPTION

- Class Size
  - Resident #: 121 (Shared with Non-resident; average of 3 semesters)
  - Non-Resident #: 121 (Shared with resident; average of 3 semesters)
- Applicant Pool (prior year)
  - Resident #: 1755 (Shared with Non-Resident; total of 3 semesters)
  - Non-Resident #: 1755 (Shared with Resident; total of 3 semesters
- International School: Yes
- Accepts International Applicants: Yes
- VMCAS Participant: Yes
  - If "No", how to apply: VMCAS Application or directly through Ross Vet

ENTRANCE REQUIREMENTS

- Pre-Requisite Chart Update
  - Date pre-reqs must be completed: Prior to enrollment.
  - Pre-requisite required grade: C
- VMCAS application: Yes
- Supplemental application: No
  - Through VMCAS: No
  - External: No
- Transcript Requirements
  - AP Policy: Must appear on official college transcripts.
  - International Transcripts
  - WES Report Required: Yes
- Experiences
  - Requirements statement
    - Minimum hours requirements: 150
- Letters of Recommendation (eLOR)
  - Your letters of recommendation should speak to your preparedness and motivation to become a veterinarian, your academic ability, and your experience in the veterinary profession. Your letters should include one academic letter from a science professor acquainted with your

academic ability and one professional letter from a veterinarian acquainted with your veterinary experience.
- Minimum number required: 2
- Veterinarian Required: Yes
- Bachelor's degree required: No
- Interview Required: Yes
  - Type of interview: Skype or in-person

ADMISSIONS PROCESS & DEADLINES
- Admissions Process Statement
  - Deadlines:
    - Application Open Date: May 9, 2019
    - Application Deadline Date: September 17, 2019 for VMCAS, Rolling (Ross Vet)
    - Transcripts Received Date: September 17
    - eLOR Received Date: September 17
    - GRE Scores Received Date: September 17
  - Interviews held: Year-round
    - Interview format statement: Skype or in-person
  - Offers released: After interview
  - Orientation held: September, January, or May
  - Deposit required: Yes
    - If YES, amount: $1,000
  - Defers granted: Yes
  - Transfers accepted: Yes

EVALUATION CRITERIA
*If applicable, please enter percentage weighted
- Academic History
- Science GPA
- Science pre-requisite GPA
- Cumulative GPA
- Last 45 GPA
- GRE Scores
- eLORS
- Experiences
- Leadership Skills
- Personal Essays
- Contribution to diversity
- Non-cognitive skills
- Readiness to matriculate
- Employment history
- Interview

ACCEPTANCE DATA (PRIOR YEAR)
- GRE Average: 304*
- GPA Average: 3.30*
- Number of applications: 1755**
- Number interviewed (or N/A): N/A
- Number selected: N/A

- Number accepted into class: 792*
- Number matriculated
- *Acceptance data is for 3 classes: January, May, and September 2018
- **Application data is for VMCAS and internal applications combined

TUITION / COST OF ATTENDANCE
*For current year (2020 matriculation)
- Resident (in-State)
  - Tuition: $20,304/semester (subject to change)
  - Fees: vary by semester
- Non-Resident (out-of-state)
  - Tuition: $20,304/semester (subject to change)
  - Fees: vary by semester

EDUCATION / RESEARCH
- Special programs / entrance pathways statement We offer a one-semester Veterinary Preparatory (Vet Prep) program for students who may benefit from specific courses that will enhance the likelihood of their success in veterinary school.
- Combined Programs statement
  - We offer a MSc by Research degree which can be combined with our DVM degree via our Dual-Degree option.
- Other Academic Programs statement
  - We have articulation agreements with 15 colleges and universities, with the purpose of helping eligible students move seamlessly from their undergraduate studies to veterinary school.
- Curriculum Statement
  - We offer an accelerated curriculum consisting of seven semesters of preclinical course work and training on our campus and three semesters of clinical training, which will be spent at an AVMA-accredited school of veterinary medicine in the US, Canada, Ireland or New Zealand that is affiliated with Ross Vet.
- Clinicals begin
  - Students will be able to start their clinical rotations in January, May or September at one of our 28 AVMA-accredited clinical affiliates in the US, UK, Canada, New Zealand and Ireland.
- Highlights
  - We offer an accelerated curriculum and three start dates (January, May and September) to allow you to start when you want and have the opportunity to potentially begin your career before your peers.

Q&A

- Top 10 FAQs

Where is Ross Vet located?
We're located on the Caribbean island of St. Kitts.

What are the requirements for consideration?
We require a minimum of 48 credits of college work in specific classes/areas, along with 150 hours of veterinary professional experience.

Will I be able to practice in the US upon completion of my degree?
Yes. As with any AVMA-COE accredited program, after completing your clinical training, you'll be eligible to apply and test for licensure to practice veterinary medicine in the US, Canada and internationally.

Does Ross Vet offer postgraduate degrees?
We offer three postgraduate degrees (MSc in One Health, and both MSc and PhD in Research), all of which can be earned alone or the MSc by Research degree can be combined with our DVM degree via our Dual-Degree option.

What is the admissions deadline?
There is no admissions deadline, as we have rolling admissions and three start dates (January, May and September).

Where can I do my clinical year?
We have clinical affiliations with 28 American Veterinary Medical Association (AVMA)-accredited schools in the US, UK, Canada, New Zealand and Ireland.

How much is tuition?
Tuition for our DVM program is $20,304 per semester.

Is financial aid and scholarships available?
Yes. We have numerous options for financing your education, as well as numerous scholarship opportunities.

What does the average Ross Vet applicant look like?
While we take a holistic approach to admissions, getting to know you and your passion, the average applicant has a 3.3 GPA and a 304 GRE.

Does Ross Vet offer online classes?
The online classes we offer are for our postgraduate MSc in One Health Degree. All other preclinical classes take place on our campus in St. Kitts.

PREREQUISITES FOR ADMISSION

Course Requirements	Number of Semester Hours
English	3
Pre-calculus, Calculus, or Statistics	3
Biology with lab	8
Cell Biology or Genetics, lab recommended	3
Organic Chemistry	4
Physics with lab	4
General Chemistry with lab	4
Biochemistry	3
Electives*	9

*One must be either Comparative Anatomy, Medical Terminology, Microbiology, Nutrition, Physiology, Spanish (or other foreign language), Public Speaking, or Introduction to Business.

ROYAL VETERINARY COLLEGE

Email Address: admissions@rvc.ac.uk
Website: www.rvc.ac.uk

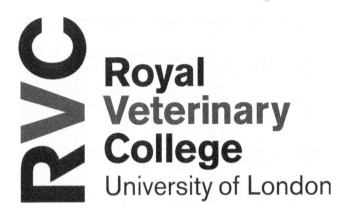

SCHOOL DESCRIPTION

Founded in 1791, the Royal Veterinary College (RVC), University of London, is now ranked as the no. 1 Vet School in the world in the QS World Rankings 2019. Throughout its history the RVC has been at the forefront of teaching, research and practice in biological sciences and veterinary medicine. The College has been behind some of the most important advances in disease control in both human and animal medicine and animal welfare.

We are an international institution, with a worldwide reputation. Our students come from 54 countries, and our staff from 95 countries. We have a successful record of training North American students and can count several hundred American and Canadian graduates as alumni.

RVC lecturers are leading researchers in their field. The College offers exciting research opportunities and provides an unrivalled learning experience to enable students to take their knowledge to the highest level.

The RVC has two campuses, one in London and one on the outskirts of London, in Hertfordshire.

Our London campus is in Camden, one of the most creative and stimulating areas of the city. Famous for its markets, vibrant culture and music venues, Camden is an exciting place to experience student life. It is also home to a beautiful canal and lock, Regent's Park, ZSL London Zoo and the iconic Roundhouse music venue.

Our historic Camden Campus is where Veterinary Medicine (BVetMed) (5 year) students spend their first two years or the first year of the graduate entry Accelerated BVetMed (4 year). Biological students study at the Camden Campus throughout their course.

You will also find on campus an anatomy museum, our first opinion small animal hospital, and the London Bioscience and Innovation Centre, the home of over forty biotechnology and life sciences companies, from small start-ups to established, global players.

The Hawkshead Campus, Hertfordshire is equipped with facilities tailored to deliver both the theoretical and practical elements of your course. It is where veterinary medicine students are based for the final three years of their course, alongside veterinary nursing students and specialists-in-training.

The self-contained Campus houses modern lecture theatres and laboratories, a large library and learning resource centre. There are also a number of specialist centres on campus, including the Centre for Emerging and Endemic Diseases, Structure and Motion Laboratory, Clinical Skills Centre and Clinical Investigations Centre.

You will also find on campus the small animal referrals hospital, one of the largest and most advanced veterinary hospitals in the world treating over 9,000 cases each year, the equine hospital, and Boltons Park Farm, our farm animal teaching facility.

Places in RVC halls of residence are available and students from overseas are guaranteed a place. The College has a number of dedicated staff who provide academic and pastoral support to students throughout the course, and we have an active and welcoming student community.

PROGRAM DESCRIPTION

- Class Size
    - Resident #: tbc
    - Non-Resident #: tbc
    - Contract # and where: tbc
    - International Seats #
- Applicant Pool (prior year)
    - Resident #: 1401
    - Non-Resident #: 611
    - Contract # and where: 12 – Ross University
- International School: Yes
- Accepts International Applicants: Yes
- VMCAS Participant: Yes

ENTRANCE REQUIREMENTS

- Pre-Requisite Chart Update
  - Date pre-reqs must be completed: all required courses should be completed by July of the year of admissions.
  - Pre-requisite required grade: C minimum, though strong grade profile advantageous.
- VMCAS application: Yes
- Supplemental application: Yes
  - Through VMCAS: Yes
  - External: Yes
- Transcript Requirements
  - AP Policy: not applicable for graduate applicants.
  - International Transcripts
  - WES Report Required: No
- Test Requirements
  - TOEFL Test Deadline: 31 July 2020
- Experiences
  - Requirements statement
    - Minimum hours requirements: at least 70 hours of experience in a veterinary setting and at least 70 hours of animal handling experience in the 18 months prior to application.
- Letters of Recommendation (eLOR)
  - Letters Guidance Statement
    - Minimum number required: 2
    - Veterinarian Required: Yes
- Bachelor's degree required: Yes, for 4-year programme
- Academic Statement
  - Required minimum cumulative GPA: 3.4
  - Required Grades
  - Required minimum of last 45
  - Required minimum science GPA
  - Required minimum GRE score: N/A
  - Other GPA requirements
- Interview Required: Yes
  - Type of interview MMI

ADMISSIONS PROCESS & DEADLINES

- Admissions Process Statement
  - Deadlines:
    - Application Open Date: May
    - Application Deadline Date: September 17
    - Supplemental Open Date Early August
    - Supplemental Deadline Date September 17

- Transcripts Received Date: September 17
- eLOR Received Date: September 17
- GRE Scores Received Date: NA
  - Interviews held: November
    - Interview format statement
  - Offers released: January-March
  - Orientation held: September
  - Deposit required: Yes
    - If YES, amount: Given when offered admission.
  - Defers granted: Yes
  - Transfers accepted: No

EVALUATION CRITERIA

*If applicable, please enter percentage weighted

- Academic History
- Science GPA
- Science pre-requisite GPA
- Cumulative GPA
- eLORS
- Experiences
- Leadership Skills
- Non-cognitive skills
- Readiness to matriculate
- Interview
- Other (please list)

ACCEPTANCE DATA (PRIOR YEAR)

- GRE Average and Range NA
- GPA Average and Range 3.38
- Number of applications 2012
- Number interviewed (or N/A) 865
- Number selected
- Number accepted into class
- Number matriculated 250

TUITION / COST OF ATTENDANCE

*For current year (2020 matriculation)
- Resident (in-State)
- Non-Resident (out-of-state)

PREREQUISITE COURSES

Required at upper level (i.e., 300-400 level): At least 8 upper-level semester credits in Biology/Biological Science. Examples include but are not limited to: Immunology, Physiology, Anatomy, Parasitology, Histology. (same as website, minus Micro and Genetics which tend to cause confusion and I'll change in April turnover).

Also required (4 semester credits each): Biochemistry, Physics, Mathematics, Anatomy/Physiology, Organic Chemistry, and Biology.

PRE-VETERINARY PROFILE: CAROLINE OTTO

Current School Name
Rowan University

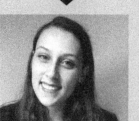

What type of veterinary medicine are you interested in pursuing, and why?
I'm hoping to become a wildlife and conservation or zoo vet after veterinary school. I want to be able to help and give a voice to animals who aren't usually taken care of by most of society.

What is/was your major during undergraduate school?
I am a biological studies major at Rowan University. I am minoring in chemistry and psychology and have concentrations in neuroscience and honors studies.

What are your short-term and long-term goals?
My short-term goal for now is to get into vet school! I'm in the application process and it's been quite a year, but I'm finally close to reaching this goal. As for the long term, I want to work toward opening a veterinary school in New Jersey. Not having an in-state school made the decision to go to vet school really difficult for me, so I'm hoping to help other students in my position so they don't to worry about that.

What are you doing as an applicant/pre-vet to prepare for veterinary school?
The biggest thing I'm doing right now is working as a veterinary technician. This has given me some incredible insight into what daily life is like as a veterinarian and some of the challenges I will face. It has prepared me for what life might be like for me after graduation, and it has confirmed for me that this is truly what I want to do with my life. I've also been volunteering at a charity wildlife refuge for the past year and a half. It's been so fulfilling to get to rehabilitate wildlife and see them released back into the wild.

What extracurricular activities are you involved in currently?
Last year, I started a pre-vet club at Rowan University. I felt like we needed somewhere for pre-vet students to meet one another and help each other out. This year we've had several guest speakers, including some representatives from vet schools, and we have talked about the application process. Next semester, we're hoping to have our first field trip to Cornell's open house and hold mock interviews for students who are interested! I am also President of the Honors Book Group, something that is so much fun for me. I've met so many fun and amazing people who just want to talk about good books with me—it's been a great stress reliever.

How old were you when you first became interested in being a veterinarian?
I think I've always known deep down that I wanted to become a veterinarian or at least work with animals, but it took me a while to really commit to it and realize that the other interests I was pursuing weren't really making me happy. It wasn't until my sophomore year of college that I really committed myself to this path.

Please describe your various experiences in preparation for applying to veterinary school.
I've made spreadsheets to try to analyze what schools I had the best chance of attending, which ones I liked the most, and which might give me the most financial aid. I've completed mock interviews to prepare myself, and I've read everything I could find on how to make myself a stronger candidate. I've also tried to diversify my experience as much as possible to find out what I really want so I can communicate a real understanding of my future career goals during the application and interview process. Oh, and lots of deep breaths and tea!

What characteristics are you looking for in a veterinary school?
First and foremost, I want a school that is trying to foster veterinarians who use medicine to give back. Whether that's through a wildlife hospital, a shelter medicine program, or helping out the local community after a natural disaster, I want to know that my school is working to help people and animals. I also want a really strong sense of community. Veterinary school can and will be very stressful, so I want to feel like my peers and professors want me to succeed and are willing to help me—just like I want to help them.

What advice do you have for other pre-veterinary students?
Work hard! If you really commit to becoming a veterinarian and give it everything you have, there's no reason you can't do it, even if it's not until your third try. I've worked harder for this than I have for anything else in my life, and no matter how long it takes, I know I'm going to get there—and you will too!

UNIVERSITY OF SASKATCHEWAN
WESTERN COLLEGE OF VETERINARY MEDICINE

Email: wcvm.admissions@usask.ca
Website: www.usask.ca/wcvm

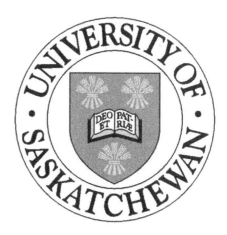

SCHOOL DESCRIPTION

The Western College of Veterinary Medicine is the premier centre of veterinary education, research and expertise in Western Canada and a key member of Canada's veterinary, public health and food safety networks. It is located in the city of Saskatoon, which has a population of about 265,000 and is the major urban center in central Saskatchewan. The city is also the major commercial center for central and northern Saskatchewan and is served by 2 national airlines with direct connections to all major centers in Canada.

The Western College of Veterinary Medicine is one of the few veterinary colleges where all health sciences and agriculture are offered on the same campus. The college is devoted to undergraduate education and has a reputation in Canada and in the northwestern United States for educating veterinarians who are well-rounded in general veterinary medicine and have good practical backgrounds. It has one of the best field-service caseloads in North America.

PROGRAM DESCRIPTION

- Health & Wellness – Student Wellness Centre - https://students.usask.ca/health/centres/wellness-centre.php
- Diversity & Disadvantaged / Accommodations – Access and Equity Services - https://students.usask.ca/health/centres/access-equity-services.php
- Class Size
  - Resident #: 58 – Saskatchewan: 20, British Columbia: 20, Manitoba: 15, Other/Territories (Yukon, Nunavut and Northwest Territories): 1, Education Equity Program: 2
  - Non-Resident #: 5-25 non-contract*
  - Contract # and where: 0
  - International Seats #: 0

* Number dependent upon current negotiations with partner provinces.
- Applicant Pool (prior year)
  - Resident # 433
  - Non-Resident # 0
  - Contract # 0
- International School: No
- Accepts International Applicants: No
- VMCAS Participant: No*

* The WCVM may expand admission for fall 2021 entry to international students.

ENTRANCE REQUIREMENTS

- Pre-Requisite Chart Update
  - Date pre-reqs must be completed: June 30
  - Pre-requisite required grade: Pass/50%
- VMCAS application: No
- Supplemental application: No
  - Through VMCAS: N/A
  - External: N/A
- Transcript Requirements
  - AP Policy: required
  - International Transcripts: N/A
  - WES Report Required: N/A
- Test Requirements
  - GRE Test Deadline: N/A
  - TOEFL Test Deadline: Dec 1
  - OTHER Test Deadlines: N/A
- Experiences
  - Requirements statement
- Letters of Recommendation (eLOR)
  - Letters Guidance Statement
    - Minimum number required: 2
    - Veterinarian Required: Yes
- Bachelor's degree required: No
- Academic Statement

- o Required minimum cumulative GPA: a minimum cumulative average of 75% is required.
- Interview Required: Yes
  - o Type of interview: Panel

ADMISSIONS PROCESS & DEADLINES
- Admissions Process Statement
  - o Deadlines:
    - Application Open Date: mid September
    - Application Deadline Date: December 1
    - Transcripts Received Date: January 31
    - eLOR Received Date: February 15
    - GRE Scores Received Date: N/A
  - o Interviews held: May–June
    - Interview format statement: The structured interview is designed to assess the applicant's ability to cope with the veterinary program and to evaluate non-academic qualities. Applicants attending out-of-province interviews will be charged a $150 fee.
  - o Offers released: on or before July 1
  - o Orientation held: Late August
  - o Deposit required: No
  - o Defers granted: Yes, case-by-case basis for extenuating circumstances.
  - o Transfers accepted: No

EVALUATION CRITERIA
*If applicable, please enter percentage weighted
- Academic History: 60%
- Interview: 40%

ACCEPTANCE DATA (PRIOR YEAR)
- GPA Average and Range: 86.4% (80.3 – 95.0)
- Number of applications: 433
- Number interviewed: 163
- Number selected: 93
- Number accepted into class: 78
- Number matriculated: 78

TUITION / COST OF ATTENDANCE
*For current year (2018 matriculation)
10% increase anticipated for 2019 matriculation
- Resident (in-State)
  - o Tuition: CAN$9,761
  - o Fees: CAN$922
- Non-Resident (Non-Contract) 2019 matriculation first year of non-contract seats.
  - o Tuition: ~$59,761
  - o Fees: ~$922

EDUCATION / RESEARCH
- Special programs / entrance pathways statement
- Combined Programs statement
  - o DVM-MBA (Masters Business Administration)
  - o DVM-MSc, DVM-PhD
- Other Academic Programs statement
- Curriculum Statement
  - o Our curriculum includes refined core courses and a wide range of third-year elective courses that allow students to focus on particular interest areas. It also provides instruction in leadership, communication and practice management to prepare graduates for their future professional careers.
- Clinicals begin
  - o Students gain hands-on experience throughout entire fourth/final year, as well as optional undergraduate summer student research program.
- Highlights
  - o **Veterinary Medical Centre** with new diagnostic complex, including pet radiation therapy centre, an equine performance centre, a fully-equipped medical imaging department and areas for specialized disciplines such as ophthalmology and dentistry.
  - o **WCVM Goodale Research Farm** - 840 hectares has more than 250 head of beef cattle, deer and bison where students learn stress-free livestock handling.
  - o **WCRM Research Wing** has two multi-functional laboratories with state-of-the-art technology in molecular research techniques, cell biology and cryobiology.

PREREQUISITES FOR ADMISSION

Course Description	Number of Hours/Credits	Necessity
English	6	Required
Physics	3	Required
Biology	6	Required
Genetics	3	Required
Introductory Chemistry	6	Required
Organic Chemistry	3	Required
Mathematics or Statistics	6	Required
Biochemistry	3	Required
Microbiology	3	Required
Electives	21	Required

ST. GEORGE'S UNIVERSITY

Website: www.sgu.edu

St. George's University

SCHOOL DESCRIPTION

Having received full accreditation by the AVMA COE in 2011, St. George's University School of Veterinary Medicine has recently been re-accredited by the AVMA through 2025 and is proud of its academic excellence exemplified by its breadth of highly regarded education, unprecedented student support services, and internationally recognized faculty. The core mission of the University is creating excellent academic programs within an international setting where students and faculty are actively recruited from around the world. St. Georges University has drawn faculty and students from over 140 countries, assembling a diverse community of disparate cultural and educational backgrounds.

Located on the southwest corner of the Caribbean island of Grenada, St. George's shoreline location offers its growing student body a serene environment in which to live, learn and create a worldwide network of friends and colleagues. Along with St. George's state-of-the-art facilities, complete with a large animal facility and, marine station, and the SGU Small Animal Clinic, St. George's University School of Veterinary Medicine prepares its students for leadership, life-long success and service in a constantly changing world.

Over 6,000 students from throughout the world are enrolled in the University's School of Medicine, School of Veterinary Medicine, School of Arts and Sciences or graduate programs which include a CEPH-accredited MPH and MBA program. SGU students also benefit from world-renowned international academic partnerships with universities, hospitals and other educational and scientific institutions.

The veterinary medical program is delivered with a number of entry options: the seven-, six- and five-year programs which begin with the preveterinary medical sciences and an option to enter directly into the four-year veterinary medical program. This enables students flexible entry points depending upon their academic backgrounds. Students accepted into the preveterinary medical sciences are placed in the appropriate program option (either the seven-, six- or five-year program track) according to their academic background and are enrolled in the veterinary medical program for five to seven years. Applicants accepted directly into the veterinary medical sciences generally complete the program in four years.

The DVM program is conducted on the University's main campus on the True Blue peninsula of Grenada, West Indies, except for the final year which is the clinical year spent at an affiliated AVMA-accredited School of Veterinary Medicine. These schools are located in the United States, Canada, United Kingdom, Ireland, and Australia.

PROGRAM DESCRIPTION
- International School: Yes
- Accepts International Applicants: Yes
- VMCAS Participant: Yes

ENTRANCE REQUIREMENTS
- Pre-Requisite Chart Update
  - Required courses must be completed prior to enrollment
- VMCAS application: Yes
- Supplemental application: No
- Transcript Requirements: must appear in official college transcript
  - AP Policy
  - International Transcripts: required, if applicable
  - WES Report Required: Yes, if applicable
- Experiences
  - Requirements statement
    - Minimum hours requirements: 500 preferred.

- Letters of Recommendation (eLOR)
  - Letters Guidance Statement: the letters should speak to one's academic ability, sense of community and team work spirit.
    - Minimum number required: 2
    - Veterinarian Required: Yes
- Bachelor's degree required: Yes
- Academic Statement
  - Required minimum cumulative GPA
  - Required grades
  - Required minimum of last 45
  - Required minimum science GPA
  - Required minimum GRE score
  - Other GPA requirements
- Interview Required: Yes

ADMISSIONS PROCESS & DEADLINES
- Admissions Process Statement
  - Deadlines:
    - Application Open Date: May 9, 2019 (VMCAS). Rolling (Non-VMCAS)
    - Application Deadline Date: September 17 (VMCAS) Rolling, April 15 of the current year for the August class, and November 15 of the preceding year for the January class (non-VMCAS).
    - Transcripts Received Date: September 17 (VMCAS) Rolling, April 15 of the current year for the August class, and November 15 of the preceding year for the January class (non-VMCAS).
    - eLOR Received Date: September 17 (VMCAS) Rolling, April 15 of the current year for the August class, and November 15 of the preceding year for the January class (non-VMCAS).
    - GRE Scores Received Date: September 17 (VMCAS) Rolling, April 15 of the current year for the August class, and November 15 of the preceding year for the January class (non-VMCAS).
  - Interviews held: Interviews are conducted on a year-round basis
  - Offers released: After the Interview
  - Orientation held: August or January

EVALUATION CRITERIA
*If applicable, please enter percentage weighted
- Academic History
- Science GPA
- Science pre-requisite GPA
- Cumulative GPA
- Last 45 GPA
- GRE Scores
- eLORS
- Experiences
- Leadership Skills
- Personal Essays
- Contribution to diversity
- Non-cognitive skills
- Readiness to matriculate
- Employment history
- Interview
- Other (please list)

ACCEPTANCE DATA (PRIOR YEAR)
- GRE Average and Range
- GPA Average and Range
- Number of applications
- Number interviewed (or N/A)
- Number selected
- Number accepted into class
- Number matriculated

TUITION / COST OF ATTENDANCE
*For current year (2020 matriculation)
- Resident (in-State)
  - Tuition: $37,898 per year
- Non-Resident (out-of-state)
  - Tuition: $37,898 per year

EDUCATION / RESEARCH
- Special programs / entrance pathways statement
- Combined Programs statement
  - Combined DVM/MPH, MSc, and MBA degree programs are available.
- Curriculum Statement
  - If English is not the principal language, the applicant must have achieved a minimum score of 600 (paper-based), 250 (computer-based), or 100 (internet-based) on the Test of English as a Foreign Language (TOEFL), or a 7.0 overall score on the International English Language Testing System (IELTS).
- Highlights
  - AVMA-Accredited Veterinary Program
  - 95% pass rate on the NAVLE (2017-2018)
  - Extensive Early Hands-On Training
  - On-Campus Small Animal Clinic and Large Animal Facility

- o Dual-Degree Opportunities
- o Student Support Services
- o Global Experience integrating the One Health, One Medicine Philosophy
- o Affiliated with 31 universities for the clinical year of study

ADDITIONAL INFORMATION

Applicants from North America

A completed bachelor's degree from an accredited university is required for direct entry into the four-year veterinary medical program. A candidate may apply before completion of the degree. Under exceptional circumstances a candidate may be considered with 60 undergraduate credit hours.

Applicants from Other Systems of Education

For direct entry into the four-year DVM program, a bachelor's degree with a strong science background is required.

Applicants with passes at the Advanced Level of the General Certificate of Education will be assessed individually and will be considered for appropriate entry into the five-year DVM program. Generally, A Level students with the appropriate courses and grades matriculate into the five-year veterinary medical program.

If English is not the principal language, the applicant must have achieved a score in the Test of English as a Foreign Language (TOEFL) of at least 600 points, 250 points computer-based or 100 points internet-based.

PREREQUISITES FOR ADMISSION

Course Description	Number of Hours/Credits	Necessity
General Biology or Zoology with Lab	8	Required
Inorganic Chemistry (general or Physical) with lab	8	Required
Organic Chemistry with lab	4	Required
Biochemistry	3	Required
Genetics	3	Required
Physics with lab	4	Required
Calculus, Computer Science or Statistics	3	Required
English	3	Required

SYDNEY SCHOOL OF VETERINARY SCIENCE

Email: vet.science@sydney.edu.au
Website: sydney.edu.au/vetscience

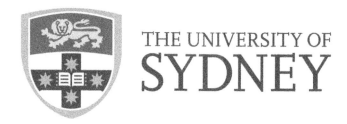

THE UNIVERSITY OF
SYDNEY

SCHOOL INFORMATION

The University of Sydney's School of Veterinary Science was established in 1910 and is the oldest continuing School of its kind in Australia. We are an international leader in veterinary and animal education and ranked as Australia's top university and equal 9th in the world for veterinary science in the latest QS World University Rankings (2019). We received a score of 5/5 from Excellence in Research for Australia (ERA) for veterinary science research. The School delivers inspirational and innovative student-centered teaching emphasizing life-long, evidence-based learning whilst also providing clinical and research excellence through creative, collaborative programs. We maintain teaching hospitals on both the inner-city Camperdown campus and the rural Camden campus, where you will work with veterinarians in a clinical teaching and learning environment. Referral and primary accession cases are seen at both sites. The University Veterinary Teaching Hospital at Camden also provides veterinary services to farms in the region, while the Wildlife Health and Conservation Clinic provides veterinary services to sick and injured Australian native wildlife; reptiles; and avian, aquatic and exotic pets. A wide range of companion animals, farm animals, racing animals, exotic and native species are seen. We have a strong global network of more than 5,000 alumni across the veterinary, agricultural, and public health sectors, including graduates in North America and Canada. Our active student societies, including VetSoc and the Camden Farms Society, ensure a rich and rewarding experience both in and out of the classroom.

PRACTICAL EXPERIENCE

During the inter-semester and intra-semester breaks you will be required to undertake placements for preparatory clinical and animal husbandry experience. The final year is free of lectures, and instead, you will participate in practice-based activities and the management and care of patients.

PROFESSIONAL RECOGNITION

Sydney graduates are immediately eligible for registration for practice with the Veterinary Practitioners Board in each Australian state and territory and are recognized by the Royal College of Veterinary Surgeons in the United Kingdom and the American Veterinary Medical Association.

PROGRAM DESCRIPTION

The Doctor of Veterinary Medicine (DVM) program aims to produce career ready graduates with excellent fundamental knowledge and skills in managing animal health and disease; and in protecting and advancing animal, human and environmental health and welfare locally and globally. Clinical exposure, clinical skills training and animal handling commence in the first semester and continue throughout the course. The program culminates in a lecture-free capstone experience year where you will be placed as an intern in a variety of different veterinary clinics and in a wide range of locations, including rotations in the University Teaching Hospitals at Sydney and Camden and in our Wildlife Health and Conservation Clinic. The program will equip you with the knowledge and skills to choose from many career options as a veterinary professional participating in the care and welfare of animals. Completion of the course will provide you with a wide knowledge of the principles associated with every aspect of health and disease in animals—domestic and wild.

PROGRAM DESCRIPTION

- Class Size
  - Bachelor of Veterinary Biology/DVM:
  - Australian Resident: 40
  - International: 40
  - Doctor of Veterinary Medicine (Graduate entry):
  - Australian Resident: 30
  - International: 30
- Applicant Pool (prior year)
  - Resident #: 145
  - Non-Resident #: 215
  - Contract # and where: 0
- International School: Yes
- Accepts International Applicants: Yes
- VMCAS Participant: Yes (DVM Entry only)
  - If "No", how to apply, or apply direct at: https://sydney.edu.au/vetscience/dvm/entry.shtml
  - BVB/DVM entry, apply direct at: https://sydney.edu.au/courses/courses/uc/bachelor-of-veterinary-biology-and-doctor-of-veterinary-medicine.html

ENTRANCE REQUIREMENTS

- Pre-Requisite Chart Update
  - Date pre-reqs must be completed – by application closing date
- VMCAS application: Yes
- Supplemental application: No
  - Through VMCAS: No
  - External: No
- Transcript Requirements
  - AP Policy
  - International Transcripts
  - WES Report Required: No
- Test Requirements
  - TOEFL Test Deadline: 31/12/2019
  - OTHER Test Deadlines IELTS – 31/12/2019
- Experiences
  - Requirements statement
    - Minimum hours requirements: 28 days
- Letters of Recommendation (eLOR) Not required
- Bachelor's degree required: Yes
- Academic Statement
  - Required minimum cumulative GPA credit average
- Interview Required: No

ADMISSIONS PROCESS & DEADLINES

- Admissions Process Statement
  - Deadlines:
    - Application Open Date: May 9, 2019
    - Application Deadline Date: September 17, 2019
    - Supplemental Open Date: NA
    - Supplemental Deadline Date: NA
    - Transcripts Received Date: September 17, 2019
    - eLOR Received Date: NA
    - GRE Scores Received Date: NA
  - Offers released: Late November
  - Orientation held: February week 3
  - Deposit required: No
  - Defers granted: No
  - Transfers accepted: No

EVALUATION CRITERIA

*If applicable, please enter percentage weighted

- Academic History
- Cumulative GPA
- Experiences
- Leadership Skills
- Personal Essays – Questions listed below only
- Contribution to diversity
- Non-cognitive skills
- Readiness to matriculate
- Employment history

ACCEPTANCE DATA (PRIOR YEAR)

- Number of applications: 360
- Number Selected (assuming from interview): NA
- Number accepted into class: 125
- Number matriculated: 60

TUITION / COST OF ATTENDANCE

*For current year (2020 matriculation)
https://sydney.edu.au/courses/courses/pc/doctor-of-veterinary-medicine.html.

- Resident (in-State)
  - Tuition
    - Indicative Fees: 58,000AUD per year (Domestic Fee Paying Places)
    - Student Contribution Amount for Commonwealth Supported places: 11,000 AUD per year approximately
- Non-Resident (out-of-state)
  - Tuition
    - Indicative Fees: 66,000 AUD per year

EDUCATION / RESEARCH

- Special programs / entrance pathways statement NA
- Combined Programs statement NA
- Other Academic Programs statement NA

- Curriculum Statement
  - The key educational aim is to produce career-ready veterinarians, able to register and work as a veterinary practitioner upon graduation.
  - The pedagogical methods employed in the programme are mixed with a combination of structured learning through lectures, tutorials, practical/laboratory classes as well as independent research and practice-related learning.
  - Learning in core units across the DVM is supported by first-hand experiences in intramural activities and extramural placements, and engagement with authentic scenarios through the School's community-engaged programmes.
  - Case-based approaches are used to enhance your engagement, foster problem-solving skills and skills in evidence-based diagnosis and clinical management.
- Clinicals begin
  - Clinical experience begins in Year 1 of the program and continues throughout the program.
  - Research and inquiry studies occur from Year 1-3 of the program, culminating in an independent research project.
- Highlights
  - Research-driven teaching to ensure you will learn from the latest developments and advances in evidence-based practice, veterinary science research, animal behaviour and welfare science and veterinary public health.
  - Benefit from a fully integrated learning curriculum with clinical exposure, clinical skills training and animal handling commencing in the first semester and throughout the course.
  - One Health framework, ensuring you understand the linkages between veterinary health, human medicine and the environment at local, national and global levels.
  - Capstone experience year with hands-on experience as an intern in veterinary clinics of all varieties and in a wide range of locations, including rotations in the University teaching hospitals at Sydney and Camden.
  - Note: DVM has semester dates that are different to the standard University calendar. Classes commence mid-

February and International students are expected to arrive atleast two weeks prior to commencement of semester. For semester dates, please visit: https://sydney.edu.au/courses/courses/pc/doctor-of-veterinary-medicine.html.

Q&A
- Top 10 FAQs
  - In terms of pre-requisites, what does "one semester of study" mean?
    You must have completed the equivalent of a standard, semester-long unit of study at the University of Sydney i.e. 6 credit points. A full time load for one year at the University of Sydney is 48 credit points. Therefore a 6 credit point unit of study at the University of Sydney is equivalent to 1/8 or 12.5% of a standard full time load for one year (0.125 EFTSL).
  - What documentation about pre-requisites is required?
    As part of your application, you must submit an official academic transcript and a detailed outline for each of the units of study you have completed in fulfilment of the pre-requisite requirements. This documentation must be submitted with your online application or your application will not be assessed.
    The unit of study outlines should come from an official publication of the Provider University, such as the Faculty Handbook. The outline and transcript together must demonstrate that each unit you have completed in fulfilment of the pre-requisites is equivalent to 6 credit points at the University of Sydney and in the correct subject area i.e. 6 credit points of biology, 6 credit points of general chemistry, 6 credit points of organic chemistry and 6 credit points of biochemistry.
  - Where will the DVM be taught?
    Years 1 to 2 will involve learning opportunities at both our inner-city Camperdown campus, and our rural Camden campus. Year 3 is primarily based at our Camden Campus. Fourth year consists of professional placements in the University Veterinary Teaching Hospitals at both campuses, as well as with our Partners in Vet-

erinary Education. The majority of placements are undertaken in New South Wales, however interstate and overseas placements may be arranged for some rotations.

○ How much and what kind of experience is expected when applying for the DVM?

All applicants for the DVM must demonstrate their interest in, and commitment to animal health and welfare and a career in veterinary practice, industry or research on the DVM Admission Statement (supplementary application form). You should provide evidence of this through relevant, documented experience in some or all of the following areas:

- Animal production industries such as sheep, cattle, pigs, goats, horses and poultry.
- Veterinary clinical practices.
- Other relevant animal industry experience including government bodies, charities and research organisations.

To be considered for admission, you must have completed a minimum of 4 weeks of experience, a substantial portion of which must have been completed within the 2 years prior to application (the equivalent of 28 working days). The experience must involve direct contact and hands-on experience with animals. Ideally, some of this experience would be completed in a veterinary practice. Offers will not be made to applicants who have not completed the minimum 28 days of hands-on animal experience and/or exposure to the profession.

Applicants who can demonstrate the following will be highly regarded:

- Breadth of experience across a variety of species or depth of experience in a particular species;
- Research experience involving animals or animal models;
- Longer experiences, spanning several weeks or months;
- Longstanding commitment to/interest in the profession demonstrated by dates of experiences;
- Rural background and any rural experiences (not only those related to animals).

○ Can I apply as a part time student?
No, only full time attendance is available for the DVM

SUPPLEMENTARY QUESTIONS
All applicants must answer the following questions

1. Describe your pursuits and interests and any associated leadership roles you have experienced outside of academia and animal related activities.

2. What are your career aspirations in the veterinary profession and how does that fit with your view of the roles of the veterinarian?

PREREQUISITE COURSES
Applicants must have successfully completed one semester of study in general chemistry (physical and inorganic), organic chemistry, biology and biochemistry at bachelor's degree level to be eligible for entry.

UTRECHT UNIVERSITY

Email: osz.vet@uu.nl
Website: www.uu.nl/en/education/veterinary-education

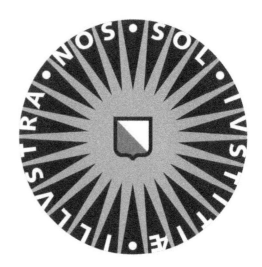

SHORT HISTORY

In 1821 a state veterinary school was founded in Utrecht. Almost a century later, in 1918, the school acquired the status of an institution of higher learning and in 1925 it was incorporated into the State University of Utrecht and thereby became the first and until to date the only Faculty of Veterinary Medicine in the Netherlands. Utrecht University, founded in 1636, is one of the 14 universities in the Netherlands. The faculty of Veterinary Medicine is now one of the 7 faculties of Utrecht University and is located at the Utrecht Science Parc just outside the city of Utrecht. The Faculty of Veterinary Medicine is housed in modern and spacious buildings on a total surface of 60.000 m.

ORGANISATION AND STAFF

The faculty encompasses 8 departments with specialized facilities, a Faculty Office and a number of general services (e.g. learning environment with audio-visual units and the library, pharmacy, experimental farms, museum, student computer rooms etc). Most staff members can communicate well in English and most lecturers have experience in teaching veterinary medicine in the English language.

VETERINARY EDUCATION

Admission of students to the 6-year veterinary training programme (taught in Dutch) is limited to 225 each year, resulting in a total yearly average of 1400 students. The veterinary curriculum leads to the 'dierenarts' degree (Doctor of Veterinary Medicine, DVM). The veterinary curriculum consists of a three-year bachelor and a three-year master program, specializing in either companion animal, equine, and farm animal/veterinary public health. After completion of the study the veterinarian is generally certified according to Dutch and European law. The 1st year of the master programme started in September 2010.

RESEARCH AND POSTGRADUATE EDUCATION

Research at the faculty of Veterinary Medicine is the responsibility of the Institute for Veterinary Research (IVR). Research which is conducted as part of PhD programmes is linked to five interdisciplinary research programmes of the IVR, plus an additional research programme called 'Applied Veterinary Research'. Additionally, all PhD students are participating in Utrecht University's Graduate School of Life Sciences.

QUALITY OF EDUCATION

The faculty of Veterinary Medicine is accredited by the American Veterinary Medical Association (AVMA) and Canadian Veterinary Medical Association (CVMA) since 1973. Furthermore, the faculty is accredited by the European Association of Establishments of Veterinary Education (EAEVE) and the Dutch and Flemish Accreditation Organization (NVAO).

PROGRAM DESCRIPTION

- Class Size
- Applicant Pool (prior year)
- International School: Yes
- Accepts International Applicants: Yes, residence permit required, Dutch language requirement.
- VMCAS Participant: No
    - If "No", how to apply: Apply using http://www.studielink.nl/

ENTRANCE REQUIREMENTS

- Pre-Requisite Chart Update
- VMCAS application: No
- Supplemental application: No
- Transcript Requirements
- Test Requirements
- Experiences
    - Requirements statement

- Letters of Recommendation (eLOR)
    - Letters Guidance Statement
- Academic Statement
    - Required minimum cumulative GPA
    - Required Grades
    - Required minimum of last 45
    - Required minimum science GPA
    - Required minimum GRE score
    - Other GPA requirements

EVALUATION CRITERIA
*If applicable, please enter percentage weighted
- Academic History: 30%
- Science GPA
- Science pre-requisite GPA
- Cumulative GPA
- Last 45 GPA
- GRE Scores
- eLORS
- Experiences
- Leadership Skills
- Personal Essays
- Contribution to diversity
- Non-cognitive skills
- Readiness to matriculate
- Employment history
- Interview
- Other (please list): knowledge test 30%, critical reasoning test 30%, personality questionnaire 10%

ACCEPTANCE DATA (PRIOR YEAR)
- GPA Average and Range
- Number of applications
- Number interviewed (or N/A)
- Number selected
- Number accepted into class

TUITION / COST OF ATTENDANCE
*For current year (2020 matriculation)
- Resident (in-State and EU & Swiss Citizens)
    - Tuition: €2083
- Non-Resident (out-of-state)
    - Tuition: €25.400

EDUCATION / RESEARCH
- Special programs / entrance pathways statement
- Combined Programs statement
- Other Academic Programs statement
- Curriculum Statement
- Clinicals begin
- Highlights

Q&A

INFORMATION ABOUT THE ADMISSION TO THE FACULTY OF VETERINARY MEDICINE FOR INTERNATIONAL STUDENTS
- Special rules apply for the study of Veterinary Medicine. The Dutch Ministry of Education has declared the so-called 'numerus fixes' applicable to the study of Veterinary Medicine. This entails that only 225 students are admitted each year. The number of admission requests largely exceeds the number of allocations. Those restrictions affect both Dutch and international students. The available places are assigned by selection.

NON-DUTCH DIPLOMAS
- Non-Dutch diplomas have to be evaluated and compared with the Dutch equivalent diplomas. This evaluation takes time and can result in the fact that you have to take supplementary exams before being accepted for selection procedure. Information about the evaluation of your diplomas can be obtained at:
- Utrecht University, Admissions Office
- P.O. Box 80 125, 3508 TC Utrecht, the Netherlands
- Phone: +31 30 253 7000
- Visiting Address: Heidelberglaan 6, Utrecht – De Uithof

DUTCH LANGUAGE EXAM
- Prior to admission to the study of Veterinary Medicine - you have to prove your (sufficient) knowledge of the Dutch language. This is a requirement under the Dutch law because the education is in the Dutch language. The owner of a non-Dutch diploma therefore has to pass the exam "Dutch as Second Language program 2" ('Staatsexamen Nederlands als Tweede Taal, programma 2'), or the Certificate of Dutch as a foreign language 'Certificaat Nederlands als Vreemde Taal: 'Profiel Academische Taalvaardigheid' (PAT) or "Profiel Taalvaardigheid Hoger Onderwijs" (PTHO)' before being admitted. More information about language requirements, courses and examinations can be found through http://www.uu.nl/bachelors/en/limited-enrolment-programmes-dutch under Entry requirements.

RESIDENCE PERMIT
- Every international student who wants to receive academic education in the Netherlands needs a residence permit. More information can be obtained at the International Office of Utrecht University.

DOCUMENTATION

- When requesting admission, the following documents have to be sent to the Admissions Office (see above):
  - o Your passport copy
  - o A certified copy of your diploma, OR a certified statement of your school, with the name of the diploma you will obtain and when, and the subjects in which you will be examined
  - o A certified copy of your transcript
  - o Official translations of your diploma and transcript (if documents are not in Dutch, English, French, German or Spanish)
  - o Proof of your proficiency in Dutch
- For further information about the admission to the study of Veterinary Medicine please contact:
  - o Study adviser
  - o Faculty of Veterinary Medicine
  - o Department of Educational and Student Affairs
  - o PO Box 80163, 3508 TD Utrecht, the Netherlands
  - o E-mail: osz.vet@uu.nl

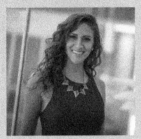

Current School Name
University of Illinois at Urbana-Champaign

Why do you want to be a veterinarian?
I am learning that your DVM degree really opens so many doors for you. I not only want the opportunity to make a difference in people's lives by healing their animals, but I also love the fact that I can be a business owner, active in legislation, involved in public health, and so much more. The possibilities with this degree are endless.

What are your short-term and long-term goals?
In the short term, I desperately want to travel abroad. I've never been out of the country and UIUC Vet Med offers so many learning experiences in other countries.

My long-term goals are always changing. As of now, I think I would like to be a practice owner or possibly a board-certified surgeon. Maybe both—who knows!

What did you do as an applicant to prepare for applying to veterinary school?
I tried to set attainable and reasonable goals for myself with my grades, and I gave everything I had in reaching those goals. I indulged in my other hobbies in extracurricular activities (a cappella was my thing), and I tried to be open-minded to different animal experiences. Say yes to things outside of your comfort zone; for me it was semen collection on the university horse farm. It was scary, but I learned and grew from it!

What advice would you give to applicants or those considering applying to veterinary school?
Your very best is the most you can ask of yourself! If you are giving your 100%, stop stressing about the other details. I spent so much time thinking that my best was not good enough, and the truth is that it will be! Take time to live life, too. Well-roundedness and a healthy outlook on life are just as important as your grades when it comes to being an excellent doctor someday!

What helped make the transition to veterinary school easier for you?
I think having a very strong sense of self, and being comfortable in my strengths and weaknesses, has helped me immensely. I chose to take some time off before entering veterinary school, so I'm slightly older than my classmates. That time off gave me time to establish confidence in myself outside of my academics. In vet school, it's so easy to get down on yourself and start to compare yourself to your classmates. Knowing my strengths and capabilities, and being comfortable in working through my weaknesses, has been such an asset in staying sane and focused.

What is your advice on student debt?
What has helped me is keeping my loan money separate from my own earned money. I keep them in two separate accounts and try to only use my loan money for educational costs and the necessities (rent/groceries). This helps me be mindful of how much "fun money" I'm spending, and it has allowed me to have leftover loan money so I can borrow less the following year!

What are you most excited about learning in veterinary school?
Surgery has always fascinated me! I'm really looking forward to junior surgery and the many opportunities to observe the extraordinary surgeons we have here.

VETAGRO SUP*

Email: international@vetagro-sup.fr
Website: www.vetagro-sup.fr

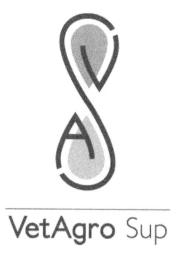

VetAgro Sup

SCHOOL DESCRIPTION

VetAgro Sup was born on January 1, 2010 from the merger of the National Veterinary School of Lyon (the oldest veterinary institution established in the world in 1761), the National School of agricultural engineers in Clermont-Ferrand and the National School of Veterinary Services.

Institute of Higher Education and Research in food, animal health, agricultural sciences and the environment, VetAgro Sup operates on both Auvergne and Rhône-Alpes regions and ranks first of its objectives training of veterinarians and engineers, production of knowledge and support for economic, social and public actors in the areas of food, animal health and welfare, agricultural sciences and the environment. VetAgro Sup trains students around multiple veterinary and agricultural occupations (animal health, public health, protection and animal safety, environmental protection, nutrition and food science, etc.).

This great institution was the first French structure created to train both agricultural engineers and veterinary doctors. This model is consistent with international models (university with two colleges), reinforcing the Structure international readability.

With 1,200 students (700 undergraduate vet students) and 120 faculty members gathered in this adventure, VetAgro Sup proposes a set of high-level training in the field of life, legible and competitive national, European and international. The veterinary teaching program is approved by AVMA and EAEVE.

The veterinary campus Lyon (Marcy l'Etoile) and the Agricultural Campus Clermont (Lempdes) are both valued because they offer recognized frameworks for the development of teaching and research. Benefits and services are available to companies and institutional and professional partners: laboratory analysis, medical devices, advice and expertise. Partner authorities (regions Rhône-Alpes and Auvergne, Lyon and Clermont Community, and departments of the Rhone and Puy-de-Dôme) here find a new link for the development of their competitiveness, their scientific potential and their international attractiveness.

FOR INFORMATION ON APPLYING TO VETAGRO SUP:

VetAgro Sup
College of Veterinary Medicine
1 Avenue Bourgelat
69280 Marcy L'Etoile, FRANCE
Phone: 04 78 87 25 25
Email: international@vetagro-sup.fr
Website: http://www.vetagro-sup.fr

AAVMC AFFILIATE MEMBER
VETERINARY MEDICAL SCHOOLS
Non-COE Accredited

UNIVERSITY OF ADELAIDE

Email: savsadmissions@adelaide.edu.au
Website: sciences.adelaide.edu.au/vethowtoapply

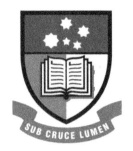

THE UNIVERSITY *of* ADELAIDE

SCHOOL DESCRIPTION

The School of Animal and Veterinary Sciences at the University of Adelaide is located in South Australia. The University of Adelaide is a world-class tertiary education and research institution committed to delivering high-quality and distinct learning, teaching and research experiences. The University was established in 1874 and is consistently ranked in the top 1% of universities worldwide. It is a member of the Group of Eight, a coalition of Australia's foremost research intensive universities. The University constitutes a vibrant and diverse community with over 25,000 students and over 3,500 members of staff across three main campuses (North Terrace, Roseworthy and Waite).

The School of Animal and Veterinary Sciences is based at the Roseworthy Campus, located approximately 30 miles (50 kilometres) north of Adelaide. Australia's first agricultural college was established at Roseworthy, in 1883. Since its establishment, the Australian agricultural industry has recognised Roseworthy Agricultural College as the premier teaching facility for the sector and close partnerships with industry and government research groups have always been a feature of Roseworthy's development. In 1991, the Roseworthy Agricultural College joined forces with the University of Adelaide. The Bachelor of Science (BSc) (Animal Science) has been taught at the campus since 2004 and the veterinary program commenced in 2008.

Roseworthy Campus is located on a 1600 ha property and includes a working farm on which students gain practical experience and training. In addition, our leading-edge Veterinary Health Centre (which includes the Companion Animal Health Centre, Equine Health and Performance Centre, Production Animal Health Centre and Veterinary Diagnostic Laboratories), provides exceptional services to the public and offers students in the Doctor of Veterinary Medicine (DVM) program real-world experience.

The campus is currently home to over 100 staff and approximately 650 students, including undergraduates, and post-graduates in both coursework and higher degree by research (Masters and PhD). The campus is a vibrant and exciting centre for undergraduate teaching, post-graduate training and clinical service and is fast becoming the major animal and veterinary research centre for the State.

PROGRAM OVERVIEW

The veterinary science program at the University of Adelaide is comprised of two degrees: the BSc (Veterinary Bioscience) and the DVM. Students satisfactorily completing the undergraduate degree will gain direct entry into the postgraduate program and completion of both degrees (6 years in total) is required to register as a veterinarian. The veterinary science program at the University of Adelaide has been granted accreditation by the Australasian Veterinary Boards Council (AVBC), the Veterinary Surgeons' Board of Hong Kong, and the Royal College of Veterinary Surgeons (UK). Graduates from this program are eligible for registration as veterinarians in all states and territories of Australia, New Zealand, Hong Kong, Singapore, South Africa and the United Kingdom. The program also has affiliation membership with the Association of American Veterinary Medical Colleges.

- Class Size
  - Resident #: 60
  - International Seats #: 20
- Applicant Pool for entry to Bachelor of Science (Veterinary Bioscience)(prior year)
  - Resident #: 412
- Accepts International Applicants: Yes
- VMCAS Participant: No
  - See: sciences.adelaide.edu.au/vethowtoapply

ENTRANCE REQUIREMENTS
- Pre-Requisite Chart Update
  - Date pre-reqs must be completed: Prerequisite courses must be completed by 31 December.
  - Pre-requisite required grade: Successful completion
- VMCAS application: No
- Supplemental application: Yes - questionnaire
  - Through VMCAS: No
  - External: Yes
- Transcript Requirements
  - International Transcripts - certified
  - WES Report Required: No
- Test Requirements
  - GRE Test Deadline: GRE not required
  - TOEFL Test Deadline: negotiated upon conditional offer
  - OTHER Test Deadlines IELTS: negotiated upon conditional offer
- Experiences
  - Requirements statement
    - Minimum hours requirements: None
- Letters of Recommendation (eLOR): None
- Bachelor's degree required: No for entry to Bachelor of Science (Veterinary Bioscience) degree; yes for direct entry into DVM
- Academic Statement
  - Required minimum cumulative GPA: 5.0 on a 7.0 scale
  - Required minimum ATAR
  - Required minimum of last 45: None
  - Required minimum science GPA: None
  - Other GPA requirement: None
- Interview Required: Yes
  - Type of interview
    - Multi-mini interview (MMI) – resident (domestic)
    - Panel interview - international

ADMISSIONS PROCESS & DEADLINES
- Admissions Process Statement
  - Deadlines:
    - Application Open Date
      - Mid-August - resident (domestic)
      - All year - international
    - Application Deadline Date: September 30
    - Transcripts Received Date: September 30
  - Interviews held
    - Resident (domestic) – late Nov/early Dec
    - International - Dates and times for the interview will be negotiated between the School and the applicant.
  - Offers released
    - Resident (domestic) – January
    - International – minimum of 2 weeks once final academic results have been received and interviews have been conducted.
  - Orientation held: March
  - Deposit required:
    - Resident (Domestic) No
    - International Yes
    - If YES, amount: $14000 - international
  - Defers granted: Yes
  - Transfers accepted: Yes

EVALUATION CRITERIA
*If applicable, please enter percentage weighted
- Cumulative GPA or ATAR – 50% resident (domestic)
- Experiences – Evaluated as part of Questionnaire
- Leadership Skills – Evaluated as part of Questionnaire
- Non-cognitive skills – Evaluated as part of MMI
- Interview
  - 50% resident (domestic)
  - 100% international with minimum GPA met

ACCEPTANCE DATA (PRIOR YEAR)
- Number of applications
  - 412 domestic
  - 95 international
- Number interviewed
  - 210 domestic
  - 40 international
- Number matriculated
  - 66 domestic
  - 17 international

TUITION / COST OF ATTENDANCE
*For current year (2020 matriculation)
- Resident (Domestic)
  - Tuition 10,275 AUD (2019)
- Non-Resident (International)
  - Tuition:
    - $47,000 AUD BSc Veterinary Bioscience
    - $62,000 AUD DVM

EDUCATION / RESEARCH
- Special programs / entrance pathways statement
  - Aboriginal and Torres Strait Islander pathway

- Curriculum Statement
  - The veterinary program at the University of Adelaide is composed of two 3-year degrees: Bachelor of Science (Veterinary Bioscience) and Doctor of Veterinary Medicine. Successful completion of both degrees is required for eligibility for registration as a veterinarian. The curriculum is a predominantly traditional style with blended learning, in the forms of flipped classroom, team-based learning, and problem-based learning, interspersed throughout the program

- Clinicals rotations begin in the final year of the DVM degree
- Highlights
  - Hands on Animal Handling throughout program, beginning in first semester Veterinary Bioscience 1
  - Clinical Research Project course in DVM 1
  - Opportunities for overseas travel to study wildlife medicine and conservation in Africa and business entrepeneurship in the UK

UNIVERSITY OF BRISTOL

Choosebristol-ug@bristol.ac.uk
http://www.bristol.ac.uk/study/undergraduate/2019/vet-science
/bvsc-veterinary-science-accelerated-graduate-ent/

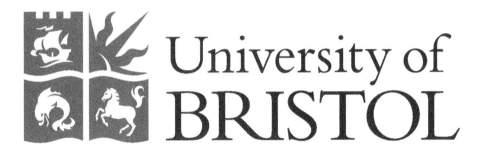

PROGRAM DESCRIPTION
- Health & Wellness / Diversity & Disadvantaged / Accommodations: The University of Bristol is committed to ensuring the health and well-being of its students. Support, both academic and pastoral, is provided at a School, Faculty and University level. Each student is assigned a member of academic staff to act as Personal Tutor and the School's Personal Tutoring System is overseen by the School's Senior Tutor (an MRCVS). Students can also access support through a range of University services including the Student Wellbeing Service, the Residential Life Services, the Student Counselling Service, the International Office, Disability Services, Financial Advice services and the Student Health Service.
- Class Size
  - Resident #: 35 (including non-resident)
- Applicant Pool (prior year)
  - Resident (UK and EU): 236
  - Non-Resident (International): 25
- International School: No
- Accepts International Applicants: Yes
- VMCAS Participant: No
  - Universities and Colleges Admissions Service (UCAS)

ENTRANCE REQUIREMENTS
- Pre-Requisite Chart Update
  - Undergraduate bachelors level degree (First or 2:1 or equivalent) in a relevant science subject. Please see http://www.bristol.ac.uk/study/undergraduate/2019/vet-science/bvsc-veterinary-science-accelerated-graduate-ent/ for detailed entry requirements. Any queries should be directed to Choosebristol-ug@bristol.ac.uk

- VMCAS application: No
- Supplemental application: No
- Transcript Requirements
  - WES Report Required: N/A
- Experiences
  - Requirements statement
    - Minimum 40 hours in veterinary practice and 40 hours in animal-related setting to be completed within 18 months prior to application.
- Letters of Recommendation (eLOR)
  - Applicants can submit one reference via UCAS, which we would normally expect to be an academic reference from a current/previous educational establishment. Full details of suggested content of references can be accessed via the admissions statement which can be found via: http://www.bristol.ac.uk/study/media/undergraduate/admissions-statements/2019/veterinary-science-graduate-entry.pdf
    - Minimum number required: 1
    - Veterinarian Required: No
- Bachelor's degree required: Yes
- Academic Statement
  - Required minimum cumulative GPA 3.2
  - Required minimum science required: N/A
  - Required minimum GRE score: N/A
- Interview Required: Yes

ADMISSIONS PROCESS & DEADLINES
- Admissions Process Statement
  - Deadlines:
    - Application Open Date September 5, 2019
    - Application Deadline Date: October 15, 2019

- Interviews held: Yes
  - Interview format statement: Shortlisted candidates are invited to an assessment day at the Langford Campus which consists of a group exercise, practical task and panel interview. Candidates will also be offered a tour of the Langford campus to see the main clinical and teaching facilities. International applicants have the option of choosing interviews in South East Asia or New York subject to available dates.
- Offers released: From January
- Orientation held: September 2020
- Deposit required: No
- Defers granted: Yes
- Transfers accepted: No

EVALUATION CRITERIA
*If applicable, please enter percentage weighted
- Academic History
- Experiences
- Interview
- Personal and Professional Attributes

ACCEPTANCE DATA (2018 Entry)
- GRE Average and Range
- GPA Average and Range
- Number of applications: 261
- number interviewed tbc
- Number selected: tbc
- Number accepted into class: tbc
- Number matriculated n/a

TUITION / COST OF ATTENDANCE
*For current year (2020 matriculation)
- Resident (Home/EU)
  - Tuition: £9,250
- Non-Resident (International)
  - Tuition: £29,100

EDUCATION / RESEARCH
- Special programs / entrance pathways statement
- Curriculum Statement: The Bristol Graduate Entry BVSc is an accelerated, four-year veterinary degree. The first two years are delivered primarily through case-based, tutor-facilitated teaching and learning. This is a distinctive student-led approach which is complemented by lectures, seminars and practicals. In the bespoke first and second years of the course you will study the integrated structure and function of animals, principles of disease, clinical veterinary science and professional studies. Years three and four will integrate with the final two years of our five-year BVSc Veterinary Science degree, which will further develop your skills in clinical sciences and professional studies. Themes running throughout the course instill the importance of professional skills, animal health and welfare, veterinary public health and evidence based medicine, which underpin all veterinary disciplines.
- Clinicals begin: The final year of the programme is spent on clinical rotations consisting of: 21 weeks of core rotations, which includes on-site clinical rotations and off-site extra-mural placements; 3 weeks of track (student-selected) rotations; and a 4-week elective period.
- Highlights: The University of Bristol is one of the UK's top ten Universities (QS World University Rankings 2019) and Bristol was ranked 11th on National Geographic's Cool List 2018. Bristol Vet School carries out world-class research and was the top for student satisfaction across the UK's BVSc courses (2015 National Student Survey). The Vet School has excellent clinical facilities, including first opinion practices and state-of-the-art referral hospitals. You will be taught by subject specialists committed to supporting student learning.

Q&A
- Top FAQs

Where will I be taught?
BVSc Accelerated Graduate Entry Programme students study at the Langford campus for the duration of their degree. Bristol Veterinary School at Langford is a rural campus that boasts first-class clinical facilities alongside farm animal, small animal and equine practices on-site, allowing you to gain experience of working on first opinion cases on farms and in clinics.

How far apart are the two campuses and is there a bus?
The Bristol city campus and the Langford campus based in the Somerset countryside are 14 miles apart. Free bus transport is provided between the campuses.

What is EMS?
Extra mural studies (EMS) is the mandatory work experience that is undertaken by all veterinary students studying in the UK. Requirements are set out by the Royal College of Veterinary Surgeons (the UK accreditation and registration body) and

students can only graduate with a veterinary degree having completed 38 weeks in total. Requirements comprise 12 weeks of preclinical EMS (in animal establishments) and 26 weeks clinical EMS.

Can I do EMS abroad?
Yes. A proportion of your EMS can be carried out abroad and guidance is provided by our dedicated EMS team.

When do I get hands on contact with animals?
Right from the start of the course. We teach practical pre-clinical and clinical skills using a combination of both live animals and models (including a haptic cow) to give you the best opportunities to develop your practical skills.

I have a medical condition or a specific learning difficulty, can I study on the veterinary program?
All offers are subject to satisfactory occupational health clearance. Applicants with a medical condition are advised to contact the university for advice prior to applying. The veterinary program can be physically demanding and requires contact with all domestic species. Approximately 10% of the students have a specific learning disability (e.g. dyslexia) and accommodations can be made (e.g. extra time in written exams)

What research can I get involved with on the program?
Summer research studentships are available and can be counted towards the mandatory work experience (EMS) undertaken on the program.

How easy is it to find accommodation?
The university offers accommodation at both campuses which you can apply for. After first year most students live in private rented accommodation in either Bristol or Langford and the surrounding villages. For more information please visit http://www.bristol.ac.uk/accommodation/

Where is Bristol in the UK and how far is it from London?
Bristol is in the South West of the UK and is 2 hours from London by train (from Bristol Temple Meads station to London Paddington station). There is an international airport in Bristol and easy access to some London airports using airport buses.

CENTRAL LUZON STATE UNIVERSITY*

Email Address: clsu@clsu.edu.ph
Website: clsucvsm.edu.ph

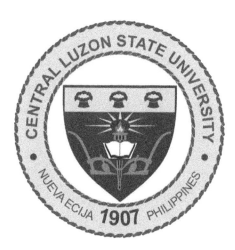

SCHOOL DESCRIPTION

Central Luzon State University (CLSU) is located on a 658-hectare sprawling main campus in the Science City of Muñoz, which is located 150 kilometers north of Manila. It also has a more than 1000-hectare site for ranch type buffalo production and forestry development up the hills of Carranglan town, in northern Nueva Ecija, 40 kilometers away from the main campus. The University is the lead agency of the Muñoz Science Community and the seat of the Regional Research and Development Center in Central Luzon. To date, CLSU is one of the premier institutions of agriculture in Southeast Asia known for its breakthrough researches in aquaculture (pioneer in the sex reversal of Tilapia), ruminants, crops, orchard, and water management researches.

The College of Veterinary Science and Medicine (CVSM) was established in 1978 through Republic Act No. 4067 enacted into law by Congress in 1964. Subsequently, CVSM offered the first ladderized veterinary curriculum in the Philippines: Bachelor of Science in Animal Husbandry (first 4 years) and Doctor of Veterinary Medicine (6 years). This was designed to produce veterinarians adept not only in disease control and prevention but in animal production as well. For many years, DVM graduates from CVSM have consistently topped the Veterinary Licensure Examinations in the country. This excellent performance has made the Philippine Commission on Higher Education (CHED) and the Professional Regulation Commission (PRC) to recognize the CVSM as one of the Top Performing Veterinary Colleges in the country. In 2009, CHED awarded the college the title, Center of Excellence in Veterinary Medicine.

PROGRAM DESCRIPTION
- International School: Yes
- Accepts International Applicants: Yes
- VMCAS Participant: No

ENTRANCE REQUIREMENTS
- Letters of Recommendation (eLOR)
  - Letters Guidance Statement
    - Minimum number required: 2
    - Veterinarian Required: No
- Bachelor's degree required: No
- Academic Statement
  - Required minimum cumulative GPA: 2.25 (Undergraduate), 2.0 (Graduate)

ADMISSIONS PROCESS & DEADLINES
- Admissions Process Statement
  - Deadlines:
    - Application Deadline Date: Last week of April
    - Transcripts Received Date: Last week of April
    - eLOR Received Date: Last week of April
  - Transfers accepted: Yes

TUITION / COST OF ATTENDANCE
*For current year (2020 matriculation)
- Resident (in-State)
  - Tuition: Php 7,000.00 per semester
- Non-Resident (out-of-state)
  - Tuition: Php 12,000.00 per semester

APPLICATION INFORMATION
The following are the admission requirements for both undergraduate and graduate programs:

UNDERGRADUATE PROGRAM

- Must have a GPA of 2.25 or better. Second courser must have at least 2.50 or better.
- Must have taken a minimum of 40 units of general education courses.
- Must not have a grade of "5".
- Grades of "4" or "INC" must be removed or completed upon filing of application.
- Must qualify in the online exam and panel interview conducted by the college admission committee.
- Submission of duly accomplished application form with:
    - A. four (4) 2x2 pictures (studio taken only)
    - B. certification of grades (1st and 2nd semester)

For Transferees

- Applicants must meet all the prescribed admission requirements of the University/College and the course applied for:
    a. Must qualify in the University/College Admission Test
    b. Must have complete and valid credentials
    (a) Copy of birth certificate
    (b) Two 2"x2" colored ID pictures
    (c) Certificate of completion of a secondary curriculum
    (d) Original transcript of records
    (e) Personal history statement
    (f) Affidavit of support
    (g) Alien certificate of registration (ACR)
    (h) Student visa
    (i) Certificate of Proficiency in English issued by the CLSU Department of English and Humanities for a fee, for students who come from coun tries where English is not the medium of instruction
    (j) Security clearance from his/her embassy
    c. Must pay a non-refundable application fee
    d. Must qualify in the physical or health examination conducted by the University physician
    e. Must present an approved application for admission
    f. Others as prescribed by the concerned College
- Applicants must meet all the prescribed requirements by the Department of Foreign Affairs and the BID.
- A foreign student may be admitted based on availability of slot in the course applied for.
- He or she must pledge to abide by and comply with the rules and regulations of the University/College.

GRADUATE PROGRAM

A DVM degree or its equivalent from a recognized institution is a requirement along with the submission of the following:

- Duly accomplished application form
- Original or authenticated transcript of records showing a grade point average (GPA) of at least 2.0 or its equivalent.
- Applicants with GPA below 2.0 may be admitted on a probationary status if recommended by the department chair and approved by the dean after thorough review of the applicant's qualification to do graduate work.
- Two letters of recommendation from former professors in the undergraduate course.

CHINA

CITY UNIVERSITY OF HONG KONG

Email cvmls.go@cityu.edu.hk
Website https://www.cityu.edu.hk/cvmls

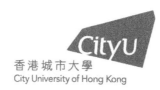

香港城市大學
City University of Hong Kong

College of Veterinary Medicine and Life Sciences
in collaboration with Cornell University

PROGRAM DESCRIPTION
- Class Size
  - Resident #: 29
  - Non-Resident #: 8
  - International Seats #: included with Non-Resident
- Applicant Pool (prior year)
  - Resident #: 255
  - Non-Resident #: 74
- International School: Yes
- Accepts International Applicants: Yes
- VMCAS Participant: No
  - If "No", how to apply: Joint University Programmes Admissions System (JUPAS) or Direct Application

ENTRANCE REQUIREMENTS
- Pre-Requisite Chart Update
  - Date pre-reqs must be completed: required courses should be completed prior to admission in the fall
  - Pre-requisite required grade
- VMCAS application: No
- Supplemental application: No
- Transcript Requirements
  - International Transcripts: Yes
  - WES Report Required: No
- Test Requirements
  - TOEFL Test Deadline: 600 (paper-based test) or 100 (Internet-based test)
  - OTHER Test Deadlines: IELTS overall band score of 7 and 7 in each category
- Experiences
  - Requirements statement
- Letters of Recommendation (eLOR)
  - Letters Guidance Statement

- Bachelor's degree required: No
- Academic Statement
  - JUPAS (Chinese L3; English L5; Mathematics L3; Liberal Studies L2; Chemistry L3; Biology L3)
  - IB Diploma (HL/SL English; HL/SL Mathematics; HL Chemistry; HL/SL Biology)
  - GCE – AL/IAL (English Language/ English Literature; Mathematics; Chemistry; Biology)
- Interview Required: Yes
  - Type of interview: Face-to-face or video conference

ADMISSIONS PROCESS & DEADLINES
- Admissions Process Statement
  - Deadlines:
    - Application Open Date: September
    - Application Deadline Date: JUPAS: 5 December; Direct application: 3 January
    - Transcripts Received Date: Before application deadline
  - Interviews held: Early March & Mid-July
    - Interview format statement
  - Offers released: JUPAS – 5 August; Direct application: March to July
  - Orientation held: End August
  - Deposit required: Yes
    - If YES, amount: HK$10,000
  - Defers granted: No
  - Transfers accepted: Yes

EVALUATION CRITERIA
*If applicable, please enter percentage weighted
- Academic History
- Science GPA

206

- Science pre-requisite GPA
- Cumulative GPA
- Last 45 GPA
- GRE Scores
- eLORS
- Experiences
- Leadership Skills
- Personal Essays
- Contribution to diversity
- Non-cognitive skills
- Readiness to matriculate
- Employment history
- Interview
- Other (please list)

ACCEPTANCE DATA (PRIOR YEAR)
- GRE Average and Range: N/A
- GPA Average and Range: N/A
- Number of applications: 255
- Number interviewed: 62
- Number selected: 40
- Number accepted into class: 17
- Number matriculated: 17

TUITION / COST OF ATTENDANCE
*For current year (2020 matriculation)
- Resident (in-State)
  - Tuition HK$42,100
- Non-Resident (out-of-state)
  - Tuition HK$140,000

EDUCATION / RESEARCH
- Special programs / entrance pathways statement
- Combined Programs statement
- Other Academic Programs statement
- Curriculum Statement
  - The CityU BVM curriculum was designed with five objectives:
    - To include the curriculum of the four-year Cornell University veterinary medicine programme
    - To include the pre-requisites of the Cornell veterinary medicine programme

- To meet the accreditation standards set by the Australasian Veterinary Boards Council
- To meet the CityU's Gateway Education requirements
- To include courses of particular relevance in East, Southeast, and South Asia and arranged in themes:
  - Animal Welfare
  - Aquatic Animal Health
  - Emerging Infectious Diseases
  - Food Safety
- Clinicals begin
- Highlights
  - The Jockey Club College of Veterinary Medicine and Life Sciences offers the first veterinary programme in Asia modelled on DVM lines that aspires to international programme accreditation, with a vision to raise the standard of animal health care and the teaching of the veterinary discipline in the region. The goal is "to be the premier provider of comprehensive, evidence-based veterinary training, research and service in Asia, with particular emphasis on Emerging Infectious Diseases, Food Safety, Animal Welfare and Aquatic Animal Health."

Q&A
1. What are the general qualities/ academic competence we are looking for?
2. Can I specialize in one type of animal if I am enrolled to the BVM programme?
3. Are there any internship opportunities available for the students admitted to Bachelor of Veterinary Medicine programme?
4. Is the Bachelor of Veterinary Medicine programme an internationally accredited programme?

PRE-VETERINARY PROFILE: EMMA WALSH

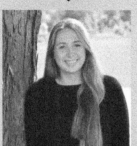

Current School Name
Hamilton College

What type of veterinary medicine are you interested in pursuing, and why?
I am interested in becoming a general practitioner at a small animal clinic or dealing with exotic animals. These interests are inspired by my dealings with animals throughout life.

What is/was your major during undergraduate school?
My intended major is biology with a minor in philosophy.

What are your short-term and long-term goals?
Short-term, I would like to gain as much veterinary experience as I can, especially with large animals outside clinics. Long-term, I would love to someday work in a shelter, helping make dogs, cats, and other species more adoptable.

What are you doing as an applicant/pre-vet to prepare for veterinary school?
To prepare for veterinary school I am gaining as much experience as I can with animals, especially observing surgeries in clinics.

What extracurricular activities are you involved in currently?
Currently I am involved in the Hunt and Dressage Club, Vegan Club, the Pre-Health Club, and 4-H. I also recently started shadowing at a local clinic.

How old were you when you first became interested in being a veterinarian?
I don't remember my exact age, but I was always fascinated with animals, and when I realized that helping them was a viable career option, I decided that was what I wanted to do.

Please describe your various experiences in preparation for applying to veterinary school.
Though I am still very early in the process, I have found that taking as many science courses as possible is a wise course of action. Seeking advice from any veterinarians is also very helpful.

What characteristics are you looking for in a veterinary school?
In a veterinary school I am looking for a willingness to work closely with students, opportunities for research that I find interesting, a focus on the animals, and a chance to study abroad.

What advice do you have for other pre-veterinary students?
I would advise getting as much experience as possible as soon as possible and devoting a lot of time to schoolwork. I would also suggest balancing pre-vet requirements with exploratory classes in completely unrelated subjects and doing any extracurricular activities that you find interesting, not just those that relate to veterinary medicine.

SEOUL NATIONAL UNIVERSITY*

Email Address: snuadmit@snu.ac.kr
Website: en.snu.ac.kr/apply/info

서 울 대 학 교
SEOUL NATIONAL UNIVERSITY

SCHOOL DESCRIPTION

Seoul National University honors the ideals of liberal education and aims to teach students a lifelong love of learning that will form the basis for continuous personal growth.

At the same time it is committed to preparing students to work and live in an increasingly competitive global environment. As South Korea's first national university, Seoul National University has a tradition of standing up for democracy and peace on the Korean peninsula.

Graduates have long served as public servants in key positions of the Korean government. In teaching, research, and public service, Seoul National University continues to set the standard of excellence.

The mission of Seoul National University in the twenty-first century is to create a vibrant intellectual community where students and scholars join together in building the future. As Korea's leading research university, Seoul National University is committed to diversifying its student body and faculty, fostering global exchange, and promoting path-breaking research in all fields of knowledge.

PROGRAM DESCRIPTION

- International School: Yes
- Accepts International Applicants: Yes
- VMCAS Participant: No
  - If "No", how to apply: http://en.snu.ac.kr/apply/info

ENTRANCE REQUIREMENTS

- VMCAS application: No
- Supplemental application: No
- Letters of Recommendation (eLOR)

  - Letters Guidance Statement
    - Minimum number required: 2
    - Veterinarian Required: No
- Bachelor's degree required: Yes
- Interview Required: No

ADMISSIONS PROCESS & DEADLINES

- Admissions Process Statement
  - Deadlines:
    - Application Open Date: February 18 (Korea Standard Time)
    - Application Deadline Date: March 7 (Korea Standard Time)
    - Transcripts Received Date: March 8 (Korea Standard Time)
    - eLOR Received Date: March 8 (Korea Standard Time)
  - Offers released: June 7
  - Orientation held: Late August

TUITION / COST OF ATTENDANCE

- Non-Resident (out-of-state)
  - Tuition: KRW 5,789,000

PERFORMANCE TEST

International admission type II (Undergraduate) applicant who received the entire education abroad applying for the following programs: Fine Arts, Music, or Physical Education, may be subject to a performance test.

*In such a case, the corresponding College/Department will individually notify the applicants for further details.

ST. MATTHEW'S UNIVERSITY

Email Address: admissions@stmatthews.edu
Website: www.stmatthews.edu

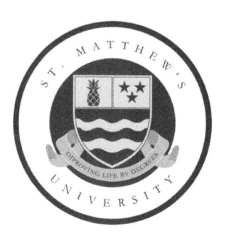

SCHOOL DESCRIPTION

St. Matthew's University School of Veterinary Medicine is located on beautiful Grand Cayman in the Caribbean. Grand Cayman is the fifth largest financial district in the world and has a highly developed infrastructure which is very comparable to the United States. It is also one of the safest islands in the Caribbean, boasting one of the lowest crime and poverty rates. Grand Cayman has hundreds of restaurants, numerous U.S.-style supermarkets, movie theaters, world-class hotels, and many opportunities for boating, diving, horseback riding, and other recreation. The island is less than an hour's flight from Miami, and also has direct flights from Atlanta, Chicago, Charlotte, Denver, Houston, New York, Tampa, Toronto, Washington D.C., and other locations.

At SMU, we are as committed to your dreams as you are. Throughout your ten semesters with us, we will do everything we can to ensure your success by supporting all aspects of your education and life, including:

Focus on Teaching: Dedicated, talented faculty whose time commitments are focused on teaching and mentoring.

Student Mentors: Student mentors understand about adjusting to life in veterinary school, and are eager to see you succeed.

Very Low Student to Faculty Ratio: With a student to faculty ratio of less than four to one, you will have an unprecedented level of faculty support and attention. We limit each incoming cohort of students to a maximum of 20.

Best Value: Most affordable tuition of any Caribbean veterinary school.

Graduate in 3+ Years: Complete your pre-clinical education on Grand Cayman in just 28 months, and then return to the U.S. or Canada for clinical training, with the ability to complete vet school in just over three years.

SMU's modern, state-of-the-art main campus is located across the street from beautiful Seven Mile Beach, and boasts wireless technology throughout the bright, air-conditioned classrooms, labs, library, and student lounges. SMU also has a Clinical Teaching Facility which hosts surgery, medicine and clinical skills training as well as anatomy and pathology laboratories. Students have the opportunity to travel to local farms with veterinary staff from the Cayman Department of Agriculture. Our students spend seven (7) semesters on Grand Cayman and their final months in clinical programs at one of our many AVMA-accredited Clinical Program Affiliate Schools in the United States and Canada.

There are significant opportunities for students to gain experience with exotic species through our collaborations with the Cayman Turtle Farm, Central Caribbean Marine Institute, Dolphin Discovery, the Blue Iguana Project, and the Marine Research Program.

PROGRAM DESCRIPTION

- Class Size
  - Resident #: 0
  - Non-Resident #: 20
  - Contract # and where: 0
- International School: Yes
- Accepts International Applicants: Yes
- VMCAS Participant: No
  - If "No", how to apply: https://applications.stmatthews.edu/

ENTRANCE REQUIREMENTS

- Pre-Requisite Chart Update
  - Date pre-reqs must be completed
  - Pre-requisite required grade
- VMCAS application: No
- Supplemental application: No

- Transcript Requirements
  - AP Policy
  - International Transcripts
- Test Requirements
  - GRE Test Deadline: None
  - TOEFL Test Deadline: None
  - OTHER Test Deadlines
- Experiences
  - Requirements statement
    - Minimum hours requirements
- Letters of Recommendation (eLOR)
  - Letters Guidance Statement: Ask for recommendations from individuals who can give a concise and thorough assessment of your personality, industry, reliability and motivation. Applicants are given the option of signing a waiver regarding the confidentiality of these letters.
    - Minimum number required: 2
    - Veterinarian Required: No
- Bachelor's degree required: No
- Academic Statement
  - Required minimum cumulative GPA
  - Required Grades
  - Required minimum of last 45
  - Required minimum science GPA
  - Required minimum GRE score
  - Other GPA requirements
- Interview Required: Yes
  - Type of interview: videoconference or in-person

ADMISSIONS PROCESS & DEADLINES
- Admissions Process Statement
  - Deadlines:
    - Application Open Date: None
    - Application Deadline Date: None. Rolling admissions. Three incoming cohorts per year.
    - Supplemental Open Date
    - Supplemental Deadline Date
    - Transcripts Received Date
    - eLOR Received Date
    - GRE Scores Received Date
  - Interviews held: After submitting the application.
    - Interview format statement
  - Offers released: Dates
  - Orientation held: Semesters begin in September, January, and May.
  - Deposit required: Yes
    - If YES, amount: $500
  - Defers granted: Yes
  - Transfers accepted: Yes

EVALUATION CRITERIA
*If applicable, please enter percentage weighted
- Academic History
- Science GPA
- Science pre-requisite GPA
- Cumulative GPA
- Last 45 GPA
- GRE Scores
- eLORS
- Experiences
- Leadership Skills
- Personal Essays
- Contribution to diversity
- Non-cognitive skills
- Readiness to matriculate
- Employment history
- Interview
- Other (please list)

ACCEPTANCE DATA (PRIOR YEAR)
- GRE Average and Range
- GPA Average and Range
- Number of applications
- Number interviewed (or N/A)
- Number selected
- Number accepted into class
- Number matriculated

TUITION / COST OF ATTENDANCE
*For current year (2020 matriculation)
- Non-Resident (out-of-state)
  - Tuition: $16,125
  - Fees: $410

Q&A
- Top 10 FAQs

What makes St. Matthew's University unique among Caribbean veterinary schools?
St. Matthew's School of Veterinary Medicine offers quality education with unmatched student support services on a beautiful, safe, modern island.

Our Basic Science campus is on Grand Cayman which is only an hour flight from Miami. Students spend seven semesters on the island completing Basic Science and Pre-Clinical classes with highly credentialed and experienced faculty. The program offers students a veterinary medical education program focused on patient-centered care as the foundation of the program. The veterinary medical education is integrated with a new surgical facility built by St. Matthew's University for the benefit of our students, the citizens of the Cayman Islands and the local animal population.

The Cayman Islands offer a unique setting for veterinary study. The island has a rich variety of wildlife, large animals and companion animals. Students spend

28 months of classroom, laboratory and surgical facility based instruction on Grand Cayman. Students then move on to a year of clinical instruction at premier veterinary schools in the U.S and Canada.

Grand Cayman boasts one of the highest per capita incomes in the world. The island is modern and has an economy similar of that of the U.S. which allows students to easily assimilate into the lifestyle of the island. Grand Cayman has one of the lowest crime rates of any country in the Caribbean, and the local residents are hospitable and inviting. St. Matthew's University is just steps away from the famous Seven Mile Beach. Students can literally walk out of their class for a quick swim, snorkel, sunset volleyball game, or even to study on the beach.

Are St. Matthew's University graduates easily able to practice veterinary medicine in the United States?
Yes. St. Matthew's University graduates are eligible to practice veterinary medicine in the United States once they pass the requisite licensing examinations. Most of our graduates are licensed and practicing in the United States or Canada.

What is the average class size?
Typical class sizes range between 10 and 20 students to ensure a high degree of individual attention from faculty.

What is the ratio of students to faculty?
The ratio of students to full-time faculty is only four to one, which affords our students an unprecedented level of faculty support and attention.

Will I gain exposure to a variety of animals and their care?
Students are provided with many opportunities to work with large and small animals throughout their education at SMU. Students in the early semesters learn animal handling techniques and participate in local projects in the community that help local businesses/farms and provide students with hands on experience with a variety of animals. At our clinical facility, faculty and students work closely with the Cayman Islands Department of Agriculture and have the opportunity to work with a wide variety of local domestic large and small animals. Students have opportunities to work up real cases with faculty and local veterinarians, gaining a wide variety of experience that only comes from exposure to actual cases in the field. Because of our location in the Caribbean,

students also gain exposure to many exotic animal species, including marine turtles, iguanas, tropical birds and fish.

Can I transfer to St. Matthew's from a U.S. veterinary program?
The SMU Veterinary Medicine program welcomes applications from transfer students in another Caribbean or U.S. veterinary program. Transfer credits may be awarded depending on grades in particular courses, references from faculty at the current/previous school, and how closely the curriculum at the current/previous school matches the SMU curriculum.

Is there an application deadline?
We do not have application deadlines. We have a rolling admissions process and we encourage student to apply no later than two months prior to the semester start date to allow students to select the semester they prefer. If an application is received after the class has closed, the application is automatically reviewed for the next available semester.

How long does it take to process an application?
Once we have received your completed application and a personal interview has been conducted, it takes approximately two (2) weeks for your complete application to be processed.

Do you accept applicants over 30 years of age?
St. Matthew's University will consider any qualified applicant for admission, regardless of age. Some of our most successful students and graduates have had prior careers, often as certified veterinary technicians or other occupations.

What is the makeup of your student body?
Although the majority of our students are U.S. residents, St. Matthew's University boasts an extremely diverse student population. 20% of our students are from Canada and around 5% are from Europe. Over 40 countries are represented in our student body.

ADDITIONAL INFORMATION
The admissions team at SMU wants to get to know you! To us, you are much more than a GPA or GRE score. We want to know about you as a person because ultimately, that is what will determine the kind of veterinarian you will be. We want to support you in your dream of becoming a veterinarian, and we welcome your application!

PRE-REQUISITE COURSEWORK

The SMU School of Veterinary Medicine requires the following pre-requisite courses:

Course

General Biology or Zoology*	1 academic year (6 credit hours)
General Chemistry*	1 academic year (6 credit hours)
Organic Chemistry*	1/2 academic year (6 credit hours)
Biochemistry	1/2 academic year (3 credit hours)
Language Arts (English)**	1/2 academic year (3 credit hours)
College Math or Computer Science	1/2 academic year (3 credit hours)

*These courses must include an attached laboratory.

** A student may substitute any course that has a writing component, such as a term paper or written project, for the Language Arts requirement.

TOKYO
UNIVERSITY OF TOKYO*

Graduate School of Agricultural and Life Sciences
The University of Tokyo
1-1-1, Yayoi, Bunkyo-ku, Tokyo, 113-8657

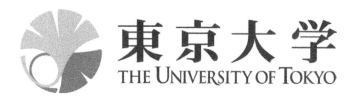

SCHOOL DESCRIPTION

Veterinary medicine covers wide areas of life sciences, not only medicine for animals but also biology of mammals and higher vertebrates. In the Department of Veterinary Medicine, most advanced research is being carried out at molecular, cellular and in vivo levels, in order to fully understand vital processes of normal and diseased animals. Veterinary medicine has two aspects of science: basic science to understand the mechanisms underlying biological phenomena, and applied science to satisfy the social demands for maintenance and improvement of human welfare and productivity of domestic animals. This depart-ment collaborates with the veterinary medical center located on the Yayoi campus. This center is facilitated with the latest and most advanced medical instru-ments, and plays an important role as an advanced veterinary hospital in this area.

FOR MORE INFORMATION

For more information about the University of Tokyo's Veterinary Medicine Program, please go to the follow-ing website: http://www.u-tokyo.ac.jp/en /admissions-and-programs/graduate-and-research /graduate-schools/agricultural.html

UNITED ARAB EMIRATES UNIVERSITY*

Email Address: servicedesk@uaeu.ac.ae
Website: www.uaeu.ac.ae/en/catalog/undergraduate
/programs/program_21931.shtml

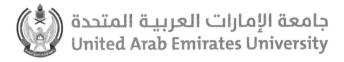

SCHOOL DESCRIPTION
The Bachelor of Veterinary Medicine Program is the only one of its kind in the United Arab Emirates. The program is five years long, after which graduates will be qualified veterinarians. Students will receive veterinary basic sciences education and intensive clinical training sorted by animal species and specialized disciplines.

PROGRAM DESCRIPTION
The Bachelor of Veterinary Medicine Program at UAE University aims to: enable the veterinary students to acquire knowledge, practical skills, and experience needed for a qualified veterinarian; enforce evidence-based veterinary medicine and problem-oriented, problem solving methods; graduate veterinarians capable of providing superior animal health care, including disease investigation and prevention, at the individual and herd or flock level; meet the growing national needs for qualified veterinarians in the public and private sectors; and demonstrate the achieve-ment of the PLOs by the graduation time and enable graduates to pursue higher academic degrees in veterinary medical sciences or other related sciences.

- International School: Yes
- Accepts International Applicants: Yes
  VMCAS Participant: No
  - If "No", how to apply: Online UAEU application portal: https://ssb.uaeu.ac.ae/prod/bwskalog.P_DispLoginNon

ENTRANCE REQUIREMENTS
- Bachelor's degree required: No

ADMISSIONS PROCESS & DEADLINES
- Admissions Process Statement
  - Deadlines:
    - Application Open Date: May 15
    - Application Deadline Date: July 15
  - Orientation held: Early January

UNIVERSITY OF VETERINARY AND ANIMAL SCIENCES, LAHORE-PAKISTAN*

Email Address: webmaster@uvas.edu.pk
Website: www.uvas.edu.pk/index.php

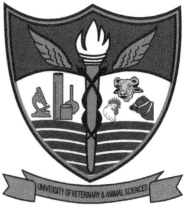

LAHORE

SCHOOL DESCRIPTION

With a marvelous history of 133 years of excellence, the University of Veterinary and Animal Sciences (UVAS), Lahore, is now positioned among the top ten Universities of Pakistan. Originally established as a school in 1882, it was later transformed into a college within the next two decades (i.e., end of the nineteenth century). Realizing the importance of livestock and poultry sectors in the economy of the country and the growing need of human resource and research work in veterinary and animal sciences and allied fields in the country, this historic institution was upgraded as a university in 2002. Presently, UVAS comprises of 23 departments in five faculties, three institutes, one constituent college, and a school, along with seven affiliated institutes at Attock, Rawalpindi, Shiekhupura, Okara, Lahore, Narowal, and Sahiwal. The UVAS reflects a unique blend of glorious history and ongoing professional advancement of the modern era. The main building of the institution, which was built 100 years ago, is still considered as the symbol of historical glory while the University has now expanded to five campuses, including its City Campus Lahore, Ravi Campus Pattoki, Avian Research & Training Center at Ferozepur Road, College of Veterinary and Animal Sciences Jhang, and the Para Veterinary School in Karor Lal Easin, District Layyah.

*This page was not updated for the VMSAR 2019/2020 edition. For updated information, visit the website located at the top of the page listing.

UVMP IN KOŠICE

Email: zas@vlf.sk
Website: http://www.uvlf.sk/en

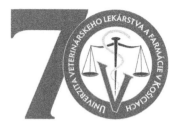

SCHOOL DESCRIPTION

UVMP in Košice is located in the Slovak Republic, in the heart of the Europe. The university was founded in 1949. It has been providing veterinary education for 70 years and veterinary education in the English language is provided for more than 25 years. The university offers General Veterinary Medicine study programmes in English: 6-year programme for secondary-school graduates and 4-year post BSc. programme for bachelors in Veterinary Sciences or Animal Sciences, Biosciences or related sciences) both leading to the title of Doctor of Veterinary Medicine (DVM). The study programmes are provided by 11 departments, 5 clinics (Small Animal Clinic, Clinic of Birds, Exotic and Free Living Animals, Clinic of Horses, Clinic of Ruminants, Clinic of Swine), University Veterinary Hospital and university special facilities (University Farm in Zemplínska Teplica, Equestrian Centre, University Facility for Breeding and Diseases of Game, Fish and Bees in Rozhanovce). All facilities ensure a high level of practical preparation and permanent contact with animals which, based on hands-on teaching at the university, leads UVMP graduates to acquire day-one skills.

PROGRAM DESCRIPTION

A profile of the graduate of the General Veterinary Medicine study program is formed during study, with particular focus on professional activities in the field of state administration, private veterinary practice, laboratory practice, private sphere of agriculture, food, pharmacy, education, scientific research and environmental protection. The study plan is compiled in accordance with Directive 2005/36/EC of the European Parliament and Council on the recognition of professional qualifications. The curriculum includes Basic Subjects, Basic Sciences, Clinical Sciences, Animal Production, Food Hygiene & Public Health, and Professional Knowledge.

Health & Wellness: Students have an opportunity to get involved in activities of various interest clubs: Aqua Terra Club, Cynological Club DARCO, Hunting Cynology Club, Breeder´s Club, Falconry and Raptor Rehabilitation Club, Small Mammal and Exotic Bird Breeder´s Club, Bee Breeder´s Club, Flora Club, Mineralogy Club, Tj Slávia Sport Club, etc. Medical and dental care is available at the UVMP dormitory. Gym is part of the accommodation facility.

Diversity & Disadvantaged/ Accommodations: The UVMP in Košice has two dormitories situated about 10 minute walk from the university. The capacity of the dormitories is over 400, with fully furnished rooms equipped with a free Internet connection. Accommodation in either a single room or double room depends on the current number of accommodated students and the availability of rooms.

Students registered in the Evidence of students with specific needs at the UVMP in Košice have, according to the extent and type of the specific need, entitlement for the support services. A student with specific needs is considered a student with sensory, physical and multiple disabilities, chronic disease, health impairment, mental illness, autism or other pervasive developmental disorders or learning disabilities.

- Class Size
  - Study program provided in Slovak language: 150
  - Study program provided in English language: 60
  - International Seats are included in the number of seats approved for Slovak and English program
- Applicant Pool (prior year)
  - Study program provided in Slovak language: 292
  - Study program provided in English language: 119

- International School: Yes
- Accepts International Applicants: Yes
- VMCAS Participant: No
  - Application is done directly through the email address zas@uvlf.sk. For the preliminary evaluation by the UVMP admission committee, the following is necessary:
    - 6-year General Veterinary Medicine (GVM) study program: high school leaving certificate entitling for the university study including passed subjects, CV, email from previous education institution confirming applicant´s obtained qualification. Email must be sent directly from the institution to zas@uvlf.sk
    - 4-year post BSc GVM study program: high school leaving certificate entitling for the university study including passed subjects, CV, official academic transcript and bachelor degree diploma, conversion formula of US credits into ECTS credits, email from previous education institution confirming applicant´s obtained qualification. Email must be sent directly from the institution to zas@uvlf.sk.

ENTRANCE REQUIREMENTS
- Pre-Requisite Chart Update
  - 6-year GVM study program – N/A
  - 4-year post BSc GVM study program – completion of specified subjects during the first level of higher education studies (Biology, Chemistry and Biophysics); upon approval of the UVMP Management, courses of Chemistry and Biochemistry and/or Biophysics can be completed during the first year of study at UVMP in Košice
- VMCAS application: No
- Supplemental application: No
  - Through VMCAS: No
  - External: No
- Transcript Requirements
  - International Transcripts: Yes
  - WES Report Required: No
- Test Requirements
- Experiences
  - Requirements statement
    - N/A

- Letters of Recommendation (eLOR)
  - Veterinarian Required: No
- Bachelor's degree required: Yes in case of 4-year post BSc GVM study program
- Academic Statement
- Interview Required: Yes, for entrance to 6-year GVM study program
  - Type of interview: written entrance examination from Biology and Chemistry

ADMISSIONS PROCESS & DEADLINES
- Admissions Process Statement
  - Deadlines:
    - Application Open Date: October (for both 6-year GVM and 4-year post BSc GVM study program
    - Application Deadline Date: July of the following year in case of 6-year GVM study program and May of the following year in case of 4-year post BSc GVM study program
    - Transcripts Received Date: Admissions are on the first come first served basis. Complete confirmation of study completion must be submitted prior to the registration to study in September, officially verified and certified diplomas must be submitted prior to the registration (6-year GVM study program) or prior to the middle of December in the first year of study (4-year post BSc GVM study program)
    - Interviews held: Dates: officially set individual dates within period from March until August
  - Interviews held: On officially set individual dates within period from March to August
    - Interview format statement: Admission of applicant to the 6-year GVM study program is conditioned by successful passing of the admission procedure, including entrance exams from Biology and Chemistry (aggregate score is at least 51%), unless different admission requirements are approved. Applicants for study shall be arranged in the

descending order by their aggregate scores achieved from tests on the entrance exams. Results from each entrance exam date are evaluated separately. Applicants for study with successfully passed entrance exams are admitted until the number of seats set for the academic year is reached. Each test consists of 60 questions.Orientation held: Dates In case of interest, university offers number of Open Days which are announced on the UVMP website.

- o Offers released: Decision on acceptance/non-acceptance is sent via email within 5 working days and via post within 30 calendar days from the date of the entrance exam. Entry requirements are released since September 20th.
- o Orientation held: In case of interest, the university offers number of Open days which are announced on the UVMP website.
- o Deposit required: No
- o Defers granted: No
- o Transfers accepted: Yes

EVALUATION CRITERIA

- Academic History: For 4-year post BSc GVM study program it is necessary to meet 100% of admission requirements.
- **General admission requirements for 4-year post BSc GVM study program:**
  - o Full secondary education or full specialized secondary education qualification entitling for the university study, attested by certificate
  - o Completion of the first level of higher education studies (i.e. Bachelor degree in Veterinary Sciences or Animal Sciences, Biosciences or related sciences)
  - o Bachelor degree certificate not older than 6 years at the time of application
  - o Completion of specified subjects during the first level of higher education studies (Biology, Chemistry and Biophysics). Upon approval of the UVMP Management, courses of Chemistry and Biochemistry and/or Biophysics can be completed during the first year of study at UVMP in Košice
  - o Documented attainment of 180 ECTS

(or equivalent) upon completion of bachelor degree

- Science GPA
- Science pre-requisite GPA
- Cumulative GPA
- Last 45 GPA
- GRE Scores
- eLORS
- Experiences
- Leadership Skills
- Personal Essays
- Contribution to diversity
- Non-cognitive skills
- Readiness to matriculate
- Employment history
- Interview: for 6-year GVM study program
- **General admission requirements for 6-year GVM study program:**
  - o Full secondary education or full specialized secondary education qualification entitling for the university study, attested by certificate
  - o Written entrance examination from subjects Biology and Chemistry

ACCEPTANCE DATA (PRIOR YEAR)

- Number of applications: 119
- Number interviewed: 87
- Number selected: 76
- Number accepted into class: 60
- Number matriculated: 46

TUITION / COST OF ATTENDANCE

- Study programs provided in Slovak language:
  - o Tuition: 720 € in case of exceeding standard duration of study
  - o Fees: 40 € application fee, other fees are available in the Internal Regulation No 38 on the UVMP website
  - o COA: individually assessed
- Study programs provided in English language:
  - o Tuition: 8,000 €
  - o Fees: 50 € application fee, other fees are available in the Internal Regulation No 38 on the UVMP website
  - o COA: individually assessed

EDUCATION / RESEARCH

- Combined Programs statement
  - o Bachelor study program Animal Science is a joint study program of Nord University in Bodø, Norway, and University of Veterinary Medicine and Pharmacy in Košice, Slovakia. The first three semesters are completed in Bodø, the next three semesters are completed at UVMP in Košice.

- Curriculum Statement
    - Curriculum of General Veterinary Medicine study program is fully in line with curriculum of EAEVE.
- Clinicals begin
    - Clinical subjects start after the 3rd year of study. They are focused on hands-on teaching leading to the attainment of day-one skills.
- Highlights
    - The UVMP in Košice received a confirmation that General Veterinary Medicine study program complies with requirements of EU Directives concerning education of veterinary graduates and practitioners. According to the Standards and based on the educational requirements of the EC Directive 2005/36, Article 38, the UVMP in Košice is an approved and accredited EAEVE/FVE Establishment. Hands-on teaching at the UVMP in Košice leads to the attainment of day-one skills. For this purpose, UVMP special facilities and university clinics are used. This allows our graduates to work in the following areas: small animals clinics, large animals clinics, exotic animals clinics and ZOOs, game reserves, food safety and quality, pharmaceutical industry, research and development, teaching and consultancy, ecology and postgraduate study.

Q&A

- Top 10 FAQs

Why study at the UVMP in Košice?

Students are particularly attracted by the high level of practical preparation and permanent contact with animals, which leads to acquirement of day-one skills.

Students of which nationalities study at the UVMP in Košice?

Students from all over the world study at the UVMP in Košice. They are students mainly from Norway, Great Britain, Ireland, Iceland, Greece, Sweden, France, Malta, Cyprus, USA, Israel, Finland, Canada, Hongkong, Germany and other countries from all over the world study at the UVMP in Košice.

I have been informed that I will be able to apply before I have completed my secondary education. Is that true?

Applicants who have not completed their secondary education at the time of application need to e-mail to the Office for foreign studies (zas@uvlf.sk) copies of their up to date study records (i.e. transcripts or any other relevant documents). After positive preliminary evaluation of their eligibility to study and successful passing of entrance examination, they may be conditionally accepted to study at UVMP. After the conditional acceptance to study, applicant's officially verified and certified copy of high school leaving certificate must be delivered to the Office for foreign studies prior to the registration day in September.

How long does it take to get results of the entrance exam?

Applicant receives an email about acceptance/non-acceptance within 5 working days and via post within 30 calendar days from the date of the entrance exam.

I would like to transfer from another veterinary university. Would any of the exams I have taken be recognised and would I be offered any exemptions from certain subjects?

Recognition of exams and exemptions are judged individually on the case-by-case basis after the applicant presents us with full academic transcript of their previous studies.

Is there a possibility for me to get any financial support for my studies?

Students are advised to apply for grants or loans in their home countries.
Conditions for such financial support from Slovak organisations might prove to be difficult to fulfill.

Do you have any open days or days to view the UVMP campus before I apply?

The Office for foreign studies organises for applicants tours around the university campus. It is necessary to inform the Office for foreign studies of intended arrival in advance.

How are dormitory rooms furnished?

Each student room is equipped with two single beds, a desk, a wardrobe, fridge/freezer and a bathroom sink. Internet access is also included in the monthly rent.

When does the application process begin and what do I need for the application?

Application process begins in October.

When is the deadline for the tuition fee payment?

Tuition fee has to be paid prior to the registration day stipulated for the given academic year.

VETERINARIAN PROFILE: CONRAD SPANGLER

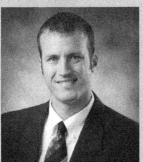

YEAR OF GRADUATION
2009

PLACE OF EMPLOYMENT
Riverview, LLP

What is your favorite aspect of being a veterinarian?
My favorite aspect of a being a veterinarian is the people I get to work with on a daily basis. The clients and caretakers of the dairy cows and calves I work with are hard-working, honest people who want the best for their families, communities, the environment, and the animals they care for. I have learned so much from them about life and animal care.

What type of veterinary medicine do you practice?
I practice dairy production medicine for a private dairy production company, Riverview, LLP.

Where did you attend veterinary school?
University of Minnesota.

How long have you been practicing as a veterinarian?
Eight years.

What advice do you have for those considering a career in veterinary medicine?
Understand the financial realities of a career in veterinary medicine and do some deep introspection to decide if you are passionate enough about this career path to overcome the financial difficulties you will face upon leaving veterinary school. Veterinary schools are admitting more students and charging them more to make up for a lack of funding, which has the potential to oversupply veterinarians and push wages down. The net present value for a veterinary education is negative for many practice types, which means it is potentially a bad investment for many students. Be sure to balance the emotional excitement of veterinary school with the financial realities and determine if you have the fortitude to truly succeed in this business.

What challenges have you faced while practicing veterinary medicine?
The two main challenges I have faced while practicing veterinary medicine are repaying student loan debt and learning how to work with and motivate clients to change. The amount of student loan debt has the potential to force one to put off other major investments in order to repay the loans, which can make savings for retirement, home ownership, and children challenging. Additionally, it can be frustrating when clients don't follow your recommendations. It is important to learn you can't be everything to everybody, and you need to adjust your strategy to motivate different personality types in order to achieve compliance with your recommendations.

POLICIES ON ADVANCED STANDING

Transfers are permitted to most colleges of veterinary medicine in the United States under specified conditions. Typical requirements include a vacancy in the class, completion of all prerequisite requirements, and compatible curricula. Following is a listing of schools and some of the conditions under which they will consider a transfer from another veterinary college with advanced standing. More detailed information may be obtained by writing to the individual schools in which you have an interest.

UNITED STATES

UNIVERSITY OF CALIFORNIA, DAVIS

Applications may be considered if available positions exist within the third-year class.

1. The applicant must have a strong academic record in their undergraduate program. At minimum, the candidate's application score used for the regular admissions process must meet or exceed the average application score for the class in which the candidate is seeking admission. This is the quantitative measure used to rank applicants—it is based on a combination of quantitative data including GPA (overall VMCAS science courses, and most recent 45 graded semester units), GRE quantitative score, and quantitative input from external letters. The average overall science GPA is 3.7; most recent 45 semester units is 3.8; 74% is the quantitative GRE.
2. The applicant must be currently enrolled in an AVMA-accredited DVM program and must be in excellent academic and ethical standing in that program. The specific minimum benchmark will be that the applicant is in the top quartile of students in the Veterinary School in which the applicant is currently enrolled as determined by GPA or class rank.
3. The applicant must have completed veterinary course work equivalent to that expected of the students in the DVM program of the School of Veterinary Medicine, UC Davis, who will be in the same academic class.
4. The applicant has a valid reason for requesting admission in advanced standing.

UNIVERSITY OF FLORIDA

1. An opening must exist in the second- or third-year class.

2. Students are only rarely considered for advanced standing based on exceptional personal circumstances.
3. Student must be enrolled in an AVMA accredited college.
4. Student must meet all prerequisites for admission as a first-year student (including GRE® scores).
5. The curricula of the two schools must be sufficiently alike to allow a student to enter without deficiencies in academic background.
6. Applicants must have a letter approving transfer from their dean or associate dean.

UNIVERSITY OF GEORGIA

1. Priority is given to Georgia residents, followed by contract state residents, then all other applicants.
2. Applicants will be considered for entry into the DVM degree program up to the third year of the curriculum, when and if space is available, as defined by the Admissions Committee.
3. Applications must include official transcripts of all completed veterinary and pre-veterinary coursework and a letter of support written by a senior administrator of the school in which the applicant is currently enrolled stating the applicant is currently in good academic standing.
4. No individual is eligible for transfer who has been dismissed or is on probation at any other school or college for deficiency in scholarship or because of misconduct.

UNIVERSITY OF ILLINOIS

1. Transfer students will only be considered for the beginning of the second year of veterinary medicine and only if transfer seats become available in that class.
2. All prerequisite science courses must be completed prior to the request for transfer.
3. Minimum grade requirements include: cumulative and science GPAs of 2.75 on a 4.00 scale (doesn't include veterinary work); results of the Graduate Record Examination General Test completed within the last two years.
4. Student must complete the same preveterinary coursework as required for students accepted to the first year of the program.
5. Student must be in good academic standing.

6. To be considered for transfer, a student must present credentials for preprofessional work that fulfill the University of Illinois College of Veterinary Medicine requirements for first-year entry.

7. Complete information and an application can be found at http://vetmed.illinois.edu/education/doctor-veterinary-medicine-degree/transfer-information

COLORADO STATE UNIVERSITY

Transfer is dependent on position openings in the year into which the student transfers (most transfers usually involve the loss of a year because of differences in school curricula). Candidate must:

1. have successfully completed at least the first year (equivalent of two semesters) of veterinary curriculum at an AVMA accredited college of veterinary medicine and be currently enrolled at the time of request.

AND

2. have obtained the equivalent of a 3.0 cumulative GPA in your veterinary program AND must not have received a D, F, or unsatisfactory grade of any kind at any time since enrolling in veterinary school.

AND

3. have a preveterinary academic record comparable to currently enrolled DVM students.

AND

4. provide evidence of noncognitive attributes comparable to currently enrolled DVM students.

5. A student who is accepted for transfer may be required to successfully complete Capstone Examinations associated with the class year into which they are transferring.

If a veterinary student with an interest in transferring to CSU's DVM program meets ALL of the above minimum requirements, he/she may apply to the DVM program. To apply for transfer to CSU's Veterinary Program, please see http://csu-cvmbs.colostate.edu/dvm-program/Pages/dvm-transfer-student-opportunities.aspx

CORNELL UNIVERSITY

1. Students are considered for advanced standing on an individual basis.

2. Transfer students will be considered if an opening exists in the second-year class. Students seeking advanced standing may enter the DVM program at two points: at the beginning of the second year of study, or mid-way through the second year, at the beginning of the fourth (Spring) semester of study.

3. Students seeking advanced standing must be enrolled in an AVMA-accredited veterinary college.

4. The curricula of the two schools must be sufficiently similar to allow students to enter without deficiencies in their academic background.

5. Students must meet all pre-veterinary requirements for first-year entry at the College of Veterinary Medicine at Cornell University (including GRE scores, prerequisite coursework, animal and veterinary experience), and may not have any failing grades on their veterinary transcript.

6. Scores from the Graduate Record Examination (GRE) or Medical College Admissions Test (MCAT) may not be older than five years.

7. Applicants seeking advanced standing must include a letter from their Associate Dean certifying that the student is in good academic standing, has not been on academic probation, and has not been subject to any disciplinary action or dismissal for any reason.

8. Applicants are required to have completed at least two full semesters at the institution from which the transfer is requested. Only veterinary coursework completed at an AVMA-accredited institution will be considered.

9. After analyzing the academic background of the applicant, the Admissions Committee will place each accepted transfer student in the semester of study in the DVM curriculum deemed most appropriate. (Veterinary course syllabi will be required at time of application).

IOWA STATE UNIVERSITY

Acceptance of students for advanced standing is on the recommendation of the Academic Standards Committee. Space must be available in the class to which the student is applying. See website, http://vetmed.iastate.edu/student/future-dvm-students/apply-to-the-college/transfer-admissions/application-process.

KANSAS STATE UNIVERSITY

Acceptance of students for transfer is on recommendation of the Admissions Committee on a space-available basis. Further information is available at http://www.vet.k-state.edu/admissions/apply/transfer-app.html

LINCOLN MEMORIAL UNIVERSITY

Transfer students are considered. Each applicant is evaluated on an individual basis. Potential transfer students can find additional information regarding LMU-CVM at the following link: https://www.lmunet.edu/academics/schools/college-of-veterinary-medicine/admissions/transfer-policy

LOUISIANA STATE UNIVERSITY

1. Transfer applications are considered on a case-by-case and space available basis.
2. The curricula must be compatible and how many semesters a student must have at their current school will be based on this compatibility.
3. The student must be in good academic standing with at least a 3.2 GPA in veterinary coursework at his/her present school.
4. Admission is limited to the second year of the program and only into the fall semester.
5. Applicants requesting a transfer must contact the Office of Veterinary Education and Student Affairs. They must be currently enrolled and in good standing and their present school must be aware of their intent to transfer. A letter of good standing will be needed as part of the transfer documentation.
6. To initiate the transfer process, please carefully read the DVM Transfer Guidelines information at http://www.lsu.edu/vetmed/dvm_admissions /how_to_apply/transfers.php.

MICHIGAN STATE UNIVERSITY

1. Admission consideration is offered only to those current matriculates in an AMA accredited veterinary curriculum, who believe that there are extenuating circumstances that would present significant hardship if they continue at their current institution.
2. Applicants requesting a transfer must contact the Dean of Academic and Student Success at the school they are currently attending and notify him or her of their intent.
3. Applicants must also demonstrate quality academic performance throughout their professional school enrollment.
4. The curricula of the two schools must be sufficiently alike to allow a student to enter the second-year class without deficiencies in academic background.
5. All selection criteria for regular applicants apply to transfer applicants.
6. Priority is given to Michigan residents.
7. Space must be available.
8. International students requesting a transfer also must fulfill all requirements set forth in the International Student Admissions Policy.

MIDWESTERN UNIVERSITY

Transfer Students

Midwestern University CVM may accept transfer students from other accredited veterinary schools on a case-by-case basis. Students requesting a transfer must meet all the standard admissions requirements. The final decision will be determined by the Associate Dean for Academic Affairs and the Dean.

Advanced Standing

All requests for advanced standing by admitted or enrolled students are processed on a course-by-course basis by the Office of the Dean. A student must submit a letter to the Office of the Dean in which the student lists the course(s) in which he or she is requesting advanced standing. The student must provide an official course description(s), a transcript, and a syllabus (syllabi) of the course(s) previously taken. All requests must be submitted prior to the start of the course being considered. The recommendation to grant or deny advanced standing will be made by the Dean in consultation with the department. It is expected that a minimum grade equal to a "B" would have been achieved in the class being petitioned.

UNIVERSITY OF MINNESOTA

1. Transfer students are accepted on a space available basis. The Admissions Committee will place each applicant in the year or semester of the curriculum deemed appropriate after analysis of equivalency of the required courses involved.
2. No academic work or standing will be accepted from DVM curricula other than those deemed accredited by the American Veterinary Medical Association.
3. All applicants must be U.S. citizens or holders of appropriate visas.
4. All applicants are required to have finished at least one full academic year at the institution from which transfer is requested and must be in good academic standing at the time of discontinuance according to written verification from the institution.
5. All applicants must have achieved a cumulative GPA of 3.00 (of 4.00) for the required courses at the initial institution.
6. Please visit the following website for more details: https://www.vetmed.umn.edu/ education/dvm/transfer-students.

MISSISSIPPI STATE UNIVERSITY

The Mississippi State University College of Veterinary Medicine accepts, on a limited basis, transfer students from other veterinary medical colleges to fill vacancies in the freshmen or sophomore classes. Transfer guidelines are as follows:

From a veterinary school not accredited by the AVMA:

Applicants for transfer into the second semester of the first year must have completed coursework equivalent to coursework taught in the first semester of the first year at MSU-CVM.

Applicants for transfer into the first semester of the second year must have completed coursework equivalent to coursework taught in the first year at MSU-CVM.

Applicants for transfer into the second semester of the second year must have completed coursework equivalent to all coursework taught in the first three semesters at MSU-CVM plus have had equivalent surgery laboratories.

From a veterinary school accredited by the AVMA:

Applicants are considered on a case-by-case basis with regard to length of time in current program.

General:

Any applicant considered for transfer admission must be in good academic standing (defined as being eligible to continue at current school from current point in the curriculum), never have failed a course while in veterinary medical school, never have been dismissed from a veterinary school and must have completed at least a full academic year at current veterinary school.

An interview is required for any applicant considered for transfer admission. Interviews via Skype are acceptable.

Typically, transfer applicants are not accepted into our program at a point later than first semester of the sophomore year. Accordingly, if a student should pursue application to Mississippi State University College of Veterinary Medicine and be accepted, it would be necessary for that student to complete at least two years at Mississippi State University to be eligible for a degree.

Students accepted for transfer are required to meet the current computer requirements of the college.

For more information, contact Tonya Calmes, Admissions Assistant, 662-325-4161, tcalmes@cvm.msstate.edu.

UNIVERSITY OF MISSOURI

1. Must be a vacancy in the class.
2. Will consider students who are U.S. citizens or holders of permanent alien visas and who have finished at least two years in a college of veterinary medicine that is AVMA accredited.
3. Students must be in good academic standing, never been denied admission from the University of Missouri for a first year position, and submit a letter of reference from the dean's office of the present college is required.

NORTH CAROLINA STATE UNIVERSITY

Effective spring 2017, the NC State CVM no longer considers transfer application requests. Changes in our curriculum and the evolution of our DVM/PhD Program make this process change necessary.

THE OHIO STATE UNIVERSITY

Transfer students are considered. Each application is evaluated on an individual basis. For questions, please email cvm-dvmadmissions@osu.edu.

OKLAHOMA STATE UNIVERSITY

Transfer students are considered. Each application is evaluated on an individual basis. See website for transfer guide: http://www.cvhs.okstate.edu

OREGON STATE UNIVERSITY

Admission of students with advanced standing is considered only in certain circumstances, and each case is considered on an individual basis.

UNIVERSITY OF PENNSYLVANIA

Penn Vet considers transfer students, on an individual basis, for entry into the second year only (September). The availability of positions will be limited and the number of seats will not be known until approximately midsummer. The following requirements will be in effect:

1. Applicants will be required to have a minimum GPA of 3.00 without having repeated a course.
2. All Penn Vet prerequisite course requirements must be completed with a "C" or above before a transfer application may be submitted for consideration.
3. All major course work required by first-year students at Penn Vet must have been completed prior to matriculation. Missing material must be made up during the second academic year and must be completed prior to starting the third year.

4. Receipt of transcripts from all previously attended institutions, GRE scores and a letter of intent describing the reasons for wanting to transfer to Penn Vet. A copy of previous VMCAS application or a copy of application to current veterinary school.
4. Receipt of a letter from the Dean or Associate Dean of the home institution, indicating that the applicant is in good social and academic standing.
5. Application materials should be received by April 1. Be certain to include your email address to facilitate communication. For those who are finishing their first term in April, please have your transcripts sent as soon as possible. For other applicants, transcripts of previous terms should be available.
6. Send all materials to: Mary Bryant, VMD - Education & Student Affairs, The School of Veterinary Medicine, University of Pennsylvania, Rosenthal Building, 3800 Spruce Street, Philadelphia PA 19104
7. Interviews will be required and will be held during the applicant's spring break, usually in April if the applicant is in an on-going program. Those applicants who have a normal summer break may choose to interview early in that period.

Curricula vary among veterinary schools. Those coming from the most similar course work will be the most likely approved for transfer.

PURDUE UNIVERSITY

1. Positions must be available in the relevant class.
2. Student must be in good academic standing in his/her present program.
3. Students must have completed 1–2 years of DVM courses with an *exceptional* academic record in those courses.
4. Veterinary medical curricula must be compatible.
5. Student must have support of the administration from the program in which he/she is currently enrolled.

For more information, please email vetadmissions@purdue.edu.

UNIVERSITY OF TENNESSEE

Admission of students with advanced standing (transfer) may be considered for unique circumstances on a case-by-case basis.

1. Position(s) must be available in the class into which one would like to matriculate.
2. Curricula of the two schools must be sufficiently alike to allow a student to matriculate without deficiencies in his/her academic background.

3. The applicant's academic dean must provide a letter approving transfer and indicating that the student is in good standing at his/her current college/school of veterinary medicine.
4. Admission is usually limited to the second semester of the first year of the DVM curriculum except for exceptional circumstances.
5. Letters of reference are required.

The Admissions Committee will review applicant credentials and interview those determined to best meet admission criteria.

TEXAS A&M UNIVERSITY

Students requesting advanced standing must meet the following requirements:

1. Must have completed all previous professional veterinary courses in an AVMA accredited college of veterinary medicine.
2. Must have successfully completed the academic term preceding the semester into which student requests admission.
3. Must comply with all requirements for transfer into the university as described in the current catalog.
4. May request transfer only into the second through seventh semesters of the professional curriculum.
5. At the time of matriculation the student must certify by letter that he/she has not been convicted of crimes in the period from first enrollment in the college of veterinary medicine from which the student desires transfer until date of matriculation at Texas A&M University.
6. To request transfer consideration, the student must meet all requirements as posted on the College website at http://vetmed.tamu.edu/dvm/future/transferring.

TUFTS UNIVERSITY

Applicants from other veterinary schools are considered. Students with advanced standing are admitted if and when space becomes available in the second-year class. The application deadline is June 1 for the following September. Please refer to our website for details: http://vet.tufts.edu

TUSKEGEE UNIVERSITY

Tuskegee University College of Veterinary Medicine has a Non-Transfer Policy with other Veterinary Schools.

WASHINGTON STATE UNIVERSITY

Admission of students with advanced standing is considered only in very specific and unique circumstances, and each case is considered on an individual basis.

UNIVERSITY OF WISCONSIN

Wisconsin does not accept advanced standing students for admission.

INTERNATIONAL

ATLANTIC VETERINARY COLLEGE AT THE UNIVERSITY OF PRINCE EDWARD ISLAND

Applicants who have completed all or portions of a veterinary medical program may apply for advanced standing to the second year of the DVM program.

Applicants for advanced standing must present evidence of educational accomplishments and may be required to address missing courses or competencies expected of our incoming second-year students. Students admitted with advanced standing must begin the college year in September.

The candidate must file a formal application and may be interviewed by the Admissions Committee and possibly other faculty. Places for admission to the college with advanced standing are limited and depend on vacancies.

It is imperative that the Admissions Committee have detailed and translated summaries of veterinary medical academic programs and accomplishments for those seeking advanced placement from schools in foreign countries.

Advanced-standing applications should be on file and completed as early as possible and no later than January 1. Candidates are strongly encouraged to visit the website http://stage.upei.ca/avcpolicies/files/avcpolicies/avcaa_adm0004.pdf.

MASSEY UNIVERSITY

Applications for admission with advanced standing will only be considered by students enrolled in a veterinary program with a compatible curriculum, and pending an available space in the appropriate stage of the program. Applicants should contact vetschool@massey.ac.nz to apply for advanced standing.

MURDOCH UNIVERSITY

Applications for advanced standing will only be considered from students whose studies have been completed in a DVM program. Applicants are required to apply formally for advanced standing and provide the necessary documentation to allow for a full comparison between the previous study and Murdoch University's unit requirements. Prior courses must duplicate or substantially overlap multiple factors including breadth and depth of content, duration, objectives, assessment, context, and academic standard (level of intellectual effort required) for exemption to be granted.

ST. MATTHEW'S UNIVERSITY

Applications for admission with advanced standing are welcomed from students from veterinary schools recognized by the American Veterinary Medical Association (AVMA) and/or the American Association of Veterinary State Boards (AAVSB). Transfer applicants must submit a complete application package to ensure a timely review. Acceptance of transfer credit is at the discretion of St. Matthew's University.

UNIVERSITY OF CALGARY

Applications for admission to advanced semesters may be considered from students who have been enrolled in DVM programs at other institutions, subject to the availability of spaces in the DVM Program and the academic standing of the candidate. When places are available, candidates may be asked to present themselves for an interview and may be asked to pass examinations on subject matter in the veterinary curriculum. Applicants are advised that vacancies are rare and that restrictions on residency and citizenship status may be applied.

UNIVERSITÉ DE MONTRÉAL

1. Transfer students will only be considered for the beginning of the second year of veterinary medicine and only if transfer seats become available in that class.
2. Applicant must be enrolled in an AVMA-accredited college.
3. The applicant must have completed veterinary course work equivalent to that expected of the students in the DVM program of the Faculté de médecine vétérinaire de l'Université de Montréal, who will be in the second-year class.
4. Applicant must be a Canadian citizen or a permanent resident.
5. Applicant must fulfill the admission process as first-year students do.
6. Applicant shall contact the associate dean of studies of the FMV.
7. Applicant must complete the CASPER test.
8. Applicants who are not fluent in French must have a score of 785/990 at the TFI.

ROSS UNIVERSITY SCHOOL OF VETERINARY MEDICINE

Students who have completed a portion of the curriculum at another approved school of veterinary medicine may apply for admission with advanced standing. Such transfer applicants must present evidence of completion of courses (or their equivalent) at a school of veterinary medicine accredited by the American Veterinary Medical Association (AVMA), comparable to those offered in the pre-clinical curriculum of Ross University School of Veterinary Medicine. Additionally, transfer students must meet all the requirements for admission.

Placement is determined by the Academic Promotions Committee and the Dean, and will depend on the courses already completed. Credit will not, however, be given for more than the first four semesters of study. Transfer students must take all of the courses offered for the semester they are admitted and may be required to repeat part or all of the curriculum.

THE UNIVERSITY OF QUEENSLAND

Applications for advanced standing will only be considered from students whose studies have been completed in a veterinary program with a compatible curriculum, and where a space is available in the appropriate stage of the program. Please refer to the University of Queensland Policy 3.50.03 - Credit for Previous Studies and Recognised Prior Learning (http://ppl.app.uq.edu.au) or contact the School directly (vetenquiries@uq.edu.au).

Current School Name
Mississippi State University

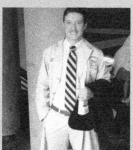

Why do you want to be a veterinarian?
Veterinary medicine unites two of my favorite things: science and medicine. Every case is a mystery, and information from many subject areas must be incorporated to diagnose and treat the patient appropriately and effectively. Fostering the human-animal bond is also very important to me, not only from the emotional perspective, but also from a one-health perspective.

What are your short-term and long-term goals?
My current short-term goals as a veterinary student are to do my best in the DVM curriculum and decipher my specific interests in vet med. I also plan to get as much hands-on clinical/surgery experience this summer before our second-year surgery lab. Regarding my long-term goals, I plan to go into small animal medicine and possibly complete a surgery or internal medicine residency.

What did you do as an applicant to prepare for applying to veterinary school?
In my sophomore year of my undergraduate studies, I called as many veterinary offices in my area as I could. I started to volunteer at three of them. One of the clinics offered to hire and train me to be a veterinary assistant. On my days off, I started to volunteer at a large animal referral center to diversify my veterinary experiences. Academically, I took summer classes and graduated in three years, making sure to satisfy all of the prerequisites for the schools I was interested in attending.

What advice would you give to applicants or those considering applying to veterinary school?
It is very important to work hard and not give up on your dream. There are going to be a lot of volunteer and study hours, but it will all be worth it in the end. Staying focused is essential as well. Everything you do needs to be related to achieving your goal. It is not going to be easy, but if you want something bad enough, nothing can stop you. It is also never too late to start getting experience and to save your GPA if you work hard enough.

What helped make the transition to veterinary school easier for you?
Making friends early in veterinary school was helpful for me to transition. Our class is very supportive of one another. My undergraduate university also prepared me for the demanding curriculum of veterinary school. I enjoy exercising and doing outdoor activities. It is very easy to stay inside day in and day out to study, but it is important to take breaks and do something recreational.

What is your advice on student debt?
It is very easy to get overwhelmed with the amount of debt vet students accrue over a four-year program. Taking advantage of your university's financial planning tools is essential to keep finances organized. Living below your means is a big part of saving money. This doesn't mean starving yourself or living under an overpass, but rather doing little things like making food or coffee rather than eating out. Every little bit counts when you are spending borrowed money. In the end, the degree is worth much more than we pay to get it.

What are you most excited about learning in veterinary school?
I am most excited to learn surgery. I think it is an essential skill for veterinarians. I am excited to learn routine spay and neuter procedures that are important in population control measures. Soft tissue surgery and orthopedic surgeries also interest me because of the difference surgeons can make in the quality of life of the patient.

	University of Adelaide	Atlantic Veterinary College of Prince Edward Island	Auburn University	University of Bristol**	University of Calgary	University of California – Davis	Central Luzon State**	Colorado State University	Cornell University	University of Edinburgh	University of Florida	University of Georgia	University of Glasgow	University of Guelph	City University of Hong Kong**	University of Illinois – Urbana-Champaign	Iowa State University	Kansas State University	Lincoln Memorial University	Louisiana State University	Massey University	University of Melbourne	Michigan State University	Midwestern University	University of Minnesota	Mississippi State University	University of Missouri	Universite de Montreal
Biology/Zoology		●	●		●	●		●	●	●	●	●	●	●		●	●	●	●	●	●	●	●	●	●	●	●	●
Organic Chemistry		●	●		●	●		●	●	●	●	●	●			●	●	●	●	●			●	●	●	●	●	
Biochemistry			●		●	●		●	●	●	●	●	●			●	●	●	●	●		●	●	●	●	●	●	
Inorganic Chemistry	●	●	●		●	●		●	●	●	●		●			●	●	●	●	●			●	●	●	●		●
Physics			●			●		●	●	●	●	●				●	●	●	●	●			●	●	●	●	●	●
Mathematics/Statistics	●	●	●		●	●		●		●	●		●	●							●		●	●	●	●	●	●
English Composition		●	●		●			●	●	●	●		●			●	●	●	●	●			●	●	●	●		
Humanities/Social Sciences		●						●		●	●		●	●		●	●	●	●			●					●	●
Genetics		●			●	●		●		●	●		●	●			●	●	●								●	
Microbiology										●	●		●					●		●							●	●
Electives		●	●					●	●								●	●		●							●	●
Speech/Public Speaking											●					●	●	●									●	
Science Electives		●						●			●					●	●		●						●		●	
Cellular Biology			●							●			●	●							●							
Physiology (Systemic)						●					●						●											
Anatomy											●						●											
Animal Nutrition			●																									
Advanced Biological Science											●	●												●				
Animal Science											●																	
Advanced Life Sciences							●				●																	
Medical Terminology																												
Physical Education																												
Ecology					●																							
Bachelor's Degree Required	No	No	Yes	No	Yes		No	No	See Details	No	No	No	No	No		No	No	No	No	No	No	Yes	No	No	No	No	No	No

** = No Data Available	● = Required Courses	● = Recommended Courses

The online version of this pre-requisites chart can be found at:
https://www.aavmc.org/assets/Site_18/files/VMCAS/prereqchart.pdf

	Murdoch University	North Carolina State University	The Ohio State University	Oklahoma State University	Oregon State University	University of Pennsylvania	Purdue University	University of Queensland	Ross University	Royal Veterinary College, University of London	Seoul National University**	St. George's University	St. Matthews University	University of Sydney	University of Tennessee	Texas A&M University	University of Tokyo**	Tufts University	Tuskegee University	United Arab Emirates University**	Universidad Nacional Autonoma	Univeriteit Utrecht**	University College Dublin	University of Veterinary Medicine and Pharmacy in Kosice **	University of Veterinary and Animal Sciences** - Pakistan	VetAgro Sup **	Virginia/Maryland College of Veterinary Medicine	Washington State University	Western University of Health Sciences	Western University of Veterinary Medicine - Saskatchewan	University of Wisconsin	Schools with common pre-requisites
		●		●	●	●	●	●	●	●		●	●	●	●	●		●	●	●		●	●				●	●	●	●	●	46
	●	●		●	●	●	●	●	●	●		●	●	●	●	●		●	●	●							●	●	●	●	●	42
		●	●	●	●	●	●	●				●	●	●	●	●		●	●			●					●	●	●	●	●	42
	●	●		●	●	●	●	●	●			●	●	●	●	●		●	●	●	●	●						●		●	●	40
		●		●	●	●	●	●	●			●	●	●	●	●		●	●								●	●	●	●	●	40
	●	●		●	●	●	●	●	●		●	●	●		●	●		●	●			●					●	●	●		●	39
		●		●	●	●	●	●	●			●	●		●	●		●	●			●					●	●	●		●	36
		●	●	●	●	●	●		●						●			●	●	●							●	●	●		●	27
		●	●	●	●		●		●			●			●	●		●	●									●	●	●	●	26
		●	●	●	●		●		●						●	●		●	●			●							●	●	●	20
					●				●									●	●		●										●	14
		●	●	●	●		●								●													●				12
			●							●				●				●														12
	●													●				●			●									●		10
			●		●									●				●										●		●		8
	●								●					●				●												●		7
		●		●			●								●				●									●				6
				●														●											●			6
																		●														2
																																2
																		●										●				2
																		●														1
																																1
	No	No	No	No	No	No	No	No	No	No	Yes	No	No	No	No	No	No	No	No	No	No	Yes	Yes				No	No	No	No	No	

The online version of this pre-requisites chart can be found at:
https://www.aavmc.org/assets/Site_18/files/VMCAS/prereqchart.pdf

General Information Chart - VMCAS - 2020
(as of 02/26/2019; subject to change)

College	Location	Contract States	Estimated Annual Tuition* Resident / Sponsored	Contract/WICHE	Non-Resident / Non-Sponsored	Available Seats* Resident / Sponsored	Contract / WICHE	Non-Resident / Non-Sponsored	Total Seats	Test Requirements	Web Address	VMCAS Participation	Accepts International Applicants	Deadline
Atlantic Veterinary College (UPEI)***	Charlottetown, PE, Canada	New Brunswick, Newfoundland, Nova Scotia	CAD 12,746	CAD 12,746	CAD 66,500	10	NB: 13; NL: 3; NS: 16	26	68	GRE	http://www.upei.ca/avc	Full	Yes	9/17/2019
Auburn University	Auburn, AL	Alabama, Kentucky	$20,366	$20,366	$47,626	41	38	51	130	GRE	https://www.vetmed.auburn.edu	Full	No	9/17/2019
University of California - Davis	Davis, CA		$36,452		$48,697				150	GRE	https://www.vetmed.ucdavis.edu	Full	Yes	9/17/2019
Colorado State University	Fort Collins, CO	WICHE**	$33,000	$33,000	$57,000	Residents: 70; UAF/CSU 05	40 - 50	20 - 35; UAF/CSU: 05	138; UAF/CSU: 10	GRE	http://csu-cvmbs.colostate.edu	Full	Yes	9/17/2019
Cornell University	Ithaca, NY		$35,966		$52,892	66		54	120	GRE or MCAT	https://www.vetmed.cornell.edu	Full	Yes	9/17/2019
University of Florida	Gainesville, Fl		$28,790		$45,500	94		26	120	None Required	https://www.vetmed.ufl.edu/	Full	Yes	9/17/2019
University of Georgia	Athens, GA	Delaware, South Carolina	$19,448	$19,448	$48,528	80	19	15	114	GRE	https://www.vet.uga.edu/	Full	Yes	9/17/2019
University of Illinois - Urbana	Urbana, Il		$27,578 plus fees		$49,402 plus fees	70	0	60	130	GRE	https://vetmed.illinois.edu	Full	Yes	9/17/2019
Iowa State University	Ames, IA	North Dakota, South Dakota, Nebraska	$23,288	varies by contract	$51,254	60	36	60	156	None Required	www.vetmed.iastate.edu	Full	Yes	9/17/2019
Kansas State University	Manhattan, KS	North Dakota	$24,975	$24,975	$54,366	45-50	5	57-62	102-112	GRE	https://www.vet.k-state.edu/	Full	Yes	9/17/2019
Lincoln Memorial University	Harrogate, TN		$46,250		$46,250				115	GRE	http://vetmed.lmunet.edu	Full	Yes	9/17/2019
Louisiana State University	Baton Rouge, LA	Arkansas	$27,400	$33,500	$56,500	60-65	9	20-40	89-114	GRE	http://www.lsu.edu/vetmed	Full	Yes	9/17/2019
Michigan State University	East Lansing, MI		$31,008		$56,470	78		37	115	None Required	http://www.cvm.msu.edu	Full	Yes	9/17/2019
Midwestern University	Glendale, AZ		$61,921		$61,921	15		105	120	None Required	http://www.midwestern.edu	Full	Yes	9/17/2019
University of Minnesota	Saint Paul, MN		$31,984		$57,490	53		52	105	GRE	http://www.vetmed.umn.edu	Full	Yes	9/17/2019
Mississippi State University	Starkville, MS	South Carolina, West Virginia	$26,200	$26,200	$47,400	40	SC: 5; WV: 7	43	95	None Required	http://www.cvm.msstate.edu	Full	Yes	9/17/2019
University of Missouri	Columbia, MO		$26,692		$62,516	60		60	120	GRE	http://cvm.missouri.edu	Full	Yes	9/17/2019
North Carolina State University	Raleigh, NC		$18,970		$45,160	80		20	100	GRE	http://www.cvm.ncsu.edu	Full	Yes	9/17/2019
The Ohio State University	Columbus, OH		$32,350		$71,494	81		81	162	None Required	http://www.vet.osu.edu/	Full	Yes	9/17/2019
Oklahoma State University	Stillwater, OK	Arkansas, Delaware	$24,050	$24,050	$50,900	58	AR: 1 (incl. in non-resident) DE: 1	48	106	GRE	www.cvhs.okstate.edu/vetmed/	Full	Yes	9/17/2019
Oregon State University	Corvallis, OR	WICHE**	$25,540	$25,540	$48,790	40	included in non-resident	32	72	GRE	www.oregonstate.edu/vetmed/	Full	Yes	9/17/2019
University of Pennsylvania	Philadelphia, PA		$44,910		$54,910	40		85	125	GRE	http://www.vet.upenn.edu	Full	Yes	9/17/2019
Purdue University	West Lafayette, IN		$19,918		$44,746	42		42	84	None Required	http://www.vet.purdue.edu	Full	Yes	9/17/2019
University of Tennessee	Knoxville, TN		$29,310		$56,576	60		25	85	GRE	http://www.vet.utk.edu	Full	Yes	9/17/2019
Texas A&M University	College Station, TX		$24,160		$37,164	142		10	152	GRE or MCAT	http://vetmed.tamu.edu	Apply Directly	No	10/1/2019 (5pm CST)
Tufts University	North Grafton, MA		$51,116		$56,116	30		68	98	GRE	http://vet.tufts.edu	Full	Yes	9/17/2019
Tuskegee University	Tuskegee, AL	Kentucky, South Carolina	$20,585 (per semester)	$20,585 (per semester)	$20,585 (per semester)	Variable	Variable	Variable	60-65	None Required	www.tuskegee.edu/vetmed	Full	Yes	9/17/2019
Virginia-Maryland College of Veterinary Medicine	Blacksburg, VA	West Virginia	$24,772	$53,305****	$53,305 (per semester)	VA:50; MD:30	6	40	126	None Required (GRE Scores Considered if Submitted)	www.becomeavet.vetmed.vt.edu/	Full	Yes	9/17/2019
Washington State University	Pullman, WA; Logan, UT; Bozeman, MT	WICHE**, Idaho, Montana, Utah	$25,530 / $24,428 / $23,657	$25,530	$61,086 / $57,658	WA:55 / UT:20 / MT:10	ID:11	25 / 10	131	GRE	www.vetmed.wsu.edu	Full	Yes	9/17/2019
Western University of Health Sciences	Pomona, CA		$54,220		$54,220	47		53	100	GRE or MCAT	http://prospective.westernu.edu/veterinary/requirements-1?	Full	Yes	9/17/2019
University of Wisconsin	Madison, WI		$30,515		$49,203	62		34	96	GRE	http://www.vetmed.wisc.edu	Full	Yes	9/17/2019
University of Calgary	Calgary, AB, Canada		CAN 10,840.20			30 - 34			30 - 34	None Required	http://www.vet.ucalgary.ca/dvmprogram	Apply Directly	No	11/30/2019
University College Dublin	Dublin, Ireland		EUR 20,070		EUR 37,000	90		40	130	None Required (GRE Scores Considered if Submitted)	vgtprogramme@ucd.ie	Only American and Canadians apply via VMCAS	Yes	9/17/2019
University of Edinburgh	Edinburgh, Scotland, UK	England, Wales, Northern Ireland	GBP 9,250		GBP 31,450	40	32	98	170	GRE	http://www.ed.ac.uk/vet	Only American and Canadians apply via VMCAS	Yes	9/17/2019
University of Glasgow	Glasgow, Scotland, UK		GBP 9,250		GBP 29,250	72		65	137	None Required (GRE Scores Considered if Submitted)	http://www.gla.ac.uk/schools/vet/	Only American and Canadians apply via VMCAS	Yes	9/17/2019
University of Guelph	Guelph, ON, Canada		CAD 10,271		CAD 66,236	105		15	120	None Required	www.ovc.uoguelph.ca	Non-Canadian applicants use VMCAS	Yes	9/17/2019
Massey University	Palmerston North, New Zealand		subsidized		NZD 64,040	100		24	124	None Required	www.massey.ac.nz/vetschool	Apply Directly OR VMCAS	Yes	11/1/2019 (Direct App) 9/17/2019 (VMCAS)

General Information Chart - VMCAS - 2020
(as of 02/26/2019: subject to change)

College	Location	Contract States	Estimated Annual Tuition* Resident / Sponsored	Contract/WICHE	Non-Resident / Non-Sponsored	Available Seats* Resident / Sponsored	Contract / WICHE	Non-Resident / Non-Sponsored	Total Seats	Test Requirements	Web Address	VMCAS Participation	Accepts International Applicants	Deadline
University of Melbourne	Melbourne, VIC, Australia	-	AUD 60,000	-	AUD 70,000	80	-	50	130	None Required	http://fvas.unimelb.edu.au/	Apply Directly or VMCAS	Yes	Rolling admission, 12/20/18, VMCAS 9/17/18
National Autonomous University of Mexico***	Mexico City, México	-	USD 500	-	USD 500	-	-	-	85	School Admissions Test, Spanish Proficiency Test	http://www.fmvz.unam.mx/	Apply Directly	Yes	Two Dates in Jan and Apr (See Website for Info)
Université de Montréal***	Montréal, QC, Canada	-	CAD 4500	-	CAD 11,250	-	-	-	96	Fluency in French	fmv.umontreal.ca	Apply Directly	No	1/15/2019
Murdoch University***	Murdoch, WA, Australia	-	-	-	AUD 29,000-81,000	-	-	45	45	None Required	http://www.murdoch.edu.au/School-of-Veterinary-and-Life-Sciences	Apply Directly	Yes	11/20/2019
The University of Queensland	Gatton, QLD, Australia	-	AUD 10,581	-	AUD 63,120	90	-	40	130	None Required	veterinary-science.uq.edu.au	Apply Directly	Yes	11/30/2019
Ross University School of Veterinary Medicine	St. Kitts	-	$20,304	-	$20,304	121	-	121	121	GRE or MCAT	https://veterinary.rossu.edu	Apply Directly OR VMCAS	Yes	Rolling Admissions (Direct Appl) 9/17/2019
Royal Veterinary College	London / Hertfordshire, England, UK	-	pending	-	pending	tbc	tbc	tbc	tbc	GRE	http://www.rvc.ac.uk	Only American and Canadian citizens apply via VMCAS	Yes	9/17/2019
University of Saskatchewan	Saskatoon, SK, Canada	Alberta, British Columbia, Manitoba, and the Northern territories	CAD 59,761	CAD 59,761	CAD 559,761	20	38	5 to 35	63 to 93	None Required	http://www.usask.ca/wcvm	Apply Directly	No	12/1/2019
St. George's University	St. George's, Grenada	-	$42,500	-	$42,500	-	-	-	110	GRE or MCAT	http://www.sgu.edu	Only American and Canadian citizens apply via VMCAS	Yes	9/17/2019
University of Sydney	Sydney, NSW, Australia	-	AUD 11,000 (Commonwealth Supported Places) AUD 58,000	-	AUD 66,000	BVB/DVM: 40 Post Grad DVM:30	-	BVB/DVM: 40 Post Grad DVM: 30	BVB/DVM: 80 Post Grad DVM: 60	-	http://sydney.edu.au/vetscience	Apply Directly OR VMCAS (US)	Yes	9/17/2019
Utrecht University***	Utrecht, Netherlands	-	EUR 2,060 (undergraduate and graduate)	-	EUR 20,767 (undergraduate); EUR 23,882 (graduate)	-	-	-	225	Fluent Dutch	https://www.uu.nl/bachelors/en/animal-information; international-students/application-procedure	Apply Directly	Yes	1/15/2019
VetAgro Sup*** Non-AVMA / COE Accredited	Marcy L'Étoile, France	▶	▶	▶	▶	▶	▶	▶	▶	▶	http://www.vetagro-sup.fr	Apply Directly	-	▶
University of Adelaide	Roseworthy, SA, Australia	-	$10,275 (undergraduate)	-	$47,000 (Undergraduate) $62,000 (graduate)	60 (DVM)	-	20 (BSc) 20(DVM)	80 (BSc) 80(DVM)	International applicants must meet the English language requirements (see website for details)	www.adelaide.edu.au/vetsci/degrees	Apply Directly	Yes	9/30/2019
University of Bristol	Bristol, England, UK	-	£9,250	-	£29,100	128	-	20	148	None Required	http://www.bristol.ac.uk/study-undergraduate/2019/vet-science/bvsc-veterinary-science	Apply Directly	Yes	10/15/2019
City University of Hong Kong, College of Veterinary Medicine and Life Sciences	Hong Kong	-	HK$42,100	-	HK$140,000	29	-	8	37	None Required	https://www.cityu.edu.hk/cvmls	Apply Directly or through JUPAS	Yes	12/31/2019 (JUPAS) 1/3/2019 (Apply Direct)
University of Veterinary Medicine and Pharmacy-Kosice	Kosice, Slovakia	-	EURO 720	-	EURO 8000	150 (Slovak Language)	-	60 (English Language)	210	None Required	http://www.uvlf.sk_en	Apply Directly	Yes	July 2019 (6 Year Program) May (4 Year Program)
Central Luzon State University***	Science City of Muñoz, Philippines	-	PHP 7,000 per semester	0	PHP 12,000 per semester	-	-	-	-	-	http://clsu.csvm.edu.ph	Apply Directly	Yes	Last week of April
Seoul National University***	Seoul, South Korea	-	-	-	-	-	-	-	-	Korean proficiency	http://en.snu.ac.kr/apply/info	Apply Directly	Yes	Feb-19
St. Matthew's University	Grand Cayman, Cayman Islands	-	$16,125 (preclinical)	-	$16,125 (clinical)	-	-	-	20 (3 times per year)	GRE Recommended	www.stmatthews.edu	Apply Directly	Yes	Rolling Admissions
University of Tokyo***	Tokyo, Japan	-	-	-	-	-	-	-	-	None Required	http://www.u-tokyo.ac.jp/en/admissions-and-programs/graduate-and-research/graduate-schools/agricultural.html	Apply Directly	-	-
United Arab Emirates University***	Maqam, UAE	-	-	-	-	-	-	-	-	-	https://www.uaeu.ac.ae/en/catalog/undergraduate/programs/program_21931.sht ml	-	-	-
University of Veterinary & Animal Sciences***	Lahore, Pakistan	-	-	-	-	-	-	-	-	-	http://www.uvas.edu.pk/index.php	-	-	-

* Subject to change; check with schools

** WICHE (Western Interstate Commission for Higher Education) contract states: Arizona, Hawaii, Montana, Nevada, New Mexico, North Dakota, Utah, and Wyoming)

*** This information was not updated for the VMSAR 2019/2020 edition. For updated information, visit the website located at the top of the page listing.

**** West Virginia Higher Education Council (WVHEC) provides scholarship money for a portion of tuition.

The online version of this general information chart can be found at:
https://www.aavmc.org/assets/Site_18/files/VMCAS/GenInfo.pdf